Luminos is the Open Access monograph publishing program
from UC Press. Luminos provides a framework for preserving and
reinvigorating monograph publishing for the future and increases
the reach and visibility of important scholarly work. Titles published
in the UC Press Luminos model are published with the same high
standards for selection, peer review, production, and marketing as
those in our traditional program. www.luminosoa.org

Intimate Communities

Intimate Communities

*Wartime Healthcare and the Birth of
Modern China, 1937–1945*

———

Nicole Elizabeth Barnes

中

UNIVERSITY OF CALIFORNIA PRESS

University of California Press, one of the most distinguished university presses in the United States, enriches lives around the world by advancing scholarship in the humanities, social sciences, and natural sciences. Its activities are supported by the UC Press Foundation and by philanthropic contributions from individuals and institutions. For more information, visit www.ucpress.edu.

University of California Press
Oakland, California

Suggested citation: Barnes, N. E. *Intimate Communities: Wartime Healthcare and the Birth of Modern China, 1937–1945*. Oakland: University of California Press, 2018. DOI: https://doi.org/10.1525/luminos.59

Library of Congress Cataloging-in-Publication Data

Names: Barnes, Nicole Elizabeth, 1975- author.
Title: Intimate communities : wartime healthcare and the birth of modern
    China, 1937–1945 / Nicole Elizabeth Barnes.
Description: Oakland, California : University of California Press, [2018] |
    Includes bibliographical references and index. |
Identifiers: LCCN 2018028775 (print) | LCCN 2018031513 (ebook) | ISBN
    9780520971868 (Epub) | ISBN 9780520300460 (pbk. : alk. paper)
Subjects: LCSH: Public health--China--History--20th century. | Women and
    war--China--History--20th century. | Sino-Japanese War, 1937-1945. |
    Public health--Political aspects--China.
Classification: LCC RA527 (ebook) | LCC RA527 .B37 2018 (print) | DDC
    362.10951--dc23
LC record available at https://lccn.loc.gov/2018028775

27   26   25   24   23   22   21   20   19   18
10   9   8   7   6   5   4   3   2   1

To Theodore Robert Fetter, love of my life and world's best husband and father.

CONTENTS

ILLUSTRATIONS

ACKNOWLEDGMENTS

It is a rare privilege to publicly acknowledge all the people, institutions, and serendipitous adventures that accumulate into a product bearing a single name. This book has taken me on a fantastic journey full of joy and inspiration, challenges and frustration. First books generally begin as dissertations, scribbled in a shaky hand and straining under the weight of towering footnotes that praise the gods of academe. I have been lucky enough to enjoy this project from the beginning because I benefitted from superb mentorship at the University of California, Irvine. Ken Pomeranz and Jeff Wasserstrom have been better than the best academic advisers a person could ask for. I am blessed to call them both colleagues and friends long after leaving the nest, and I am deeply grateful to them for modeling not only excellent scholarship and superb collegiality, but also the far more valuable lessons of humility, dedication, and integrity. I am grateful that they did not fear the prospect of advising a project that lies somewhat outside their (many!) arenas of expertise but granted me full freedom to explore my intellectual self. Hu Ying gave me constant encouragement and valuable perspectives. Many other UCI faculty supported and stimulated me, including Vinayak Chaturvedi, Keith Danner, Doug Haynes, Guo Qitao, Susan Klein, Mark Levine, Laura Mitchell, Kavita Philip, Serk-Bae Soh, Anne Walthall, and Bin Wong (then at UCLA). My fellow students at UCI made graduate life fun and inspiring. Thanks to Nick Bravo, Maura Elizabeth Cunningham, Pierre Fuller, Chris Heselton, Giovanni Hortua, Erin Huang, Miri Kim, Young Hee Kim, Kate Merkel-Hess, Hyun Seon Park, Juily Phun, Shi Xia, Wang Guo, and Wang Wensheng.

I have too many friends in my academic family to name everyone, but I thank all of you from the bottom of my heart. This work would be neither possible nor fun without you. John Robertson Watt deserves special mention since he has been a consummate gentleman from the beginning, sharing everything he knows with me and warmly inviting me into the field of wartime medicine. Recently, after completing his magnum opus *Saving Lives in Wartime China*, he packed up several heavy boxes of books and donated the bulk of his precious personal library to me. I have done little to deserve such generosity. I would also like to thank by name the following colleagues who organized workshops that helped me think through parts of this work: Bridie Andrews, Mary Brown Bullock, James Cook, Tina Phillips Johnson, Michael Shiyung Liu, Tehyun Ma, Rebecca Nedostup, Caroline Reeves, Helen Schneider and Joanna Waley-Cohen. Zhang Jin made Chongqing a second home.

This book is the product of research undertaken at twenty-seven archives and libraries in China, Taiwan, Canada, the United States, and England. There are too many archivists and library staff to thank individually, but specific thanks do belong to Luo Zhou of Duke Libraries, He Jianye of the UC Berkeley C.V. Starr East Asian Library, and Tom E. Rosenbaum of the Rockefeller Archive Center. I received generous funding from multiple sources, including a University of California, Irvine (UCI) Humanities Center Research Grant, two University of California Pacific Rim Mini-Grants and one Dissertation Research Grant, a UCI Center for Asian Studies Research Grant, an Association for Asian Studies China and Inner Asia Council Travel Grant, a Rockefeller Archive Center Grant-in-Aid, a UCI Center for Writing and Translation Summer Research Grant, a Taiwan National Central Library Center for Chinese Studies Research Grant for Foreign Scholars, a U.S. Department of Education Fulbright-Hays Doctoral Dissertation Research Abroad Fellowship, and a UCI Summer Dissertation Fellowship.

The Faculty Book Manuscript Workshop supported by Duke University's Franklin Humanities Institute offered crucial assistance at the right time in this book's path to completion. I am most grateful for the insight that Helen Schneider and Sean Hsiang-lin Lei provided at the workshop and thank my editor, Reed Malcolm, for dedicating his time to that event. I am heavily indebted to colleagues from the Triangle region and the National Humanities Center who read the entire manuscript and offered their invaluable critique: Judith Farquhar, Nathaniel Isaacson, Pamela Winfield, and Michelle King. Jennifer Ahern-Dodson and Monique Dufour deserve warm praise for the work that they do to support our writing community at Duke. Ruth Rogaski and Sonya Grypma read the full manuscript as readers for the press; their comments helped me to improve it considerably. After receiving all of this gracious assistance, I take full responsibility for all remaining faults and omissions and look forward to the scholarship within these pages being challenged and built upon by my colleagues.

Duke University generously funded the subvention for open-access publication of this book. I am grateful to the Offices of the Dean of Social Sciences, the Asian/

Pacific Studies Institute (APSI), the Office of the Dean of Humanities, and the Duke University Center for International and Global Studies (DUCIGS) for their support. It is a pleasure to share this book in a manner that everyone with computer access can enjoy. Thanks to the University of California Press for leading the way with Luminos. Reed Malcolm and the UCP editorial team also deserve praise for their swift and thorough work.

My career began in a loving community of scholars and friends at Boston College, where I had the pleasure of living with my precious Newton family: Franziska Seraphim, Steven West, and Sophia and Elena West. Thanks to each of you for keeping me well fed, entertained, and in good spirits for so long. I am tremendously grateful for my intellectual community at Duke. My colleagues here have consistently provided hearty inspiration and provocative insight. Deepest thanks to Anne Allison, the late Srinivas Aravumadan, Ed Balleisen, David Boyd, James Chappel, Leo Ching, Eileen Chow, Rey Chow, Sarah Deutsch, Prasenjit Duara, Barry Gaspar, the late Ray Gavins, Margaret Humphreys, Reeve Huston, Deborah Jenson, Alicia Jimenez, Matt Johnson, Ranji Khanna, Hae-young Kim, Aimee Kwon, Daphne Lamothe, Adriane Lentz-Smith, Ralph Litzinger, Nancy MacLean, John Martin, Sucheta Mazumdar, Eli Meyerhoff, Jessica Namakkal, Diane Nelson, Tobias Overath, Jolie Olcott, Simon Partner, Lillian Pierce, Sumathi Ramaswamy, Bill Reddy, Carlos Rojas, Gabe Rosenberg, Karin Shapiro, Pete Sigal, Harris Solomon, Phil Stern, Karrie Stewart, Susan Thorne, Kris Troost, and Luo Zhou. All of you have helped me to write a better book, to have more fun while doing it, and to feel part of a community as I work. Thank you.

The adage that all scholarship is biographical is certainly true in my case. My maternal grandmother received her nurse's training from the United States Armed Forces during World War II and was head nurse of the public hospital where my older brother and I were born. The day my mother went into labor with me she was off duty but rushed to work in order to see her first (and only) granddaughter into the world safely. My paternal grandmother lost five of her siblings to disease— three died in infancy from the kind of unnamed disease that used to seize children before they were christened with a full name, and her twin sisters contracted tuberculosis at the age of 17. My grandmother nursed her beloved sisters on their deathbeds just months before performing the same ministrations for her mother. It seems impossible to overestimate the impact of developments in healthcare and medicine on my family, whose members embody the seismic shift from acute to chronic disease morbidity. My grandmothers also taught me about the role of women in medical care both within and outside the home, as well as women's role in holding the family together. At the same time, my grandparents' and parents' love of learning made me who I am: a woman who cannot feel at home without stacks of books all around me.

Another aspect in which personal biography shapes this work is how the westward move of a generation of China scholars denied access to the No. 2 National Archives in Nanjing (which closed soon after I entered graduate school in 2006) has uncovered the importance of the Nationalist government's westward move during the War of Resistance against Japan. Shifting our research to municipal and provincial archives in other parts of the country by necessity, we have mirrored a similar shift that took place in the 1930s and gave shape to modern China. Quite unintentionally, archivists have introduced a generation of scholars to new ways of seeing China.

World War II was a terribly dark time in human history. Tears have rolled down my face countless times as I read the stories and records of people who lived and died in wartime China, and I am filled with admiration for the people who survived the hardships that invasion, epidemics, starvation and political corruption forced them to suffer. The conviction that their stories must not be forgotten fuels this study.

Theodore Robert Fetter has served as my guiding light and source of joy throughout it all. He makes me smarter and happier in every way possible. I treasure every moment we have together and dedicate this book to him.

PROLOGUE IN TRIPTYCH

ONE

"Can you conceive of the disasters of a war when even in peace time the Chinese people live on the verge of starvation? The rich may not suffer so much, but 95 percent of the people will suffer dreadfully and countless of them will die."[1]

—AGNES SMEDLEY, WRITING FROM YAN'AN, SHANXI PROVINCE, SEPTEMBER 5, 1937

TWO

Be Gone!
Of pesky pest infections
there's a plethora of kinds,
but the worst of the lot
is malaria, you'll find

You pop pills,
take your shots,
waste all your strength;
still you're in knots

Our marvelous cure:
an external plaster
takes one day to stop and
root out all disaster

Send it packing -
save your countrymen and friends;
come in to the store yourself
and it doesn't cost a cent

Protect your tummy,
turn things to your benefit;
come and get it for others
and it's only 10 cents

Comes in a nifty pack,
could even call it convenient;
add another 10
and have it mail-sent

If you've yet to be cured
and Western drugs have set you back,
let us show you the facts:
our prestige can illuminate

Come to People's Avenue
number 178:
our National Medicine Pharmacy
is the brightest bloom of the state.[2]

—NATIONAL MEDICINE PHYSICIAN XIONG LIAOSHENG,
ADVERTISING IN *DAGONGBAO* NEWSPAPER,
CHONGQING, 1942

THREE

The Japanese bomber pilot (red-robed skeleton) and his Rising Sun airplane (an outsized mosquito) bring the scourge of death, the proboscis and legs of his mount tracing the trajectories of bombs (malaria *Plasmodia*) aimed at the very heart of Chinese civilization (a Buddhist pagoda and farmland). We must eliminate this enemy of life!

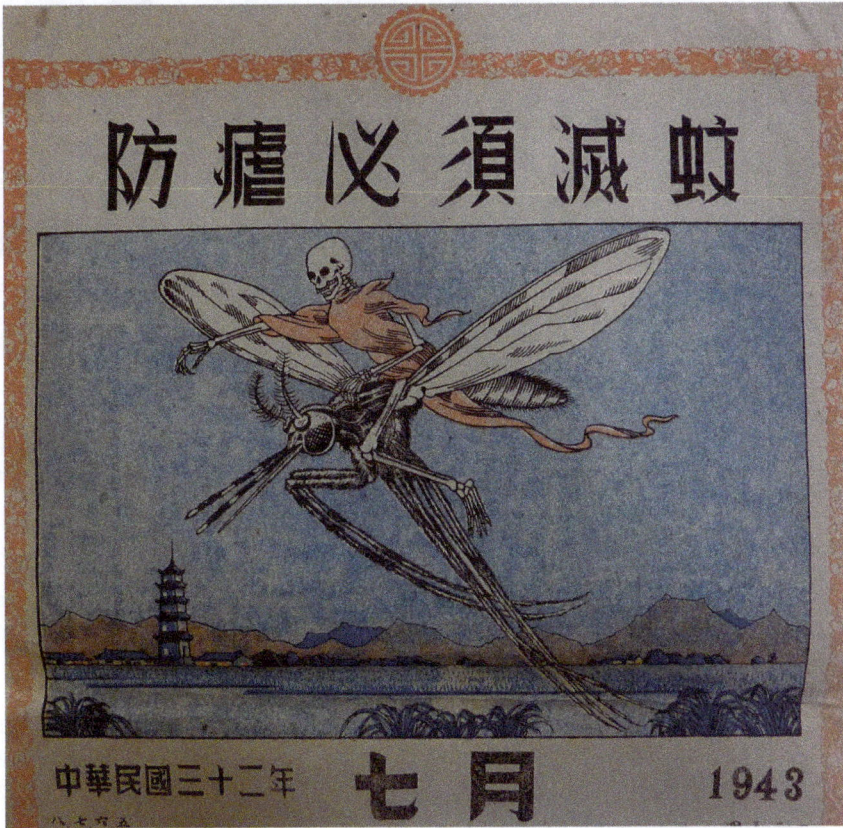

FIGURE 1. July 1943 page of the National Institute of Health public health calendar, labeled "To Prevent Malaria We Must Eradicate Mosquitoes." NLM ID 101171294, History of Medicine Division Collection. Courtesy of the United States National Library of Medicine.

Introduction

The female comrades in our war area service group came from all over the country, but we all got along very well together.

—YAO AIHUA, RECALLING HER LIFE AS A VOLUNTEER MILITARY NURSE

In July 1937, when China's War of Resistance against Japan (1937–1945) began, sixteen-year-old Yao Aihua had been a student for one year in the missionary school where her father taught in Baoding, Hebei, ninety miles southwest of Beijing. The Baoding YMCA and Red Cross immediately organized a military service corps for which many middle school students volunteered, most of them girls. They trained in a local hospital for a single week before reporting to the provincial hospital, where they faced the horrors of the war head-on. Chinese soldiers had run out of ammunition and were fighting one of the world's most formidable armies with broadswords. The number of wounded soldiers overwhelmed the hospital to such an extent that Yao and fellow volunteer nurses—indicated as healers by a single strip of white cloth around their upper arms—used sticks to coax maggots out of the wounds before applying bandages. As the battle lines shifted, the nurses traveled with the army, and Yao followed with nothing but a single blanket and one *mao* of money (one-tenth of one yuan). During the War of Resistance she moved with her unit no less than seventeen times, then seven more times during the ensuing years of the Civil War. Having lived in a single town until that point, Yao traveled throughout the entire country during the two wars. She and her fellow nurses worked day and night until dead on their feet, usually ate a single, meatless meal per day, and received no pay. They supported one another through these hardships and worked closely together—the men treating the lightly wounded, the women treating the gravely wounded—to provide medical care, entertainment, and personal support for the soldiers. Yao recalled that "during our rest time we would write letters home for the soldiers, and we used a gramophone

1

to play War of Resistance songs for them. We also bought watermelons for them to eat." In several instances she befriended the soldiers for whom she provided care.[1]

The intimacy that Yao Aihua and other nurses developed in their own ranks and with their patients can help us answer an enduring question in modern Chinese history: When did China become a nation? That is, when did the Chinese people begin to coalesce into a national community of individuals who felt bonded to each other?

Modern China presents a conundrum. After the Qing empire collapsed in 1911, the next quarter century witnessed constant warfare perpetrated by competing warlords that left millions dead and millions more on the brink of starvation.[2] The so-called Nanjing Decade (1927–1937), often celebrated as a time of peaceful state building, brought no end to warfare in the interior provinces, and in fact marked a high tide in the civil conflict between communist guerrilla fighters and the Nationalist Party's National Revolutionary Army (NRA). It ended when the Imperial Japanese Army (IJA) invaded China in 1937, launching an eight-year war in which an estimated eighteen million people died, China lost control of nearly one-third of its territory, and the national capital moved from Nanjing to Wuhan, then to Chongqing.[3] When that war ended in 1945, the conflict between the Nationalists and Communists that had simmered throughout the Second United Front (1937–41) exploded into full-fledged civil war. Yet when the Communists achieved victory in 1949 and founded the People's Republic of China, they immediately established a strong state with a complex bureaucracy, robust institutions, and formal laws, and began to lift millions out of poverty.[4] How did they manage to create a functional state so quickly after decades of warfare and social upheaval? The mere cessation of fighting certainly improved people's livelihoods a great deal. Assistance from the Soviet Union also helped (at least until 1962). Committed revolutionaries might point to the strength of communist ideology or the economic benefits of land reform. The truth is likely a combination of these factors and many more, all of which merit detailed analysis.

This book pays close attention to one such factor. Volunteer female medical workers like Yao Aihua, and others who received some pay, did far more than save the lives of soldiers and civilians during the war. They simultaneously performed both the medical labor that kept military and civilian medical institutions functioning through a period of crisis, and the "emotional labor" that cemented the bonds between civilians.[5] Having undergone training courses founded on the belief that women possessed a unique ability to soothe their patients with sympathetic care, female medical professionals provided the intimacy of healing touch to a variety of people in pain. Taught to work with a smile and more willing than men to work in the lower rungs of a hierarchical profession, women repeatedly treated discarded members of the population—soldiers and refugees—as dignified people worthy of affection and reincorporation into the productive social body. Working on the edges of the self-designated members of the "civilized," women enveloped the vulgar into the warmth of the nation's intimate communities.

The confluence of several social factors placed women in a position to heal bodies and build the nation. First, Japanese soldiers' advance down the coastline inspired a massive westward exodus of millions of refugees and an eastward countermovement of soldiers.[6] For most of these people, any medical experiences they had took place in the context of their first exposure to the vastness and diversity of their country, priming them to communicate across cultural and linguistic differences. Second, the estimated sixty to ninety-five million internal migrants who fled inland included many of the best-educated health professionals, primarily graduates and faculty of Peking Union Medical College (*Beijing xiehe yixueyuan*) (PUMC), the country's preeminent medical school. They created an unprecedented concentration of skilled health workers and administrators in the southwestern provinces. Third, the lack of concerted government programs at the beginning of the war left room for these highly educated individuals to play roles of outsize importance in creating functional medical programs at the moment of national crisis. Fourth, an influx of foreign charitable donations supported almost every single health organization in China. Members of the PUMC group capitalized on their fluency in English and familiarity with American culture to cultivate personal relationships with overseas investors to support public health at a time when the Nationalist government had lost nearly 80 percent of its tax base.[7] Fifth, the hefty influence of (predominantly American) foreign funding and the PUMC furthered the indigenization of scientific medicine, which in turn increased women's access to professional positions (if usually in lower-status positions than men), since the scientific medicine community had been actively recruiting women into nursing since the mid–nineteenth century. All of these forces combined during the war to produce a complete feminization of Chinese nursing.[8]

Although women's appearance in public, physical proximity to male strangers, and assumption of authority all constituted significant transgressions of social norms, the country needed their labor so badly, and so many women eagerly served, that a sea change in women's public roles occurred during the war.[9] Thousands of women attained formal education, assumed medical authority over patients' bodies, gained a measure of independence from their families, developed common bonds, transformed nursing and midwifery into modern professions, and developed home-based care practices.[10] Their work contributed to the formation of the modern Chinese nation in a most crucial way: they formed relationships of trust with their patients—moving across boundaries of region, gender, social class, and language—and brought into the national community people who had not previously learned how to relate to one another.

Investigating the process by which people from all over this vast and diverse country came to know, learn about, and identify with each other brings some clarity to the question of when China became a modern nation with a strong community of compatriots. Attention to personal relationships that blossomed between medical workers and patients places the focus on the lived experiences of a largely illiterate population, rather than the writings of the literate minority. This analysis employs Benedict Anderson's model of nationalism as an expression of "imagined communities" that formed in people's minds and hearts, such that "nations inspire love, and often profoundly self-sacrificing love." At the same time, the analysis departs from Anderson's (and subsequent scholars') primary focus on intellectual elites and print culture—newspapers and novels—to question how *illiterate* people imagined themselves as members of national communities.[11] We should not expect the national community of an agricultural society to have taken an urbane form, yet, given the predominance of urban studies in the field of modern Chinese history, we remain at a loss to understand the lives of the majority of Chinese people, whose rural reality far surpassed the imagination of city dwellers.[12]

The story told here counters the findings of Keith Schoppa and Parks Coble, who have both doubted the strength, or even the existence, of nationalist sentiment in wartime China. In his study of war refugees in Zhejiang Province, Schoppa remarks that they frequently reminisced about their own homes and villages while writing virtually nothing of the dangers that the war posed to the nation as a whole, and acted to preserve themselves and their families, or at most their townships or counties, without expressing any desire to act on behalf of the nation.[13] Yet one form of attachment does not preclude another, and lack of writing about feelings for the nation does not confirm their absence. Coble, in his study of wartime journalism, notes that when Chinese journalists traveled to rural areas, they frequently remarked that villagers had little to no news of the war and did not seem to care much about fighting the Japanese. He cites Xie Bingying, a famous writer and organizer of volunteer female military nurses, who bemoaned the fact that when she had mobilized people during the Northern Expedition (1926–28) "tens of thousands dropped their ploughs and came to welcome us," but those same areas became "cold and desolate" when she began recruiting volunteers for the War of Resistance ten years later.[14]

In the case of wartime China, written records, and their authors, can prove a deceptive guide to historical events. Xie's comment ignored a key difference between the Northern Expedition on the one hand and the War of Resistance against Japan on the other. The former was a battle against local warlords, most of whom had devastated rural China with their constant warfare and onerous taxation schemes to fund militias.[15] The latter was a battle against what to most people in 1937 was a distant, foreign enemy they had yet to meet. At a time when losing a single healthy worker could plunge a family into abject poverty, mobilizing war-weary farmers to resume fighting yet again naturally would have been quite difficult.[16]

Xie's was a failure of class consciousness that kept her unduly devoted to her own perspective and unable to understand that of others. Many intellectuals of her era believed that all Chinese ought to feel stirred by lofty ideals such as nationalism and Republicanism. Even if they realized that the rural poor suffered more than anyone else from state failure, they often assumed that this would catalyze desire for a stronger state rather than resentment of a state that continued to demand sacrifices before offering services. Precisely because Chinese modernity took shape in a period of humiliating defeats and torturous failures of a weak state, the literate people of that era endlessly documented their intense longing for a strong state and their disappointment with their less privileged compatriots for "failing" to want the same thing. Even the work of rural reconstructionists, designed to uplift rural communities through empowerment of individuals, had "underlying elitist tendencies" that frequently undermined the movement's impact.[17]

Scholars of modern China need not adopt the same stance. Prasenjit Duara argues that from 1900 until at least 1942, the weakened central state created "involution" in rural areas—a process whereby state agents simultaneously lost their ability to control, and increased their ability to extract revenue from, local society. For villagers, this created the experience of being charged higher taxes and fees for fewer services, delivered (if at all) by a stranger rather than a known community member.[18] The stronger the state, the greater its extraction, even as services declined because the nonlocal leaders cared much less about their communities than had local elites. Since *local* state representatives consistently abused their power throughout this period, villagers grew skeptical of *central* state power and resisted urban elites' suggestions that they devote themselves to a theoretical nation-state. Ignoring the rationality of this behavior, elites instead called it irrational (often using words like "superstitious" and "backward"), and continuously asked their rural compatriots to trust that a stronger central state would act responsibly toward them, even though none of them had the power to guarantee such a thing.

One way to think through the puzzle of how the national community took shape in a time of turmoil is to consider people's relationships with one another as primary and their relationship to the state as secondary. The war created the conditions under which new human relationships formed. To see the energy and optimism that built modern China, we must turn our gaze away from the central state and toward volunteers and low-paid medical workers who approached the suffering poor with empathy and lifesaving care. This adjusted gaze reveals the human relationships that medical encounters spawned between people who spoke mutually unintelligible dialects and lived in distinctly different versions of the same country, yet during the war could openly lament their suffering from the same problem and help each other through it. For example, many young women, themselves often refugees living in a strange environment, learned the heartbreaking stories of wounded soldiers while recording their words in letters destined for distant family members, gaining simultaneously, for the first time, an awareness of the soldiers' sufferings and of their own privilege. While urban intellectuals often assumed that only the poor needed to learn, true community formed in moments when *both* parties learned how to be part of a national community by learning about one another and, therefore, themselves.

INTIMATE COMMUNITIES: HOW FEMALE MEDICAL PROFESSIONALS SHAPED THE NATION

This book looks to human relationships to understand the creation of modern China's national community. In order for people to feel a sense of belonging to and with each other, they must learn to sympathize and identify with one another. They must develop a feeling of closeness, even if fleeting or fabricated for a particular situation. The Chinese term for compatriot, *tongbao*, meaning literally "[from the] same womb," expresses this intimacy, and does so in a manner that reifies the role of women in creating the national community. Yet given China's vastness, the population's diversity, and the divisive politics that had begun to tear the new republic asunder long before the IJA arrived, that closeness remained elusive until the very event that brought the country to its knees, precisely because it also brought people together.

Chapter 1 employs gender analysis to locate the failures of health administration in male state officials' employment of disciplinary power to control and shape citizens' behavior. The methods of what I term "the masculinist state"—which granted all positions of authority to men and prioritized political sovereignty and municipal aesthetics—produced an adversarial relationship between enforcers and enforced, to the extent that many health regulations backfired and produced the opposite of the desired effect. Chapter 2 shows how women, working within the structures of the masculinist state, altered the means and modes of delivering health services to anchor the national community in relationships born of trust and intimacy.

A variety of concepts from feminist studies and the history of emotions inform this analysis. The terms "intimacy" and "intimate" signal not straightforward affection or love, but rather the construction of emotional attachments within the confines of behavioral prescriptions that, during the war, were defined first and foremost by gender. Intimacy functioned to create closeness through the reification of gender roles, even as individuals engineered liberatory possibilities therein. In other words, intimacy "signif[ies] relations of power," though not always in expected ways.[19] Chapter 3 employs Achille Mbembe's theory of necropolitics to argue that women's intimate healing powers and men's killing powers constituted two sides of the same military force that defended the state's right to determine who can live and who must die. By adhering to gendered expectations that they must care for wounded soldiers and cajole them into returning to battle, female military nurses played an essential role in affirming men's duty to sacrifice themselves for the nation.

Barbara Rosenwein's concept of "emotional communities" informs an understanding of the national community as one founded on affective bonds between people. Rosenwein defines emotional communities as "precisely the same as social communities," determined by what the individuals therein "define and assess as valuable or harmful to them; the evaluations that they make about others' emotions; the nature of the affective bonds between people that they recognize; and the modes of emotional expression that they expect, encourage, tolerate and deplore."[20] Emotional communities overlap and break off into subcommunities, and people frequently move between different emotional communities; but too much distinction between them precludes such movement. Chapter 3 employs this concept to show that two distinct versions of the nation as emotional community took shape—one based on inclusion and one on exclusion. The political party that espoused the inclusive vision won the country in 1949.

Chapters 2 through 5 argue that female medical professionals and volunteers used emotional labor to produce feelings of closeness between themselves and those they served. Combining this with "intimacy" as an analytic concept makes room for physical contact between people—affective labor involving the body as well as the mind—in the story of building the nation as an emotional community. New forms of emotional and physical intimacy between people—particularly between non-kin women and men—brought together erstwhile strangers in the spaces of medical encounter. Women working in medicine and public health made the most essential contribution to building the national community: developing the personal relationships that comprised it.

This analysis builds on key concepts from two important studies of emotions in modern China, though in both instances it departs from the original authors' focus on the urban literate to consider how the same processes occurred among the rural illiterate. In order to think through scholarship that posited rational discourse as the basis of civil society, Eugenia Lean has introduced the concept of "public sympathy" (*tongqing*): "a new communal form of ethical sentiment" that arose in the mid to late 1930s in ardent public discussions of a famous female assassin.[21] She finds that the Confucian ideal of filial piety anchored the passions of an urban reading and consuming public that evoked a civil society on emotional rather than strictly rational terms, and asserts that by the 1930s, "the social had become not merely one factor in creating national vitality, but its most fundamental condition."[22] Though this new concept of "public sympathy" sparked intense debate throughout the 1930s, by the time the War of Resistance began in 1937, the Nationalist government capitalized on it in order to mobilize women's contributions to the nation, as chapter 4 makes clear.[23] Haiyan Lee's analysis of literature to elucidate the role that sentiment played in the construction of modern Chinese subjectivities informs a basic premise of this book: that a national community cannot arise without sentiment at the center of public discourse and understandings of the self. At the same time, this book departs from Lee's focus on literature to consider the processes by which illiterate Chinese learned to love their brethren as modern subjects. Lee traces the evolution of different versions of the modern sentimental subject, from the "Confucian structure of feeling . . . preoccupied with 'virtuous sentiments'" in the late Qing, to the Enlightenment-informed independent new man and woman practicing "free love" in the May Fourth era, to the "hegemony of the collective project" in the Nationalist period, in which the "romance of revolution" hijacked previously individualist sentiment for the sake of the national collective.[24]

Chinese people's experience of the war evoked powerful emotions. In Norman Kutcher's analysis, formulaic expressions of emotion are one of three central themes in the Chinese history of emotion. While "fully scripted" emotional expressions show up most clearly in funeral rites, Chinese language reinforces the role of the formulaic in daily life through stock phrases, especially the ubiquitous four-character phrases known as *chengyu*.[25] Generally embedded in a historical story that underscores a moral lesson, many *chengyu* became defining expressions of the War of Resistance, repeated with such frequency at the time that they gave shape to the profound grief that the invasion triggered. In recognition of this, Diana Lary used *chengyu* to structure her recent study of the war's social effects. Phrases such as *qiangzu jianguo* ("strengthening the race and building the nation"), *kangzhan daodi* ("resist to the end"), *jinzhong baoguo* ("loyally serve the country"), and *yuecuo yueyong* ("defeat breeds courage") saturated official documents and, to return to Haiyan Lee's words, expressed Nationalist officials' desire to instill a "hegemony of the collective project" during the national crisis. The oft-repeated rallying cry *huanwo heshan* ("return my mountains and streams") gave voice to the profound pain of losing one's land in an agricultural society. A variety of expressions gave people means to express the loss of family: *jiapo renwang* ("family destroyed, people dead"), *wujia kegui* ("no home to return to"), and *liuli shisuo* ("roaming with nowhere to go") described the actual situation of millions of people who lost their homes and loved ones. The intensity of the violence found expression in phrases like *qianxin wanku* ("untold suffering"), *sharen ruma* ("killing people like flies"), and *xueliu chenghe* ("blood flowing in rivers"). In the end, *bei bu zisheng* ("uncontrollable grief") and *chiku nailao* ("eat bitterness and endure hardship") vied for supremacy on the tongues and in the hearts of the survivors.[26] In recognition of the centrality of emotion in China's war experience, I exclusively employ the evocative name used for the war at the time—the War of Resistance against Japan (*KangRi zhanzheng*)—rather than an anodyne textbook phrase such as the Second Sino-Japanese War, the China War, or World War II (of which the latter in Chinese refers to the war in Europe).[27]

Taken together, these concepts inform a gendered history of emotion and of medicine that can help us understand the surprising formation of a national community in a time of territorial and political division.[28] This development has escaped attention for several reasons, not the least of which is the apparent contradiction of the birth of new things during a profoundly deadly war. Even according to the most conservative estimates, twice as many Chinese civilians died in the War of Resistance as European civilians died in the Holocaust.[29] China's combined combatant and noncombatant death toll exceeded comparable figures for Japan, the entire British Empire, and the United States *combined,* and were second only to that for the Soviet Union.[30] *Intimate Communities* upturns this narrative by examining the war as productive chaos.

GENDERING HYGIENIC MODERNITY

The War of Resistance had a profoundly cultural dimension. Fought on battlefields and in bathrooms, it became a concluding chapter in the story of Japan's imperial expansion. Ruth Rogaski demonstrated in her groundbreaking work that the Japanese anchored their empire on their presumed "hygienic modernity," predicated on the successful adaptation from Western imperialist nations of a government bureaucracy of centralized healthcare, medical education, and population management. They employed "hygienic modernity" (Rogaski's translation of *eisei/weisheng*) as part of an "apparatus to dominate Asia's future," and with it gained important recognition as the world's only Asian overseas empire. Yet during the occupation of China's treaty-port city of Tianjin beginning in 1900, Japanese colonialists also modeled exactly how to achieve this "technology of empire," and many elite Chinese took the lesson to heart.[31] Among the nearly twenty thousand Chinese students who obtained their educations in Meiji Japan (1868–1912), a high percentage studied Western medicine. The first large group returned to China in the early twentieth century armed with the knowledge and tools necessary to fashion China's own version of "hygienic modernity" so as to resist both Western and Japanese imperialisms.[32]

By the time the war began in 1937, China was ready to beat Japan at its own game, and women's labor was essential to this process. The Japanese had performed their own preemptive self-colonization at home, wherein they integrated Western medical principles and practices into the state bureaucracy in the 1870s and 1880s in order to prevent colonization by a Western empire.[33] They believed that physical fitness and the possession of science, particularly knowledge about tropical diseases, rendered them politically fit to "control the native people in the colonies."[34] In China, therefore, the Japanese envisioned a speedy victory over what they deemed to be a culturally backward country with little political direction. Instead, their invasion sparked the very process by which China developed a national community strong enough to withstand this pressure. Whereas in the early twentieth century "the absence of state control and direction . . . fostered division," the War of Resistance against Japan provided a common enemy and a need for unified resistance.[35] The threat of total conquest made the fractured nation much stronger.

This occurred because the colonial politics of hygienic modernity had placed much of the contest over political sovereignty in the realm of public health and medicine—precisely the arena in which Chinese could make the most successful appeal both to foreign donors and to their own citizens during a war that challenged all belligerent nations' health services. The knowledge that warfare spreads disease by triggering the movement of troops and refugees—together with traumatic memories of the global influenza pandemic of 1918–1919—inspired great fear and generous charitable donations from around the world, beginning with overseas Chinese. At the same time, the conditions of total war enabled the Nationalist state to make greater progress than ever before in expanding its control over the people, particularly in the southwest.[36] The greatest advances in state power occurred in the realm of public health, wherein female health workers opened the intimate space of the body to new medical practices and new state institutions. Gender politics of the era gave women special access to hearts and homes, and women played an instrumental role in escorting the state patriarch into spaces previously under control of the family patriarch.[37]

Intimate Communities argues that when Chinese resolutely took up the mantra of hygienic modernity on their own terms and for their own purposes, all of the discourses and decisions revolved around gender. When Chinese elites learned from the Japanese to craft their own hygienic modernity, the process had important class dimensions that illustrate why gender so definitively determined the ultimate outcome. In the late Qing, male Chinese elites self-identified with Japanese elites because they believed themselves responsible for reforming the behavior of lower-class Chinese, and they admired how Japanese elites had done the same in their country.[38] Chinese political culture had long charged male elites with the responsibility of caring for their social inferiors, and granted elites the right to treat them as just that: inferior beings (*xiaoren*; lit., "little people") in need of the cultural and moral guidance of the Confucian-educated literati.

Just as Japanese politicians used health as another means of policing the poor, male Chinese elites dreamed of being able to discipline the impoverished masses into a "modern" mentality and "hygienic" behavior. They witnessed the constant application of force in the foreign concessions of treaty-port cities, and concluded that only weaponry could transform the foreign occupiers' public health measures from alternative to obligatory modes of being—the *condicio sine qua non* of modernity.[39]

Chinese elites decided that they, too, would resort to force in order to police their poor, and in 1902—only two years after the eight allied foreign armies quelled the Boxer Uprising, stormed the imperial palace in Beijing, and occupied Tianjin—the Qing court established its own police force and embarked on its own "civilizing mission."[40] This process of internal colonization, distinguished by elite males' self-identification with foreign elites in the service of reforming their own nonelites, characterized the masculine approach to hygienic modernity. Because male elites' approach to achieving hygienic modernity hinged on state power born of class privilege, they subscribed to a belief that the poor should be passive recipients of health reforms and policies because only in submitting themselves to this civilizing mission could they win the right to call themselves citizens. This left many health officials without effective recourse in instances in which the targets of health reforms turned out not to be so passive. As chapter 1 explains, such methods in fact encouraged more resistance than compliance.

The supreme leader of the Nationalist Party, Chiang Kai-shek, best embodied the approach of the masculinist state. Chiang, who had received part of his military training in Japan, had a deep respect for rigid discipline and sought to instill it not only in the soldiers and officers of his army, but also in all citizens of the Republic of China. In February 1934 he inaugurated the New Life Movement (*Xin shenghuo yundong*) (NLM) in the hope of achieving this goal. Proponents of the NLM—who included the first lady, Song Meiling, as a woman representing the masculinist state—believed that "the key to China's national salvation lay in hygienic activities to purge the unhealthy habits of body and mind of the Chinese people."[41] Clearly a response to Japan's use of hygienic modernity as a tool of empire, the movement remained an essential part of social organization throughout the war and achieved a high degree of success in "foster[ing] the connections between government agencies and Chinese society."[42] Nonetheless, the successes of the NLM—and of the Nationalist state in general—remained at the level of bureaucracy. Male officials created an infrastructure of state health but failed in the implementation of health measures and therefore failed to render Chongqing, the wartime capital, hygienically modern. This book therefore makes no claim that Chinese *completed* the task of building their health infrastructure during the war. By all measures, wartime China's health services lagged far behind actual need.

Gender analysis of public health work in the wartime capital and the greater southwest shows that a profound and decisive shift nonetheless occurred during the war. This success owed not to the top-down administrative structure or disciplinary agenda of the masculinist state, but to the modes and means by which women enacted its goals among the people. Women working as doctors, nurses, and midwives established the requisite connections with their patients that made them feel cared for rather than despised, and grateful for the services they received rather than resentful of an imposition on their lifestyle. Women entered medical work in unprecedented numbers and performed the jobs that made them the first contact for wounded soldiers, sick refugees, air-raid victims, and expectant mothers. Instructed to utilize their "innate" skills of caring tenderness, and operating within a society that viewed them as naturally affectionate, female medical workers provided the type of care that sealed bonds between citizens.

These emotional ties between individuals proved to be the essential ingredient in producing a new vision for China's future, an optimistic hope that Chinese might be able to embody their own hygienic modernity. The results of women's work therefore contrasted greatly with the results of Chiang Kai-shek's disciplinary police state: rather than treat the people as objects of reform, sparking animosity and resistance, female medical workers treated wounded soldiers and refugees as subjects in need and actualized a change in people's minds—that ever-elusive space of dreams and hopes and desires. Women's medical work, funded in part by an outpouring of global philanthropy and in part through voluntarism, fostered a new vision of a China that *could become* clean enough, hygienic enough, and strong enough to claim its own modernity and author its own destiny.

The expansion of roles for women in medicine changed the shape of the Chinese state, both physically and metaphorically. In her reflections on the state of the field of Asian gender studies, Elizabeth Remick asks that scholars, rather than restricting themselves to top-down analysis of how state policy shaped the people, consider how "new visions of gender and sexuality" enforced across Asia with the rise of the modern nation-state "shaped the states themselves." Responding to this, I analyze wartime public health as a gendered activity that changed the shape of the Chinese state and the nature of the national community. Women whose labor fueled the southwestern expansion of health services created "new possibilities for control and increased state capacity" to access people's bodies.[43] Women who occupied caretaking roles—including nurses, doctors, midwives, and volunteers of all sorts—were enthusiastic accomplices in state projects of population management. Through this work, they became recognized nation builders who simultaneously extended the territorial reach of state institutions as well as the emotional reach of the nation-state as an affective community.[44]

The prewar concentration of health infrastructure in the southeast—particularly around the Nationalist Party's capital, Nanjing, and in the communist-controlled Jiangxi Soviet region—developed into a much more even coverage across the southeast and southwest during the War of Resistance.[45] The expansion of state-sponsored health services incorporated what is now China's southwestern heartland into the nation's territory. In order to understand how the chaos of the war *caused* rather than *prevented* this expansion, I interpret the War of Resistance through the lens of opportunity and employ gender as an analytic framework to render women's labor visible.[46] The dynamism of wartime society resulted directly from the destruction of coastal cities. Japanese occupation of all the major cities in eastern China forced health professionals to abandon their country's best facilities and take refuge in the internal provinces that many of them deemed cultural backwaters. They took part in transforming a handful of urban areas that had previously achieved only dot-on-the-map status into centers of intellectual ferment, hosts to influential public and private agencies, testing grounds for new health practices, and reservoirs of human capital. This included Lanzhou, capital of Gansu Province, in the sparsely populated and arid northwest; Kunming, the capital of Yunnan Province, in the deep southwest bordering Burma, Laos, and Vietnam; Guiyang, capital of Guizhou Province, with a majority non-Han population; and Chengdu and Chongqing in Sichuan Province, which, as provincial capital and wartime national capital, respectively, hosted the Nationalist state throughout the war.[47] Men—and a few notable women (Zhou Meiyu, Nieh Yuchan, and Yang Chongrui)—built a military and civilian health infrastructure in these provinces that expanded the presence of the central state. In so doing they drew on a new pool of resources; the IJA's rapid advance forced the reluctant Nationalist state to commit its scant resources to civilian and military medicines.[48] Foreign charitable donations—millions of dollars and pounds sterling—joined state funding to keep health organizations afloat despite an economic blockade and skyrocketing inflation.

Women expanded the reach of these health institutions into people's homes and hearts. Since women had long tended to family members at home, their entrance into positions of medical authority allowed them not only to cure strangers in public, but also to enter people's homes with medical bags and advice for expectant mothers and young children. As representatives of state institutions, women who gathered the wounded after air raids, delivered vaccines on the street, and tended to soldiers in military field hospitals accessed people's bodies. Their work drew people into the nation as newly constituted citizens of the Nationalist state. Thousands of daily interactions with healthcare workers modeled a new relationship between the state and the citizenry, one in which each party shouldered new responsibilities vis-à-vis the other. Since "the ideological forms of the state are an empirical phenomenon, as solid and discernible as a legal structure or a party system," the disciplinary work of the masculinist state also played a role in delivering this lesson.[49] Through accumulated participation in seemingly innocuous, quotidian processes such as gathering for vaccinations and cleaning the public lavatory on rotation, people learned a new way to relate to the state as provider of personal goods and enforcer of intimate laws. Even if they resisted that enforcement, they could not deny the renewed force of the central state in their lives. Whereas before the war independent warlords had controlled Yunnan, Guizhou, and Sichuan, after the war there could be no question that these provinces belonged to the nation. Wartime public health helped to determine the physical shape of modern China.

Submitting a central discourse of modern China—the "Sick Man of East Asia"—to gender analysis further illuminates how female medical workers fundamentally changed the shape of the nation during the War of Resistance. This discourse located national weakness in Chinese women, but simultaneously posited women as the saviors of the race through their ability to perform "motherly" duties such as childbirth, homemaking, taking care of orphans, and healing the sick.[50] Thus women shouldered many responsibilities that granted them the opportunity to create a vision of power and hope for the nation: the "Sick Woman of East Asia" became its healer.

THE "SICK WOMAN OF EAST ASIA" AND THE GENDERED POLITICS OF CHINESE MODERNITY

East Asian cultural and political power began to shift from China to Japan for the first time in over a millennium after the Qing empire faced the greatest challenges to its power: devastating defeats in the Sino-French War (1884–85) and the First Sino-Japanese War (1894–95). This eastward shift of the Asian empire's center—further reinforced when Japan won the Russo-Japanese War in 1905 and claimed the first Asian victory over a "white" people—delivered a mortifying blow to the Chinese ego and inaugurated the phrase "Sick Man of East Asia" to describe the Qing empire as the Asian version of the doddering Ottoman Empire (known at the time as the "Sick Man of Europe"). Initially applied to the Manchu court, journalistic repetition in both Chinese and foreign presses during an era of overt racism quickly transformed the expression into a universal epithet for all Chinese.[51]

Reformist intellectuals, predominantly men, immediately interpreted this phrase in gendered terms and reacted to it in gendered ways. Therefore, "Sick (Wo) Man of East Asia" (*Dongya bingfu/fu*), rather than the exclusively masculine "Sick Man" phrase used at the time and repeated in both Chinese and English language scholarship, more accurately reflects the gendered assumptions about men's and women's respective failings and potential contributions to the project of national strengthening. Through an unspoken plural, this phrase spoke more properly of *bodies*, male and female, each with a distinct and distinctly gendered means of contributing to the nation at war: men as brawny soldiers, women as mothers of plump children to replace all the men lying prone on yesterday's battlefields.

During the Republican era (1912–1949), two leaders of the Nationalist state, Song Meiling (1897–2003) and Chiang Kai-shek (1887–1975), represented this gendered division of labor in popular and political discourse. Calling himself "the Generalissimo," Chiang always appeared in public in full military uniform to deliver jingoistic speeches or survey his troops, modeling a form of military discipline that, ironically, he had learned from the armed forces of his Japanese and German adversaries and continued to admire throughout the war. Meanwhile, Chiang's wife, Song Meiling, worked tirelessly for refugees, orphans, and wounded soldiers, and inspired thousands of other women to follow her lead. Less than one month after the war started she declared in a national telegram that "women constitute half of our citizenry, and it is incumbent upon us to accept our natural duties of fund-raising, nursing the wounded, and comforting the afflicted, none of which responsibilities can be shirked."[52] Song Meiling did not limit herself to words but played a key role in all the activities she deemed the "natural duties" of her sex. In fund-raising, she frequently traveled to the United States to gather donations from Christian churches and other social organizations, and on February 18, 1943, she became the first Asian and second woman to address both houses of the US Congress, where she delivered impassioned pleas for increased aid to China.

At the same time, within this duality the "Sick Woman" shouldered the greatest burden because male elites sidestepped their shame by locating China's weakness in its women. They articulated the concept of the frail, bound-footed woman producing and rearing degenerate children as the principal source of national weakness.[53] "Sick Woman of East Asia" therefore *most* accurately describes this discourse, which "reversed the positive valence that late imperial thinkers had assigned to the family as the foundation of the state" and described the home as "a source of national pathology rather than of national health."[54]

Scholars have theorized this as an Asian response to Western imperialism, arguing that Asian nationalisms were distinctly gendered because male anticolonial nationalists attempted to delineate a domain over which they could exercise control while they engaged in a power struggle with imperialist states. In countries across Asia, male nationalists designated the home and women's place therein as their "domain of sovereignty," and conceptualized women as the bodily representations of and keepers of cultural and spiritual "traditions" that they articulated as superior to Western material power. They refuted Western claims to superiority by claiming indigenous cultural purity, but in constructing this idea they assumed intellectual and discursive—if not actual or absolute—control over women's bodies and roles in society.[55]

Male Chinese nationalists used these ideas to create a model of the "self-sacrificing woman as a symbol of national essence" and to grant precedence to state building; they argued that only women living in a powerful country would experience true emancipation.[56] Women who wished to design the parameters of their own lives were certainly constrained by this social ideal. At the same time, the idea that women produced the race and therefore the nation also gave them power to control the national body. The scholar and translator Yan Fu (1854–1921) articulated this means of redemption in his 1902 Chinese translation of Herbert Spencer's 1874 text *A Study of Sociology*. Spencer's Social Darwinism drew on Jean-Baptiste Lamarcke's theory of inheritable traits to posit that an individual's struggle for survival triggered a process of self-improvement, the positive results of which could be passed on to one's offspring. The argument that frail women produced a degenerate racial stock but strong women constituted the foundation of a robust race convinced a generation of male intellectuals to support women's education and the emancipation of bound feet. These ideas soon became laws: the Qing court outlawed foot binding in 1902, and mandated education for girls and women in 1907.

The ideal of "mothers of citizens" (*guomin zhi mu*) encapsulated women's simultaneous subjugation and uplifting through these concepts. Since "a mother of citizens was, by definition, a woman who inculcated her sons with patriotism," women could produce "not only patriotic offspring but the nation itself."[57] This formulation granted women a powerful place in the new nation, but it also subjugated women to heteronormative sexuality and constituted a double evacuation of both mother and child from their own life value.[58] It treated women's education and liberation not as ends of their own, but rather as the means to the presumed greater end of strengthening the nation through bearing and rearing healthy *male* children. At the same time, a son gained his right to existence as a national subject only through his dutiful performance of patriotism, expressed most clearly during the war as the willingness to join the military to kill (and perhaps die) for the country, rather than because of the inherent value of his life.

Thinking of them in terms of "mothers of citizens" granted women the power to create the nation itself and rendered women's work in homemaking and child-rearing equally as important to the nation as men's work in state making.[59] The masculinist focus on the home as a site of *de*generation slowly shifted back toward a positive valuation of the home as a site of *re*generation. "Sick Woman" discourse triggered both shifts, first by identifying Woman as an idealized embodiment of cultural purity and national weakness. When flipped on its head, this same discourse posited Woman as the savior of the weak nation. Once actual women shouldered responsibility during the crisis of war—particularly in fields like healthcare, which adhered to gendered expectations of "feminine" caretaking behavior—they entered a social space in which their actions had both tangible and ideological repercussions. This assertion does not reify the female gender as productive of an innate kindness, nor does it deny the fact that many men performed the work of nurses, stretcher bearers, and medical orderlies. Rather, it is to argue that the gendered discourse of hygienic modernity scripted women's involvement in the nation in a particular way, and most women played into that script.

As they entered this script, women discovered that not only could they save lives—a powerful action in its own right—but they could also transform lives in ways that created the national community. Female medical professionals and volunteers forged trusting relationships as they traveled the country healing wounded soldiers. Soldiers developed bonds with one another through their experiences in the army, but in medical encounters they learned to trust the nurses who changed their dressings and the young women who delivered their vaccinations. These re-lationships, however brief, transgressed gender, class, and regional divides to knit together a new national community of people learning to relate to each other. One young college student who volunteered to help wounded soldiers in a village in the southwestern province of Guangxi during her summer break noted that her class-mates "returned very happy and excited, since within a month they had grown very close to the local women." She also declared that their work transformed "the local Guangxi villagers with whom we could not speak" from cold strangers warily regarding the college students from a distance to warm friends, happily chatting with them about their lives and dreams for postwar life. This young woman con-cluded, "[T]he work is small, but the results are far from it."[60]

A similar process also occurred in the civilian community through women's public health work. In the decade preceding the war, the National Health Admin-istration (NHA) prioritized the training of public health nurses and midwives. The roving public health nurse, in particular, came to serve as "the point person in the extension of preventive health care and public medicine into rural China."[61] Public health nurses and midwives traveled by foot, bicycle, pedicab, and wheelbarrow to reach their patients' village homes, inspiring confidence through their steadfast dedication and willingness to accommodate people's needs and desires. Tracing the travels and relationships of this veritable army of diligent women, who had ab-sorbed and accepted their country's demand for self-sacrificial hard work, reveals an intricate web of interpersonal bonds that tied the national community together. These delicate strands of human connection did much more to sustain a nation of poor farmers than could the lofty ideals of the intellectual elite.

This book shifts the focal point to highlight the experiences between the people themselves, and thereby enhances our understanding of the Chinese nation. It argues that the national community was built on not one but two planes, with medicine a key component in both instances. The relationship between citizens and the state, solidified in part through public health regulations and services, constituted but one of these planes. Here the masculine version of hygienic mo-dernity enforced through disciplinary action dominated, and mostly failed to achieve its immediate objectives. On another plane, horizontal rather than verti-cal, the war forged new relationships between and among the people. Here the version of hygienic modernity that female nurses, midwives, physicians, and vol-unteers enacted through medical care dominated, and created a national com-munity of people learning to understand one another. Thousands of seemingly inconsequential encounters accumulated to form a network of personal ties that allowed illiterate soldiers and refugees to imagine themselves as members of a community larger than their own villages. This occurred while they traveled over the greatest distances of their lives, often on foot (refugees in flight, soldiers on the march), gaining an intimate awareness of their country's vastness and diversity as they moved. Millions of people met compatriots from distant regions with whom they could not even communicate at first. Yet often a short time later, in recognition of the need to work together to fight a common enemy, they learned how to share personal stories and intimate moments.

After centuries of living at the political and cultural center of East Asia, Chinese balked at being pushed aside at the point of a bayonet. They fought back with astonishing zeal and tenacity. Japanese politicians and militarists underestimated the capacity of the Chinese people to resist domination. During the War of Resistance against Japan—a war whose Chinese name and iconic slogan "resist to the end" (kangzhan daodi) should have tipped the Japanese off to this inner strength—the "Sick Woman" trope produced a surprising result. The IJA sought to bring China under Japanese control, but the invasion accomplished the precise opposite: modern China took shape in the crucible of the war. The desperate need to fight off a more powerful enemy provided a politically sound justification for the expansion of public health organizations across the southwest. The work of women in these organizations cemented bonds between people from across the country and knit together a national community. Working from dawn to dusk as civilian and military nurses, doctors and midwives, women repaired the war-torn nation as they mended broken bodies.

Intimate Communities fashions a national story of wartime China from a global archive. As with any country, the birth of modern China was an international story, and its contours emerged from records collected from archives and libraries in Asia, Europe, and North America. These sources include records of specific organizations such as the Sichuan Provincial Health Administration, the Chongqing Bureaus of Public Health and Police, public and private hospitals in Chongqing, the PUMC School of Nursing, and foreign charitable organizations. Personal stories come from written records of oral histories, memoirs, missionary letters, foreign funding agencies' correspondence, and wartime newspapers. Novels and short stories written during the war further enrich the picture of wartime society.

The historian faces a daunting task. We aim to re-create the whole experience of the past, including those elements that people long dead took entirely for granted and therefore never recorded. Every trace of that past contains an inherent bias; like blind people touching an elephant, we must infer from the tusk what the tail is like, and vice versa. We must navigate around missing pieces and do our best to fill in the gaps. Incendiary bombings destroyed entire months of Chongqing Bureau of Public Health records. Other records never existed in the first place because health officials and hospital staff were so overworked during the air-raid season, and military medics followed troops as they moved across the country. I have employed multiple techniques to address these challenges. I have read and interpreted hundreds of documents, comparing them against one another, treating each new piece of information as partial and incomplete. I have interpreted the actions and beliefs of the citizenry through a backward reading adopted from the field of Subaltern Studies.[62] Through such a "mirror reading," the same records that clearly state the values that health officials and police officers assigned to sanitation and hygiene can also reveal that citizens adhered to rather different definitions of the same.

Several things emerge clearly from the sources: millions of dollars in foreign aid poured into China and fueled a surprising amount of medical work, even though many challenges remained insurmountable until the fighting stopped. Although many Chinese collaborated with the Japanese or with puppet regimes, many others, especially women, risked their lives and accepted personal hardship to serve their fellow compatriots. Undoubtedly, far more people would have suffered and died without this assistance. In addition to saving lives, this work also affirmed and extended the indigenization of an erstwhile foreign medical system in China. For this reason, this book employs the term "scientific (bio)medicine," rather than "Western medicine," to describe the care rooted in germ theory, laboratory research, and anatomical knowledge of the human body. By the end of the war if not before, scientific medicine was an indelible part of modern China's medical system, which also included a robust, if forever altered, community of Chinese medicine.

No one can know what people of the past actually felt, but a historian can interpret clues that indicate the parameters of their lived experiences. Epidemiological data about the risks to health, emotional expressions in contemporary literature, the language with which people communicated their responses to enemy soldiers in their land, stories of how midwives and nurses earned peoples' trust, tales of military nurses urging young men back to battle, and exaggerated narratives of war heroes all serve as barometers of the emotionally possible. The universal human experience of desiring life also informs my analysis. People who saw death's hungry eyes in the middle of the night as they lay in the sick wards likely rejoiced when the morning light reflected a smiling nurse at their bedside. If the funerary rituals that Chinese people have performed across space and time to honor their dead and repair the social can be said to be the glue that keeps them together in all their diversity, then the work of keeping people out of the grip of death was a force that bound them to one another in their hour of greatest need.[63]

Although the war lasted only eight years, it fundamentally changed China's public health system and national community, as surely as a quickly laid foundation determines the shape and parameters of a sturdy house. Like a refugee, *Intimate Communities* follows the Nationalist Party to Sichuan to observe Chinese history from the southwest. It employs gendered medical history to narrate the birth of modern China: the fight against the Japanese invoked women to contribute to the war effort as health professionals, and their labor of healing built a network of intimate relationships across the previously independent and fractious southwest that gave human meaning both to institutionalized medical care and the idea of the nation. Looking back on the history of this terrible war, it seems that these women helped modern China to rise like a phoenix from the flames of cities destroyed by incendiary bombs and bodies cremated for entrance into early graves.

Policing the Public in the New Capital

*[T]he shifting of the capital has brought a wave of new life to the hitherto
neglected and backward interior. . . . Chungking may well be regarded as the
symbol and focal point of this process by which a nation is seeking, spiritually
as well as physically, to re-discover itself.*

—KHWAJA AHMAD ABBAS, *AND ONE DID NOT COME BACK!* (1944)

In 1938 Chiang Kai-shek likened the Nationalist Party to the nation's arteries
and described members of the Three People's Principles Youth Corps as the
"new corpuscles within the arteries."[1] If the nation was a body, during the War of
Resistance, Chongqing was its heart. How that heart looked and functioned had
direct implications for the Nationalist Party's reputation with both its own citizens
and its foreign allies. Home to the Nationalist government in retreat as well as
to foreign ambassadors, reporters, and eventually US Army commanders, the
wartime capital had special significance as the proving ground of Chinese
modernity. If the nation could succeed in "re-discover[ing] itself" both spiritually
and physically in Chongqing, then the Nationalist state could prove its geopolitical
worth and survive the Japanese invasion.

Precisely because the stakes were so high, throughout its time as wartime
capital Chongqing served as a stage upon which male officials of the Nationalist
state self-consciously performed their modernity and demonstrated their political
sovereignty to both Chinese and foreign audiences. Public health was a crucial
component of that modernity. Chiang Kai-shek had spent years achieving his
position at the helm of the still-divided Nationalist Party, and had won that power,
however tenuous, on the basis of a promise to regain complete sovereignty over
China, partly through public health regulation.[2] On July 7, 1927, one decade to the
day prior to the start of the War of Resistance, Chiang declared the following at
the convocation ceremony installing the new mayor of the Chinese-ruled section
of Shanghai:

> All eyes, Chinese and foreign, are focused on the [Chinese-ruled] Shanghai Special
> Municipality. There simply has to be a successful completion of its construction.

If all is managed according to the way described by the [Premier], then it will be even more perfect than in the foreign concessions. If all of the *public health,* economic, and local educational affairs are handled in a *completely perfect way,* then at that time the *foreigners will not have any way to obstruct the recovery of the concessions.*[3]

In 1927 all eyes had turned to Shanghai—where in the concession territories foreigners ran their own governments and police forces—and then to the prewar capital of Nanjing, where Nationalist officials first developed urban hygiene regulations.[4] In 1938 all eyes turned to Chongqing, the city where Chiang's government would either fall or hold its own against the Imperial Japanese Army (IJA). That army belonged to a nation that had occupied part of Chongqing—China's westernmost treaty-port city—from 1901 to 1931.[5] Policing the public and enforcing hygienic modernity, the Nationalist leadership wagered, would accomplish far more than keeping Chongqing clean; it would also prove it a capital city worthy of a modern, sovereign nation.

Yet Chongqing lay at a physical distance of fifteen hundred miles from Shanghai, and at an apparent temporal distance from "the Paris of the Orient" that manifested itself in out-of-date sartorial fashions and dirt roads filled with rickety rickshaws and carts drawn by mangy steeds. The Chongqing Bureau of Public Health (*Chongqingshi weishengju*) (CBPH), formed in November 1938 to work under the direction of the central government's Executive Yuan in close concert with the Bureau of Police, faced a mandate to clean the capital. A majority of its orders had to do with aesthetics; municipal and central government officials alike treated health officials like urban janitors. CBPH staff accepted these orders because, they reasoned, "picking up old trash piles" would help them "avoid the danger of seasonal diseases" that often hit in the spring and summer: cholera and smallpox.[6] Their intimate knowledge of the city's health challenges rendered health officials willing to cooperate with state mandates, despite the fact that central state officials provided paltry support; Chiang Kai-shek delivered orders to Minister of Health Jin Baoshan through an intermediary, and never once granted Jin a personal audience.[7] Trained in elite medical colleges in China and abroad, health officials began their work in a city where most of the residents drank water pulled straight from the river by shoulder-pole carriers; no municipal trash collection occurred; Japanese planes regularly dropped bombs on residences, schools, and hospitals; no quarantine service monitored the voluminous river traffic; and both endemic and epidemic diseases routinely claimed victims.[8]

While disease microbes have a concrete reality, they also trigger behavioral responses that are highly dependent on culture. Gender—the culturally determined aspect of biological sex—had special consequence in Chinese health politics. All of the leaders who employed the disciplinary power of the state to institute public health reforms in Sichuan were men—from Yang Sen, Zhou Shanpei, and Yang Wei in the late Qing, to Lu Zuofu and Liu Xiang in the early Republic, to Chen Zhiqian,

Yan Fuqing, Mei Yilin, and Jin Baoshan in the war years. As representatives of the state, whether consciously or not, these men contributed to a larger program for attaining modernity that included not only public hygiene, but also developing advanced weaponry and creating "a disciplined, martial citizenry."[9] Their work reinforced male priorities within the realm of the state. They accepted the assertion that achieving a cleaner city required enforcing hygiene regulations, which in turn required disciplining the populace. They therefore passed health regulations that empowered other men who worked as police officers, military police, soldiers, and *baojia* neighborhood association heads to enforce people's compliance with medical mandates. For example, the 1943 public health calendar created by the National Institute of Health (NIH) included this phrase on its page for June: "Cholera is a contagious disease that runs rampant [*changjue*]; it is imperative to mobilize the local troops immediately for earnest and strident prevention."[10] Men with political control granted other men control over people's bodies, all in the name of preventing disease. While tactics such as compulsory vaccination did save lives, the direct value of many other health regulations was much less evident.

Male health officials employed the language and logic of class to enforce the new hygienic order. With few exceptions, the elite possessed the right to control other bodies, while the poor possessed only the right to *be* controlled—or, as stories in this chapter show, to resist. Chiang Kai-shek and Song Meiling expressed the intersection between class politics and health politics most clearly in their signature program, the New Life Movement (*Xin shenghuo yundong*) (NLM). First launched in 1934 and continued in wartime Chongqing, the NLM charged health officials with enforcing regulations that often facilitated the universalizing of middle-class aesthetics through compulsion, rather than addressing the real health needs of the poor.[11] Nonetheless, as health workers sought to protect people's lives by touching and controlling their bodies, their small actions had great consequences for a state that predicated its sovereignty on its ability to enforce hygienic standards.

The work of protecting the national body therefore unfolded on two fronts during the war—one intimate and one public, both political. State health officials aimed to protect individual bodies from disease, but central government officials wished to use health regulations to solidify the relationship between civilians and the state and thereby assert political sovereignty in Sichuan (i.e., draw it into the national body). Many Chongqing residents felt the presence of the central government in their city most consistently and forcefully through the activities of the Bureau of Public Health. Following orders from the Executive Yuan, health officials directed and regulated people's most quotidian practices, such as where they relieved their bladders and placed their garbage, and what kinds of food and drink they could buy on the street. New rules entered parts of life theretofore subject only to social convention—including when to bury loved ones, when to gather in large crowds at public theaters, and where to give birth. This formulated a relationship between the people of Chongqing and the Nationalist state characterized by disciplinary power and resistance thereto. Health officials severed the centuries-old relationship between town and country through the night soil trade, robbing thousands of their employment, and ironically leaving the capital mired in filth. They employed police enforcement in the hope of making health regulations become new dictates of public movement and daily habit.

The War of Resistance marked a new stage in the process of imprinting individual bodies with national concerns, and gender determined how this process unfolded. An investigation of public health practices in the Nationalist state's wartime capital illustrates not only how the war affected civilian life, but also how the principles of hygienic modernity spread throughout the country and contributed to its formation as a modern nation-state. All of this occurred in a unique urban space nestled between the mountains and rivers of Sichuan Province.

SIGHTS AND SMELLS OF WARTIME CHONGQING

The story begins in a striking yet somewhat inelegant city in the heart of the southwestern province of Sichuan. Most people arrived in Chongqing by boat to witness a forest of bamboo pilings supporting the city's famous *diaojiaolou* ("hanging foot buildings") that crowded the muddy riverbank. (See fig. 2.) Reluctantly shifting their eyes from this arresting sight, they gazed up a long column of steep steps, worn smooth with the ages, snaking up from the riverside mud to a careworn city shrouded in mountain mist. Visitors with some pocket change saved themselves the sweaty toil and hired porters to carry them up these steps in palanquins, a luxury they especially enjoyed in the summertime, when the heat reached near lethal temperatures, flies and mosquitoes gathered in swarms, and noisome offal gushed from gutters at the porters' feet. One Canadian missionary described Chongqing as "a city of steps and swear-words."[12]

The wharf equipped with this majestic yet irksome entryway lay at the confluence of the mighty Yangzi and one of its largest tributaries, the Jialing River. This metropolis, hewn from limestone, experienced dizzying change and explosive growth as the wartime capital. To most refugees arriving from points east on the Yangzi (which earned them the name *xiajiangren*, "downriver people"), the city looked like a muddy backwater where gauche locals dressed in traditional-style long gowns, ate intolerably spicy food, and spoke in strange accents with mixed-up tones. Accustomed to the cosmopolitan cities of the coast, they felt that their new home "did not even look like a city, much less a national capital."[13] For their part, the locals often resented *xiajiangren* and their haughty manners, and chided their inability to cope with the delicious local chili peppers and Sichuan peppercorns.

Visitors and sojourners remembered Chongqing by both its sights and its infamous smells. In the early 1930s people described it as "notoriously dirty,

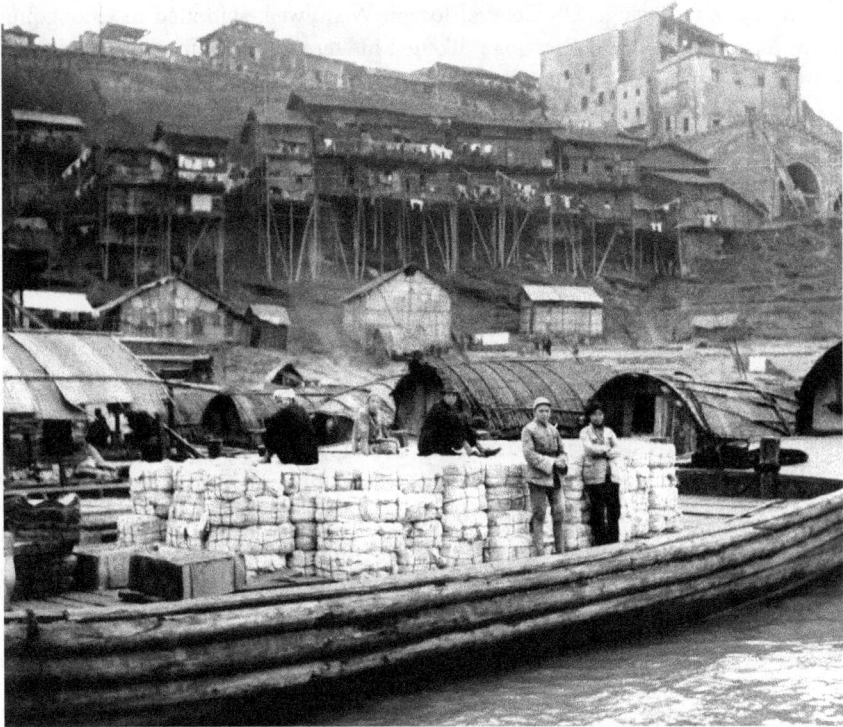

FIGURE 2. A delivery of cotton bales to Chongqing's river port, showing the famous riverside *diaojiaolou*, or "hanging foot buildings." January 15, 1944. Chinese Official Ministry of Information photograph, ID 440116045, Associated Press. No. 3615A, New York World-Telegram and the Sun Newspaper Photograph Collection. U.S. Library of Congress, Prints and Photographs Division, LC-USZ62–131087.

overcrowded, and opium-ridden," with "deplorable" public health—and a surfeit of "prostitutes, singing beggars, and ordinary beggars," known locally as the "three plenties" (*san duo*).[14] This reputation followed Chongqing into the war, when it attracted visitors from all over China as well as the world. One downriver immigrant, writing under a pseudonym, recalled of her first arrival in 1942, "[S]emi-liquid black filth drained along open ditches on either side of the road. Huge dump heaps spread down the cliff; dogs and beggar children dug in the refuse."[15] The American Martha Gellhorn, also in Chongqing in 1942, found the lepers "impossible to bear," and bemoaned the general "lack of sanitation."[16] Foreign war correspondents Theodore White and Annalee Jacoby wrote that "[s]ewage piled up in the gutters and smelled; mosquitoes bred in the stagnant pools of water . . . and malaria flourished. Dysentery grew worse; so did cholera, rashes, and a repulsive assortment of internal parasites. The smallest sore festered and persisted."[17] In his poem "Lyric to Spring," US General Joseph W. Stilwell, stationed in Chongqing from March 1942 to October 1944, likened his temporary home to an "odorous sewer" smelling of "flowers and birds, with a sprinkling of turds," and wrote, "[T]he garbage is rich, as it rots in the ditch, / And the honey-carts scatter pollution." His short, six-stanza poem contained seven synonyms for excrement.[18]

Yet Chongqing underwent a dramatic transformation as wartime capital; it gave safe harbor to a blend of people from every part of China, and some began to find it quite pleasant. It became a city where local women copied the dress of stylish downriver ladies, roadside shacks served Shanghai snacks, and financiers parlayed foreign currencies into staggering personal fortunes.[19] In the late 1930s, American traveler Graham Peck described Chongqing as "full of a traffic that was almost Occidental in quality and speed," and when Captain de Muerville arrived in the early 1940s to command the French flotilla on the Yangzi, he mentioned that "the city roads are clean and paved."[20] In late 1941, when British Army Captain Freddie Guest escaped from a Japanese POW camp and arrived in the wartime capital on foot, he remarked, "[N]o one took the slightest interest or showed surprise as I walked among them. One could immediately feel the international, cosmopolitan atmosphere of any big city in the world."[21] As the primary site where the nation began "to re-discover itself," Chongqing took on a newly hygienic mien, and presented a more modern face to the world.

A closer look reveals cracks in this facade. Many of the attempts to clean up the city failed—one disastrously so—and residents successfully resisted the health regulations that they disliked. Anecdotal accounts cannot confirm whether Chongqing was clean and cosmopolitan or grimy and gauche, but they do suggest that it was a city of contrasts whose geography reflected a clear social hierarchy. The most elite section lay outside city limits to the north, in the model factory town Beibei, which Lu Zuofu (1893–1952), magnate of the Minsheng Shipping Company, founded in 1927 to serve as an idyllic residence for his employees. Home to the Western China Academy of Sciences and harbor for elite universities during the war, Beibei was a haven of intellectual and political freedom. This made it the choice destination for famous actors and actresses, as well as other notables such as literary scholar Liang Shi-chiu (1903–87) and authors Lao She (1899–1966) and Lin Yutang (1895–1976).[22] Within Chongqing, foreigners lived across from the main city on the southern banks of the Yangzi, where they had tennis courts, pool tables, and a library. (See fig. 3.) Warlords traveled through town in limousines and lived in sprawling villas on its edges, one reputedly home to a glassed-in tennis court.[23] Meanwhile, disheveled and hungry beggars mingled with the working poor in the Lower City, the portion nearest the riverbanks where destitute people constructed makeshift homes—known colloquially as War of Resistance shacks (Kangzhan peng)—that were annually swept away in torrential rains, sometimes taking their occupants with them.[24] If they survived these floods, fires ignited by

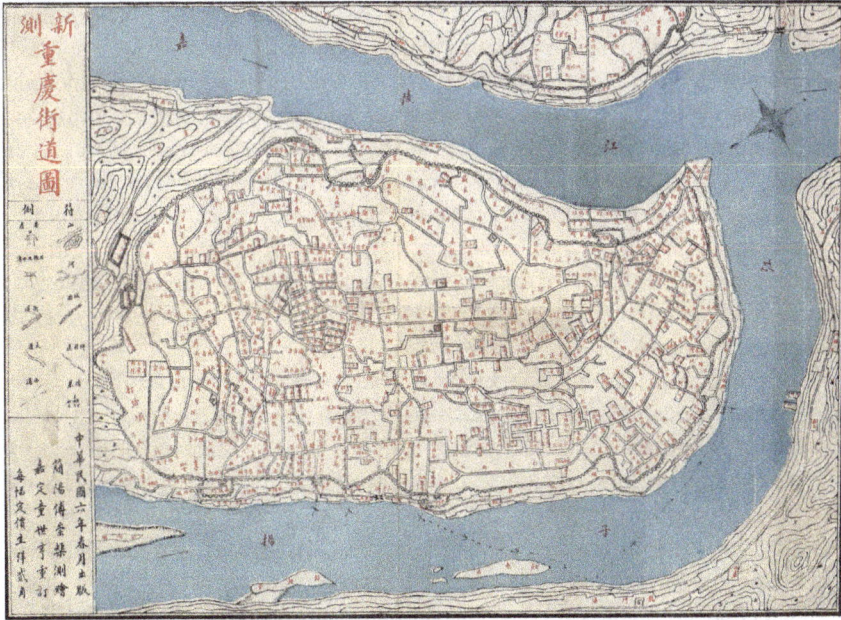

FIGURE 3. Map of Chongqing from 1917 showing the main city on the isthmus, with the northern and southern riverbanks flanking its sides. By the 1930s, those areas would become home to the more elite residences. Drawn by Fu Chung-Chii. Map 62089(1). The British Library.

incendiary bombs could consume thousands of the shacks in an instant; in April and May 1938, riverside residents suffered flood and fire back-to-back, leaving thirty thousand people homeless and more than one hundred dead.[25]

As wartime capital, Chongqing suffered more air raids than any other city in China, and was in fact the most bombed capital in the world.[26] The Japanese employed a terror bombing campaign in an effort to weaken Chinese resolve and force capitulation after Chiang Kai-shek's retreat to Sichuan signaled a shift to a multifront war of attrition.[27] Chongqing's "rain of terror" began with two calamitous attacks on May 3 and 4, 1939. These "strategic bombs," deliberately aimed at civilian targets in the heart of the city, destroyed the National Health Administration (NHA) offices, and Minister of Health Yan Fuqing barely escaped with his life.[28] Minister Yan and other health officials immediately gathered to draw up a comprehensive air raid relief plan. This included a map of all the city's hospitals and clinics, a list of the number of wounded that each unit could accept, and the order in which nurses would evacuate the wounded to hospitals in the outskirts whenever possible. Their meeting began on May 3 and adjourned on May 12.[29]

Beginning before city leaders had time to prepare, the shower of bombs on those two days alone killed 3,991 people, wounded 2,323, and destroyed 4,871 homes.[30] Chongqing did not have London's luck; whereas the British government enjoyed a full year of planning between the war's beginning in Europe in September 1939 and the beginning of the Blitz in September 1940, the Chinese government was taken by surprise. China first shocked the world in August 1937, when news coverage of Japan's brutal air strikes on the civilians of Shanghai served as a ghastly harbinger of other nations' coming fate.[31] The May 1939 attacks on Chongqing began just seven months after the fall of the first provisional capital, Wuhan, and while government officials and thousands of refugees were still moving into their second wartime stronghold.

After this tragic lesson, Chongqing followed a strange rhythm for the duration of the war. Throughout the fall, winter, and spring the city was packed with both locals and temporary residents from all over the nation. Then when the radiant summer sun blazed long enough to burn through the omnipresent fog and lay the skies bare to Japanese bombers, the city exhaled its crowds and thousands scattered to surrounding villages, seeking safety in densely foliated mountains and quiet hamlets. In order to reduce losses in property and lives, all organs of the municipal government and many social organizations urged people to leave the city, and thousands who had the means to obey did so.[32] The normally bustling city fell quiet. The poorest residents could afford neither to leave nor to pay for medical care, paying instead with their lives.

Chongqing air raids were so frequent and so closely linked to weather patterns that they became their own season, subjecting civilians to the gloomy boredom of dank air raid shelters, and health workers to the frenetic exertion of treating the unlucky victims in endless hours tainted with the stench of blood. People suffering from shrapnel wounds, severe burns, and limbs lacerated by falling debris crowded into local hospitals, where health workers placed sickbeds in hallways, foyers, and supply rooms in order to accommodate the maximum number of patients. The loss of a single hospital in the bombing season could set the region's medical staff behind for months. Disease prevention and air raid defense kept CBPH staff so busy throughout the summer that they neglected routine duties.[33] This comes as no surprise given the intensity of the air raid season. In the single month of June 1940—during the peak of terror bombings—a total of 1,515 Japanese planes attacked Chongqing on twelve out of thirty days, destroying over one thousand buildings and homes, and wounding or killing over eight hundred people.[34] The bombs frequently left Chongqing looking like a skeleton of its former self. (See fig. 4.)

Air raids posed a serious physical threat to Chongqing residents, not least because Japanese pilots deliberately targeted hospitals.[35] Raids frequently occurred on clear nights because even when city officials enforced complete blackout,

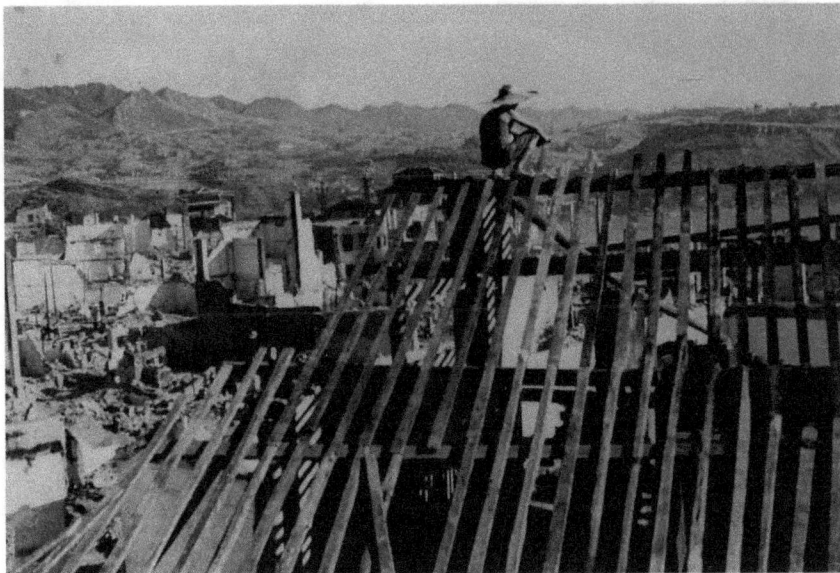

FIGURE 4. A lone man, observing the destruction of Chongqing, perches atop the home he is planning to rebuild. LOT 11511–7, WAAMD #131, U.S. Library of Congress, Prints and Photographs Division.

moonlight reflecting off Chongqing's rivers betrayed the city's precise location to Japanese pilots. (See fig. 5.) Some people began to suffer from nightmares, insomnia, and debilitating anxiety, and local health clinics hired mental health specialists. Yet most people showed a certain amount of resolve and did their best to accommodate the "new normal." When an air raid alarm sounded at mealtime, many people finished eating before heading to the nearest shelter.[36] Despite their horrific intensity, the raids failed to produce their desired outcomes: to cripple the Chinese economy and demoralize the people. In fact, Japanese bombing of China, American bombing of Japan, and Allied bombing of Europe alike all failed to achieve these goals, leading to a serious reconsideration of the value of air strikes in warfare.[37] Unfortunately, this meeting of the minds occurred only after the war, in the midst of the dusty rubble that had once formed majestic cities. By that time Chongqing topped a list of hundreds of destroyed cities around the world. From February 18, 1938, through August 23, 1943, when the ferocity of the Pacific War diverted the Japanese Army and finally granted Chongqing a respite, a total of 9,513 Japanese planes dropped 21,593 bombs on the city on 218 separate occasions, killing 11,889 and wounding 14,100 civilians.[38]

While in other belligerent nations air raids fundamentally altered the structure of governance and jump-started the creation of welfare states, in China this

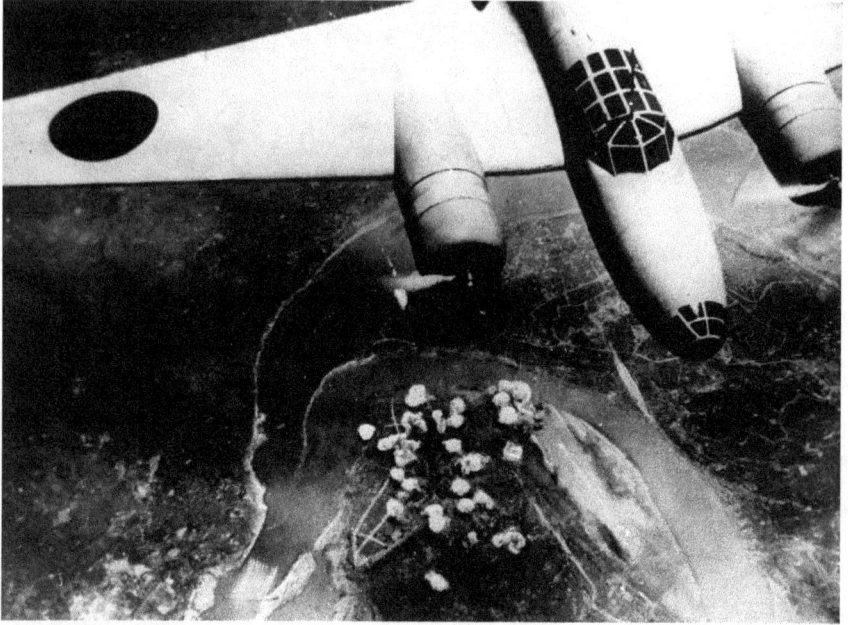

FIGURE 5. A Japanese bomber looms over Chongqing on September 14, 1940, guiding itself to the triangular isthmus formed by the meeting of the Yangzi and Jialing Rivers. Photograph by Hulton Deutsch, Corbis Historical Collection, Getty Images. Acme Newspictures, New York World-Telegram and the Sun Newspaper Photograph Collection. U.S. Library of Congress, Prints and Photographs Division, LC-USZ62–131086.

process was muted by three openly reported tragedies in the wartime capital.[39] On these occasions the air raid shelters became death traps: June 11, 1939; August 13, 1940; and June 5, 1941. Death tolls ranged from eight to four hundred in the August 1940 incident, and untold hundreds—some say thousands—in the June 1941 "18 Steps" incident (named after the location of the shelter's main entrance).[40] In all three cases the victims died not from enemy bombs, but from asphyxiation in overcrowded shelters. Sadder still, the lack of air was a result of human error. A newspaper reporter wrote of the June 1939 event, "[T]he military police posted at the entryway did not let the sufferers leave, even opening fire and killing people." Not having learned their lesson yet, in August 1940 when people once more tried to leave the shelter for a bit of air during an hours-long air raid, police officers and medical relief personnel stationed at the site "blocked their passage, creating conflict, so people [panicked and] trampled on each other, killing many." These people ran out of air because, although electric fans had been installed in the shelter for better air circulation—authorities *had* learned this lesson—they were all still: the electricity company had shut off power in that area for maintenance but failed to report the scheduled outage.[41] State officials' response included a detailed report from a seven-person investigative committee and the discharge of Liu Qiying from his position as air raid defense minister, but none of this took place until after the *third* tragedy, in June 1941.[42] The lethally disciplinary response to civilians' demands for air, as well as the belated and punitive means of "solving" the problem, both indicate the Nationalist state's general attitude toward governing civil society: control through didactic militarism, best embodied in the NLM.

THE NEW LIFE MOVEMENT AND MIDDLE-CLASS AESTHETICS IN NATIONALIST CHINA

Faced with the challenge of defending the nation from their new residence in Sichuan while under constant siege, Nationalist Party leaders resorted to their strongest ideological tool: the New Life Movement. Chiang Kai-shek inaugurated the NLM in Jiangxi Province in February 1934, in the midst of his campaign to "exterminate" the Communist "bandits" whose stronghold lay in that province (the famed Jiangxi Soviet). The Communists utilized literacy programs and public health education to fight rural poverty and attract villagers to communism. At the same time, Christian leftists in the Rural Reconstruction movement conducted similar programs in rural China to fight poverty and alleviate suffering, though often with different politics.[43] Once the war began, circumstances forced both the Nationalist and Communist parties to demand even more from their civilian base. Accordingly, party leaders on both sides entered a new kind of political competition, striving to offer more and better services to the people as a means of demonstrating the usefulness of their respective politics and states.[44] To counter the work of his political adversaries, Chiang created the NLM to increase the visibility of and loyalty to the Nationalist Party.

Chiang envisioned the NLM as a unified social movement based on the philosophies that had long constituted the twin principles of Chinese statecraft: militarism and Confucian moralism. Its foundation in moral pedagogy marked the NLM as a movement of its time. An integral part of China's grappling with modernity, conversations on morality knew no political bounds. Even the radical May Fourth movement included the lesser-known "moral revolution," with "Miss Moral" serving as its poster child.[45] In the early 1900s, prominent anarchists and other leftists established morality societies requiring members to abstain from visiting prostitutes, gambling, smoking, drinking alcohol, and eating meat. In the case of radical feminist Qiu Jin (1875–1907), the "will to self-extinction" marked her as a consummate anarchist so morally committed to her cause that it superseded her ego.[46] In this sense the Nationalist officials' obsession with morality placed them squarely within the trends of modern Chinese intellectual and social life, and the NLM was "a modern response to a modern problem."[47] While right-wing Nationalists certainly did espouse the most conservative version of feminine morality—and reviled Communists in part for their more-radical gender politics[48]—even the most progressive organizations and individuals asked women to make sacrifices on behalf of a larger, male-led collective, be it the nuclear family, the nation-state, the international proletariat, or a political party. The NLM succeeded in part because intellectuals also supported its primary goals. Long after the sea changes of late-nineteenth-century political culture and the abolition of the civil service examination system in 1905, the Confucian belief in "public morality" (*gongde*) as the bedrock of a strong nation persisted.[49]

As the guiding light for the Nationalist social agenda, the NLM also had a distinct class politics that posited middle-class behavior as the standard of modernity, and all other modes of being as deviant and inferior. Layered on top of, and affirming, the class dynamic was a gender politics that Generalissimo Chiang Kai-shek and First Lady Song Meiling epitomized in their division of state labors. Briefly stated, Chiang championed the masculine approach that emphasized military discipline and national defense, while Song led the feminine approach that emphasized social services and moral suasion. In actual practice, Chiang wrote the orders to the National Health Administration, but delegated to his wife the real public health work of meeting with health officials, accepting overseas medical donations, visiting wounded soldiers in hospital, talking with soldiers' mothers, and courting support for orphans—all of which she performed in elegant dress, with extensive media coverage.[50] Each side needed the other in order to function, and the cultivation of political loyalty lay at the heart of their movement, serving as ballast for the centripetal force that kept the two in a harmonious spin, like figure skaters on ice.

Both leaders played their respective roles well. For Chiang Kai-shek militarism was not merely an ideal but a way of life. In his inaugural NLM speech, delivered on February 19, 1934, Chiang claimed that foreigners' strength derived from their "proper way of life," and the "instillation of discipline" would ensure that China could follow the examples of Germany and Japan—two countries from which the Generalissimo had received some of his own military training, and which he continued to admire even when they became his adversaries. Chiang imagined this discipline to come from improving one's personal hygiene and eating habits, instituting a regimented schedule, keeping one's living environment spick-and-span, and abstaining from all drugs, alcohol, and tobacco.[51] As a self-professed Christian and military man, Chiang ruled his own life in this manner, rising at the crack of dawn every morning, wearing a starched military uniform and polished leather shoes whenever he appeared in public, performing calisthenics to keep his body trim, and reading the works of Confucian philosophers to guide his moral compass.

Chiang expressed faith that Chinese people could discipline themselves into the "proper way of life" that he believed foreigners already inhabited, but the way he framed the goals of the NLM suggests that he allowed foreign eyes to direct the gaze of his state toward its offending subjects. In the prewar capital of Nanjing, as well as in wartime Chongqing, Western attitudes toward prostitutes and beggars as vectors of disease and troublesome vagrants who willfully eluded state power influenced the Nationalists' drive to get such people off the capital's streets and out of the foreigners' line of vision.[52] In Chongqing, the Bureau of Police worked alongside NLM activists in projects that targeted shantytown residents, beggars, vagrants, prostitutes, and street-side peddlers alike for removal from the city. This squared Chiang's state with a political tradition in China; the Qing (1644–1911), Nationalist (1927–49), and Communist (1949–) states all treat(ed) poor people like criminals "guilty of indigence."[53]

Police officers played a dominant role because what Chiang Kai-shek understood as self-discipline could not be enacted upon an entire population without recruiting biopower—state mechanisms used to police bodies, such as rigidly enforced public health regulations, and disciplinary measures that defined and restricted how the modern body could look and act.[54] In Chongqing this manifested itself in an obsession with "municipal appearance" (*shirong*), to which health officials also adhered. Their reports repeatedly denigrated poor people's residences as "ugly alleys and disgustingly dirty, unkempt areas." They also created a demonstration residence at the National Institute of Health and other promotional materials that held a middle-class home as the standard and demarcated poor living quarters as outside the pale of civilization.[55] In January 1943, this sentiment became law when a new municipal regulation outlawed the construction of the so-called War of Resistance shacks (*Kangzhan peng*) due to their obstruction of traffic, shopkeepers' rights, and "municipal appearance." The law displaced an estimated ten thousand people who lived in such makeshift homes built by war refugees, primarily on the riverbanks.[56]

Two women who attempted to live in these shacks described how this law affected them. Wang Shufen and Li Shuhua, poor peasants born near Chongqing in 1920 and 1913, respectively, experienced Nationalist government officials as adversaries. From their perspective, not only did the government fail to provide relief to the capital's poorest residents; it also refused to let them construct the only homes within their means. Li Shuhua and her husband joined with other poor families in a group of "guerrilla residents" who stayed in their makeshift bamboo shelters only until an official discovered them, then moved along quickly to avoid punishment. In the early war years, Li and her husband moved at least fifty times in an ongoing effort to dodge state officials. Wang Shufen had much less luck at avoiding reprimand; security police regularly beat her with leather belts and called her a "stupid woman," but she overcame her fear and "cursed them," addressing them as "you bastards!"[57] In their oral history interviews, both women gave voice to the implicit war on the poor within the government's urban aesthetic. The focus on municipal appearance, and dedication to middle-class values as a universal standard, taught state officials to treat poor people as dangers to the social order rather than individuals in need of care, and inspired both overt and covert resistance.

Emphasis on appearance increased dramatically after November 1943, when Chiang Kai-shek designated Chongqing a "demonstration district" (shifanqu) for the New Life Movement, stating, "Cleanliness and hygiene shall be the most emphasized elements."[58] This new plan included dozens of municipal mandates that ostensibly related to public health but evinced greater concern for how the city looked. Recognizing that implementation would require a great deal of force, Chiang linked his new health policies to the larger goal of disciplining the people. He drew a decisive link between public health and personal hygiene practices on one side and maintaining social order through building national and racial strength on the other. The Generalissimo charged the Chongqing Bureau of Police and the Chongqing Military Police with enforcement and sent a flurry of orders to the Bureau of Public Health.

Now that they lived in a demonstration district of the NLM, people in Chongqing were not allowed to sell tea, snacks, or towels in any public establishments, lest these items end up on the ground and create a mess. Nor could they relieve themselves outside at will (renyi daxiaobian). People in military uniform could not accept a ride in a rickshaw, and no rickshaw drivers could operate within city limits, since they tainted the city with an overly rustic air (though two photographs dated January 1944 show rickshaws in the center of town, displaying the chinks in Chiang's armor).[59] It is worth noting that Wang Shufen's husband pulled a rickshaw, and they needed his income desperately.[60] The national flag was to hang only at regulation height lest it obstruct pedestrians' passage, allowing the heads of passersby to stain the sacred national symbol. The regulations held the "ugly alleys" and the "disgustingly dirty areas of poor residents" to the same cleanliness standards as the city's main thoroughfares and required that local police or baojia heads assign their residents, on a rotating basis, to clean the public toilets each morning and night and regularly sweep the streets. Horse cart drivers had to keep their carts clean and their horses healthy and strong. Chiang tasked the mayor with serving as his eyes and ears, betraying a lack of trust in local health officials and police. At least once a week, the mayor toured the city with the directors of each respective bureau, paying special attention to those "disgustingly dirty" areas where poor people lived and ensuring that everyone obeyed the regulations.[61]

Chiang's decision to make Chongqing a New Life Movement demonstration district in 1943 undoubtedly related to the fact that the city had become command center of the Pacific Theater of World War II, and both the US and British militaries—Chiang's key allies—stationed top personnel there. The wartime capital also swarmed with foreign reporters who frequently dispatched stinging criticisms of the Nationalist state or army, which Chiang always took as a barb. Government officials policed the poor and took out the trash in order to present themselves as rightful rulers of a nation at war to an army of skeptical onlookers.

And yet, as Li Shuhua's crafty evasion and Wang Shufen's brazen retorts demonstrate, enforcement alone cannot guarantee compliance. People also have to police themselves and must therefore internalize the desirability of certain behaviors and the repugnancy of others. Michel Foucault theorized that the stage of convincing people to police their own behavior occurs when, through stringent and consistent application of law, biopower accumulates to the point that it instills "governmentality"—his word to describe the mentality of a citizen who has developed an internal self-control mechanism to police him- or herself well before active state interference.[62] In this way, biopower has a positive charge: regular exercise of overt discipline encourages people to police themselves, so as to avoid direct confrontation with agents of the state. In other words, biopower re-creates itself inside the bodies and minds of the people, thereby saving state actors time and effort.[63] An overwhelming body of evidence suggests that biopower failed to reproduce itself in the wartime capital. Male state officials who interpreted the lifestyles of the poor as a character flaw rather than as a result of poverty itself wasted their time policing people who consistently resisted to the best of their ability. The poor shouldered the heaviest burden of the war effort but lived a skeletal existence, crushed between their own government's demands and an invader's dreams of conquest.

CLEANING THE CAPITAL: THE WORK OF THE CHONGQING BUREAU OF PUBLIC HEALTH

When the Chongqing Bureau of Public Health opened in November 1938, its staff faced a seemingly impossible agenda: to ensure a high standard of cleanliness in one of the country's most crowded cities—one to which new refugees arrived on a regular basis, where little public health work had previously taken place, and where enemy planes regularly terrorized the population. With four hundred thousand yuan in seed funding from the central government, the new bureau supported the already established Municipal Hospital and its new branches, as well as the new Sanitation Team and Lead Cleanliness Team, two health offices, four Maternal and Child Health clinics, the Infectious Disease Hospital, the Opium Addicts' Treatment Hospital, and a health laboratory.[64] Although financial shortfalls frequently interrupted construction, by May 1944 Chongqing had twenty-one hospitals and numerous clinics, almost all of them new or newly expanded.[65]

CBPH Director Mei Yilin (1896–1955), a trusted appointee of then Minister of Health Yan Fuqing, typified the May Fourth generation of highly educated men and women who came of age in the first two decades of the twentieth century and displayed a commitment to leveraging their privilege for the greater social good.[66] The eighth child of ten in a prosperous scholar-gentry family claiming heritage with Ming dynasty founders, Mei was born in Tianjin in 1896 and belonged to the first generation of gentry to be educated at top-tier, modernized, Western schools. He attended Nankai Middle School in Tianjin (graduating in 1916, one year ahead of close family friend Zhou Enlai), Qinghua University in Beijing (class of 1920; his elder brother Mei Yiqi later served as its president), the University of Chicago (PhD in Medicine, 1925), and Johns Hopkins University (PhD in Public Health, 1926). After completing his two doctoral degrees, Mei researched tropical diseases at the London School of Hygiene and Tropical Medicine through 1927. Upon his return to China, Mei worked at the Central Field Health Station, directed the Nanjing Bureau of Public Health, and rose to the position of vice commissioner and then commissioner of the Army Medical Administration (*Junyishu*) (AMA) before the war started.[67]

A family portrait taken on the occasion of his mother's seventieth birthday shows Mei Yilin as the sole brother wearing a western suit rather than a traditional long gown, and his wife, Jiang Lan (a nurse at the Peking Union Medical College Hospital), as the sole woman of all the daughters and daughters-in-law to sport glasses, pearl earrings, and a jaunty smile. While all members of the Mei family's younger generation were "new men" and "new women," this young couple appears distinctly self-confident. The differences in their attire and bodily stance illustrate an important point about public health workers in Nationalist China: they joined a new profession that marked them as innovators, possessed with the passion and conviction that they could make China anew by making the country stronger, individual by individual. A rhetoric that permeated wartime culture and eclipsed personal goals for the sake of the collective informed their professional lives—the rhetoric of hygienic modernity, which infused even the most mundane acts of personal hygiene with patriotic importance.[68] Mei Yilin and Jiang Lan also fit the profile of the quintessential refugee intellectual: a highly educated and upper-class transplant from another part of China, where people spoke a different dialect, ate different food, and followed different customs from the people of Sichuan. Such people obtained at least a portion of their education abroad—many spoke fluent English, German, or Japanese—and their experiences overseas made them even more culturally distinct from the majority of their compatriots.

As director of the CBPH, Mei Yilin worked within a structure that set him apart. China's modern public health had its roots in an event that defined the state and public as adversaries: a pneumonic plague epidemic that struck Manchuria at the tail end of the Qing dynasty (1910–11). The Cambridge-trained Malaysian

Chinese physician Dr. Wu Lien-teh (1879–1960) successfully controlled the epidemic that killed an estimated sixty thousand people, but only by employing an unprecedented degree of coercion. He enforced *cordons sanitaires,* removed people from travelers' inns for baths and weeklong quarantines, confiscated and burned the effects of sick residents, and implemented compulsory cremation of the plague dead (which so contradicted usual practice that it required an imperial edict to enforce). This manner of disease control "polarized the dichotomy between the state medical elites and the general public. For the sake of containing the plague, state bureaucrats and medical officers were forced to treat the Chinese people as ignorant, unreasonable, and even immoral . . . [they] felt obligated to put into practice policies that even they regarded as brutal and extreme."[69]

This adversarial relationship between educated men who desired to protect people's lives and the people they served was not only a tragedy. It was also a tremendous victory for state power. Because the epidemic occurred in a world in which "only western medicine counted,"[70] Dr. Wu's successful control of the world's first known epidemic of *pneumonic* plague, with a pathology distinct from that of bubonic plague and completely misunderstood at the time, also "allowed China for the first time to face the world as a country performing cutting-edge scientific research" when it hosted the International Plague Conference in April 1911. This in turn secured Qing power over the contested region of Manchuria, where both Russia and Japan controlled the railroads and jockeyed for power, and set the state on a determined course toward biomedicine.[71] The imperative that the Chinese state control disease with force in order to win geopolitical respect established a definitive connection between public health—care for the people's lives—and the disciplinary power of what I term the masculinist state, concerned first and foremost with its political sovereignty.

This same dynamic—securing sovereignty through health regulation—defined the conditions in Chongqing. In the wartime capital the masculinist state exclusively employed men in positions of high authority, prioritized political jurisdiction, used its resources to discipline people into "proper" behavior, and collected information as a means of control. In its first full month of operation in December 1938, the CBPH conducted a comprehensive survey of all medical professionals in the city, including physicians of Chinese medicine and biomedicine, pharmacists, and midwives. The local survey complemented a national one performed in 1937 but included much more detail, including name, age, sex, hometown, education, clinic location and hours of operation, starting date of practice, and medical license number for those already registered.[72] This information gave health officials the means to oversee all medical professionals in the city and force them to register with the government. They also demanded that doctors and nurses perform free labor—such as conducting emergency rescue work or serving on seasonal vaccination teams—and threatened to revoke the licenses of those who refused to serve.[73] Physicians of Chinese medicine must have felt threatened indeed, because in 1929 opponents of Chinese medicine who worked in the Ministry of Health (*Weisheng bu*) had deliberately used revocation of professional licensing in an attempt to push such practitioners out of the field entirely (though they succeeded only in spurring organized resistance).[74]

Results of the medical personnel survey, published in February 1939, reported 310 physicians of Chinese medicine, 122 physicians of scientific biomedicine, 58 midwives, 12 pharmacists, and 8 herbalists practicing in Chongqing.[75] The survey shows clearly that migration into Chongqing after the October 1938 fall of Wuhan, the first provisional capital, precipitated a dramatic change in the wartime capital's medical marketplace. Over one-third of Chongqing's biomedicine physicians (44 of 122) arrived between October 1937 and December 1938, peaking in the four months around Wuhan's fall. On the other hand, just 39 percent of the biomedicine physicians, and fully 76 percent of Chinese-medicine physicians, were Sichuan locals. The balance of power had shifted, but Chinese-medicine physicians still constituted the majority and had the most powerful local networks. However, they now outnumbered biomedical physicians roughly two and a half to one rather than four to one.

Chongqing health officials continued to survey the city, illustrating their "passion for facts" and commitment to data as a new form of incontrovertible truth, which itself signaled an ontological shift from late-imperial understandings of reality.[76] The central bureau in charge of health wanted to centralize information. In the same month of December 1938, CBPH staff also completed a school health survey that the municipal education bureau distributed to all schools, and launched a citywide health program for schoolchildren. They also formed the Chongqing Municipal Rescue Team (*Chongqingshi jiuhu dui*) for air raid relief, consisting of one lead team and eight branch teams to be assigned to the city's clinics and hospitals; conducted a factory health survey and distributed it to all factories in the city, many of them newly arrived; surveyed the city's public toilets and planned to build ninety-eight new ones; surveyed the condition of residents' drinking water; made plans for trash incineration and night-soil processing; and requested six hundred vials of cowpox from the NHA to institute the first smallpox vaccination campaign.[77]

CBPH staff employed two strategies to maintain a productive working relationship with central government authorities: utilizing politically savvy language to describe their work, and prioritizing projects that simultaneously satisfied their own agenda and that of Nationalist officials. Ever cognizant of the need to court state support, CBPH staff cleverly employed central government language in their reports, framing everything from aseptic midwifery to staving off disease in the language of "strengthening the race and building the nation" (*qiangzu jianguo*) and "increasing the power of resistance and nation building" (*zengqiang kangjian liliang*).[78] Projects such as trash collection and rat control simultaneously slowed the spread of disease and improved the city's looks, allowing health officials to balance central government priorities (hygienic aesthetics) with their own (lowering disease morbidity and mortality).

Nonetheless, records suggest that as the war progressed, maintaining people's health needs at the core of CBPH work became increasingly difficult. State authorities fixated on rapid results and forced health officials to cooperate with multiple entities that used disciplinary power to win compliance through force rather than by persuasion. This was abundantly clear during epidemics. Very few threats to public health worried state officials as much as did infectious diseases. The Ministry of Health, precursor to the NHA, identified nine legally notifiable contagious diseases in 1930: typhoid, typhus, dysentery, smallpox, plague, cholera, diphtheria, cerebral meningitis, and scarlet fever. In the same month that the war began, the NHA published a pamphlet stating that infectious disease caused forty-two of every one hundred deaths each year.[79] Moreover, throughout the war no effective treatment or vaccine existed for three of the nine notifiable diseases: typhus, plague, and scarlet fever. (Vaccines or serum shots did exist for typhoid, smallpox, cholera, cerebral meningitis, and diphtheria.) The CBPH conducted mass vaccination campaigns every spring and autumn for both smallpox and cholera/typhoid (the latter diseases often prevented through the administration of a combined vaccine), beginning with an inaugural smallpox vaccination campaign in December 1938, with vaccine from the NHA and staff from the various health clinics, the Municipal Hospital, Bureau of Police, and the Household Registration Police (*kouji jing*) providing free inoculations.[80]

The first instance of vaccinations by force occurred when a cholera epidemic began unseasonably early in 1939—arriving on the heels of the city's horrendous May air raids—and had already claimed nearly twenty lives before the CBPH could enact the plan it had drawn up for summertime cholera prevention. Once the bureau confirmed that the cholera vibrio had caused these deaths, the Chongqing Garrison headquarters decided to implement compulsory vaccinations (*qiangpo zhushe*) across the board. The Bureaus of Public Health and Police composed teams of vaccinators who went door-to-door giving mandatory shots to all residents.[81]

Compulsory vaccinations constituted only one arm of state intervention, and most activities entailed politely asking for cooperation rather than violently demanding it. Health officials assembled forty vaccination teams that administered shots at wharfs, bus stations, teahouses, refugee asylums, and densely inhabited neighborhoods. They delivered free vaccines to all public and private hospitals, medical clinics, and social organizations throughout the city. (Bureau personnel went to the latter sites to administer the shots.) The AMA vaccinated all troops stationed in the city, while police inspected all food, drink, and fruit stands to ensure that they installed fly screens and did not serve any cold foods or drinks or cut-open melons. Meanwhile, the CBPH informed the public about cholera prevention via leaflets, posters, radio and newspaper announcements, public speeches, and lantern shows. To provide treatment to cholera victims, the municipal government hastily set up a makeshift hospital that opened its doors on May 25 inside the Liziba Beggar Asylum.[82]

Extant records do not indicate how many people the bureau managed to inoculate against or otherwise treat for cholera, but the 1939 epidemic demonstrated that cholera could come well before summer. The following year, the CBPH had vaccinated over 10,000 people by the end of May (and over 150,000 by the end of September). This method proved effective: in 1940 both the CBPH and the NHA reported victory in controlling cholera, with not a single case over the entire year.[83] However, a sharp gender disparity in recorded vaccinations provides good reason to doubt these claims; unless women possessed natural immunity or suffered less exposure to cholera, campaigns in which more than four times as many men as women received vaccines could not possibly have eradicated the disease entirely.[84]

In 1941, health officials vaccinated over 150,000 people against cholera and reported only seven cases of the disease.[85] In 1943, the next year for which records exist, the CBPH vaccinated over 200,000 residents against cholera and reported no epidemic.[86] Financial shortfalls resulting from severe inflation hampered the vaccination campaign of 1944, and the CBPH inoculated a grand total of only 125,753 people—a far cry from the original goal of 600,000.[87] Still, these vaccinations averted disaster. In July 1944, the CBPH received word that cholera was spreading in Henan Province as well as in one of Sichuan's neighboring provinces, Yunnan. By early October, fifty-six cases had been reported in Guiyang, capital of neighboring Guizhou Province. People in Chongqing grew alarmed, and a story spread that two bank employees had contracted cholera and died, but the CBPH investigation proved it to be a false rumor.[88] Eventually cholera did arrive in Chongqing, killing one Trauma Hospital patient in early November, and several people in the Jiangbei district by midmonth, at which point the CBPH sent personnel out to disinfect the area and vaccinate nearby residents by force.[89] No total annual death toll was reported for cholera, but this handful of cases and the bureau's response suggest that they managed to keep it to a minimum. Not so in 1945. That year, the CBPH reported nearly three thousand cases of cholera and created seventeen mobile medical teams, each with a vaccinator and a police officer, to enforce compulsory vaccinations throughout the city and its suburbs. Despite these thorough control efforts, the dreaded disease returned in 1946.[90] None of this work could have been accomplished without the labor of vaccinators—often women, whose work is described in the next chapter—and male law-enforcement officers.

GENDARMES OF GERMS: "CRIMES AGAINST HYGIENE" AND ENFORCING HYGIENIC MODERNITY

The ubiquity of male police officers, *baojia* neighborhood association heads, and sanitation men on the streets of Chongqing illustrated Nationalist officials' desire to perfect the art of policing the public in their wartime capital. While the process of hygienic discipline began under foreign rule in treaty-port cities such as Tianjin and Shanghai, in wartime Chongqing, Chinese policed fellow Chinese to demonstrate their control over one another and independence from foreigners. Having risen to dominate the Nationalist Party during China's hypercolonial period and regained control over tariffs in 1930, Chiang Kai-shek assumed that containing Chongqing's filth and policing its bodies would demonstrate his political mastery at once to Japanese invaders, Communist adversaries, and foreign diplomats. Beginning in prewar Nanjing and Shanghai, the Nationalist government's obsession with making "useful" and "productive" citizens out of gamblers, beggars, adulterers, indigents, and people deemed "unclean" crafted an indelible link between the concept of modernity and specific types of behavior.[91]

Men so frequently enforced hygienic regulations that their work constituted a central aspect of the masculinist state. Nationalist state officials granted social space and political power to male groups, chief among them the military but also paramilitary groups—the Three People's Principles Youth Corps and military police—as well as the civilian police and quasi state bodies. Men in these groups possessed disciplinary power over the bodies of their fellow citizens.[92] At the same time, multiple levels of coercion undergirded the masculinist state, complicating the role of individual men therein. Despite their status as local working-class men, Chongqing police officers possessed a statist mentality; they identified with the state's desire to control people and willingly served as enforcers of state law. Yet it is impossible to know whether any policemen may have wished to resist state decree, for their jobs came with a mandate, and had they refused to enforce regulations they would have lost their source of employment in a time of hunger and privation. They therefore also belonged to the controlled; they enforced compliance with the state among the poorer of their brethren lest they too plummet to the even lower—and hungrier—class.

Science provided the logic for the masculinist state. As the international scientific community began to embrace germ theory in the late nineteenth century, awareness of bacteria and its ease of travel through large populations transformed disease from "a private misfortune [to] an offense to public order" and justified treating a sick person like a criminal to be reported, disinfected, and isolated from the healthy.[93] Though bacteriology initially served to justify states' attempts to control their citizenries during disease outbreaks, as the push for modernization increased, scientific proof of contagion justified state control of daily life even in times of health. While many people assume that the aim of scientific medicine is to find cures for sick individuals, "[i]n fact, its role in the modern era . . . has been to safeguard the collective national health."[94] Therefore, the pursuit of aggressive health policies both for and against the populace accords with the foundational philosophy of state-directed public health. Hygienic discourses hold physical coercion at their core; they invite the state into people's personal lives and "locat[e] the body of the modern at the intersection of the public and the private," making individual bodies "subject to negotiations with the state."[95]

Science and the modern state developed in tandem, each reinforcing the other, and male mastery of the unruly public made wartime Chongqing look like any other city in the world. "Hygiene police" were a quotidian phenomenon in many countries from the late eighteenth through mid–twentieth centuries. In an era of frequent disease epidemics, police officers had the power to enforce *cordons sanitaires,* isolate the sick, inspect private homes, seize personal goods, and, once vaccinations were available, deliver them by force. In both Italy and France medical officers with emergency powers intervened in disease outbreaks as early as the late fifteenth century, but the precise idea of "medical police" dates to 1764, when Austrian physician Wolfgang Thomas Rau first used the phrase.[96] Implemented first in the Prussian empire, medical police also operated from the late eighteenth and into the nineteenth centuries in the United States, England, Austria, Italy, and France, where in 1802 the Paris police prefect established the Health Council (Conseil de Salubrité).[97] In 1893, medical police began to shape public health in Japan, where the Meiji government, following the French model, transferred public health administration to the Board of Police.[98] In China, medical police had by the late nineteenth century established themselves in key cities, including Chengdu and Chongqing, following the Franco-Japanese model of urban law enforcement.[99]

The Chinese state also called upon heads of *baojia* neighborhood associations—divisions of a hundred households—to operate as informal police. The Nationalist state had adapted the imperial-era *baojia* system in the early 1930s to increase public security and mutual surveillance within communities. Originally designed to facilitate census taking, self-defense, law enforcement, and tax collection, during the war the *baojia* system was used by the state to improve social cohesion and enforce the military draft. As home to the wartime capital, Sichuan had the most intensive *baojia* recruitment, and eventually housed nearly one-fifth of the entire country's population incorporated into the *baojia* system.[100] In the Republican era members of the *baojia* elected their heads, who would serve on a rotational basis and held the responsibility to collect taxes, decide which men to draft into the military, lead community fund-raising drives for refugee relief and war bonds, mediate disputes, report potential disease outbreaks, and spread Nationalist Party propaganda in their communities.[101]

Baojia heads in wartime Chongqing, occupied Beijing, and colonial Taiwan all played key roles in public health work. They occupied the lowest rung in the state medicine system and served as local representatives of state authority, augmenting the perception of public health as yet another manifestation of the state's disciplinary control over the populace. They reported outbreaks of epidemics to the local authorities, conducted physical checkups of their residents, and served as a reserve labor force for the CBPH, which asked local *baojia* heads to: assign their members to rotational lavatory cleaning duty, ensure compliance with all health regulations, examine local food and drink stalls, facilitate trash collection, assist with seasonal vaccination campaigns, and participate in health exhibitions. During most of these activities *baojia* heads accompanied district police constables in an ingenious combination of the two parties' effort and local knowledge.[102] In other words, *baojia* heads worked as policemen, draft officials, tax collectors, firefighters, community judges, neighborhood watchmen, and health workers—all on behalf of a state that paid them nothing.

Although upon its opening the CBPH had dissolved the Police Bureau's health department to reduce administrative redundancies, the labor of police officers and *baojia* neighborhood association heads extended the power of the short-staffed bureau into people's homes and onto their bodies. Serving as the eyes and ears of the CBPH, they performed much of the physical labor required to enforce its regulations and police the daily lives of Chongqing residents. Health officials wrote the laws in their offices, while disciplinarians working the beat actualized them. The creation of compulsory cleanliness occurred in thousands of interactions between representatives of the state—sanitation men, vaccinators, police officers, *baojia* heads—and local residents. Perhaps inevitably, people resisted such control of their bodily functions and consumption habits.

No category of crime in wartime Chongqing revealed the punitive and disciplinary logic of the masculinist state more clearly than "crimes against hygiene" *(fanghai weisheng an)*. In 1941, six such cases went all the way to the court, including that of one man who was tried for "relieving himself at will" on the street.[103] The cash-strapped state cared so much about public urination that it devoted precious funds to penalize it in a court of law. The punitive state defined the boundaries of proper behavior so tightly that many people committed "crimes against hygiene" simply by going about their daily business. Yang Xuegao, a forty-three-year-old chicken farmer from Sichuan's Anyue County, paid the handsome fine of 420 yuan for placing his chicken's excrement at his doorway, thereby spreading a noxious smell around the neighborhood and "obstructing public health."[104] In October 1942, police fined Long Jiugao between ten and thirty yuan (the precise amount was not specified) for letting his pigs roam free to eat—a common practice at that time—and thereby harming public health since the pigs pooped as they roamed.[105] In March 1944, police fined fourteen-year-old He Bingzhang thirty-five yuan for throwing dirty water onto the street.[106] In June 1944, district police confiscated a sugarcane press from thirty-five-year-old Mrs. Yu Liang from Hechuan County. Claiming that her equipment was so filthy that it constituted a danger to public health, the police officers impounded the machine and made Yu write and sign a statement that she would abandon her métier.[107] On September 25, 1944, police officer Cai Zhixian discovered that the twenty-year-old restaurateur Chen Guowen, of Wan County in Sichuan, had failed to place screen lids (*shazhao*) over the food in his establishment, and also sold illicit pork despite a ban on this product. Both Chen and his chef paid a fifty-yuan fine and were required to put another five hundred yuan into a public savings account.[108]

One case illustrates two police officers' adherence to the logic of the masculinist state. On March 10, 1944, Li Dianju, an eighty-eight-year-old restaurateur from Shandong, "relieved himself at will right at the police post, then did not submit to the regulations outlawing [such behavior], but rather cursed at the police officers." The authors of this report, officers Chen Yingming and Xu Lin, asserted that Li "not only obstructed public health, but also *insulted national policemen [guojing]*," and asked that their chief officer "deal with him severely."[109] Their bureau chief fined Li Dianju thirty-five yuan—far less than what beat cops Chen and Xu believed fitting. But the true source of the officers' ire demonstrates the significance of the ideological connection between personal hygiene and the national community in wartime Chinese society. Li, perhaps oblivious of the fact that two years prior a Chongqing man had been tried in court for the same offense, or that two decades prior a Chengdu man had likewise been arrested for the same act, refused to accept the policemen's rebuke of his behavior, and rebuked them in turn.[110] In other words, he rejected the association between his bodily habits and his respect for social order and national sovereignty—the very concept that formed the foundation of the Nationalist state's public health administration.[111] The behavior of officers Chen Yingming and Xu Lin, who called themselves *national* policemen and took personal offense at Li's resistance, demonstrates that they approached their job with this concept in mind, and believed themselves responsible for ensuring that people living in their jurisdiction behaved according to the principles of the Sanitation Nation.

Cases of "crimes against hygiene" continued to pile up in Chongqing's district police offices in the postwar years.[112] They reveal an obsession on the part of police officers and health officials with the filth and stench of excrement, both human and animal. The ongoing accumulation of the same genre of complaints betrays a certain level of inadequacy on the part of local police, who failed to achieve full compliance with public health regulations despite years of effort. The police cannot take all the blame, however; the fluidity of Chongqing's population, the newness of knowledge about disease transmission, and the attitude of resistance, so clearly demonstrated in the behavior of Li Dianju, all contributed to this phenomenon. Yet the long criminal record indicates a certain failure in the logic of the punitive masculinist state, which tended to foster its nemesis—sustained resistance—rather than compliance.

The obsession with excrement produced an undesired outcome that most clearly illustrates the pitfalls of the masculinist state. Health officials' attempts to transform the city's night soil business ended in tragicomedy. Following municipal orders, CBPH staff ignored the local Night Soil Porters' Guild and instituted their own collection system with covered buckets to prevent stench and accidental spillage of the human waste.[113] In response, fifteen members of the guild went above local authorities and sent a beautifully crafted petition written in perfect calligraphy to the governor of Sichuan (at the time Chiang Kai-shek himself), claiming that they had registered their guild with the state and therefore had a legally protected right to their métier. Demanding that their collection rights be returned to them, the petition's signatories used the language of the state to make their case, claiming in one instance, "[W]e have undergone training with the Public Security Bureau several times, and like police officers at all times and places we urge people to pay close attention to cleanliness and hygiene." Representing twenty thousand now unemployed porters, the petitioners ended with a veiled threat that "we cannot die peacefully with this grudge in our hearts."[114]

This petition became a dead letter within the official channels, and ultimately the city lay drowning in its own excrement. Some of the night soil porters may have become water carriers; air raids destroyed most of Chongqing's plumbing, and in 1940, the year of the petition, city officials counted eight hundred water porters, all men.[115] Others may have delivered on their threat and harassed CBPH collectors until they no longer felt safe entering neighborhoods to clean the public latrines. Still others may have applied for the CBPH jobs and then, as an act of resistance, refused to perform them. Whatever their form of resistance, it succeeded; the bureau's night soil collection system began to break down immediately, and by 1943 the contents of most of Chongqing's public toilets flowed out into the streets for lack of cleaning.[116] Government officials, myopically focused on a particular interpretation of hygienic modernity, had forced their own public health personnel to replace a functional system with a dysfunctional one, thereby creating a health hazard. In the battle of wills with the populace, the disciplinary state had lost again.

Health officials in wartime Chongqing, caught in the crossfire between government mandates and popular resistance, devoted an inordinate amount of time to custodial duties. They heeded requests to clear specific piles of unsightly trash outside the British Embassy (illustrating the power of foreign eyes to direct the attention of the Chinese state) and shielded the chief of police from Chiang Kai-shek's wrath by devoting special attention to the sidewalk directly facing central government offices.[117] They sent the local police constable to make daily inspections of an area in Xiaolongkan (now a region of the Shapingba district) where people allegedly burned large trash piles by the roadside, thus emitting a "nostril-stinging stench" (chouqi hengbi).[118] They designed a regulation trash can, square and with a slanted lid, emblazoned—in black—with the phrases "Pay Attention to Cleanliness" (*zhuyi qingjie*) and "Do Not Toss [Garbage] outside the Bin" (*wu dao kouwai*).[119] In August 1939, they passed regulations requiring all residents and shopkeepers in the city limits to sweep up their trash daily. They divided the city into six districts, each with a cleaning corps (*qingjie zongdui*), itself divided into groups of fifteen to twenty-five sanitation men who swept the streets in their beat twice each day and rang a specific bell to alert residents to bring out their refuse for free collection. They mandated that trash be transported in wooden boats down the Yangzi to the bottom of an empty mine or to a low-lying marshland.[120] The cleanliness regulations and CBPH work reports created an impression of a tidy city humming with the daily perambulations of a sanitation brigade.

Yet one need not look too hard to notice cracks and fissures in this orderly image. The very same regulations contained provisions that illustrated city officials' a priori expectations of passive noncompliance and active resistance, while other documents confirm people's resistance. Health officials instructed residents and shopkeepers not to accumulate garbage, throw it around their premises, or discard trash in gutters or on riverbanks. They particularly beseeched residents not to throw fruit peels, vegetable detritus, and rotten food items onto the street. Beat cops who discovered anyone violating the new trash regulations could fine offenders one to five yuan, and detain repeat offenders for up to five days.[121] Despite all the best efforts of CBPH staff—who transported nearly one million tons of trash down the Yangzi in 1940 and again in 1941[122]—documentation of refuse spilling over hygienic bounds piled up in the CBPH office as quickly as trash piled up on the city streets. The bureau's sanitation men, no match for the sheer volume of waste, had to enroll police officers as fellow urban janitors; beat cops placed rubbish bins in strategic sites throughout the city and instructed citizens to use them, while sanitation men swept up the piles that resulted from people's persistent habit of tossing trash on the street and deposited them neatly into the regulation trash cans.[123] Police constable Guo Zhaoxi reported that soldiers gathered in the capital for training formed a trash pile "as tall as a mountain," and refused to listen to the police officers' requests that they observe directives.[124] That a man charged with enforcing the cleanliness regulations pled inadequacy to his superiors demonstrates the severity of the problem.

Training the residents of a city that had never had centrally organized trash collection to understand the need for such services, and acclimating them to using these services, proved to be an uphill battle. As the capital's population swelled with immigrants from virtually every province and social stratum, the Bureaus of Public Health and Police could no longer stem the tide of ever increasing and always unruly trash. Eventually the Bureau of Public Works, Civilian Militia Corps, Chongqing municipal government, and even military police got involved in the task. Even then, some locals did not know that their municipal government now had a trash-collection system. Li Shuhua washed people's clothing and collected trash for businesses during the war. Li reminisced, "Back then, Chongqing did not have any public sanitary service to take care of trash for private businesses. They had to hire people to carry their garbage in bamboo baskets to be dumped outside the city. During the 1930s and 1940s, Wang Jiapo, a hilly area outside the city proper, was where garbage and the bodies of dead people were dumped."[125]

Li Shuhua did not know that Chongqing had a garbage-collection system because in actual operation, each party simply transferred the dirty duty down the social hierarchy until the onerous task lay on the shoulders of a woman like herself who could not refuse to handle refuse. Those with the power to determine cleanliness regulations never had to touch filth. Municipal officials ordered health officials, who ordered police officers, who ordered *baojia* neighborhood association heads to order the people to do the work themselves, without compensation.[126] In turn-of-the-century Tianjin, health officials had hired coolie laborers to transport trash.[127] In wartime Chongqing, after skyrocketing costs and chronic lack of personnel thwarted their first, earnest efforts to employ a veritable army of sanitation men to scour the city clean, officials merely demanded that *baojia* heads force all the residents to do the work for free. By early 1944, the CBPH could not even afford to purchase proper equipment for the job; its plans to purchase six new wooden boats for transporting trash and night soil down the river never materialized, thwarted by the prohibitive price of 650,000 yuan.[128] Hundreds of pages of work reports for 1944 mention garbage collection only once, as a step on the way toward building new plumbing lines for the municipal water service.[129] Trash piles and the citizens who made them won. State officials had given up on trash collection in the New Life Movement Demonstration District.

Other failures stemmed from wartime realities rather than officials' incompetence. In an effort to control malaria, the CBPH ordered people weekly to empty the large water jugs that they kept at their doorways in order to combat fires ignited by incendiary bombs—a regular occurrence during air raid season. These barrels of standing water, health officials argued, became mosquito breeding grounds perched at the very doorways of businesses and residences throughout the city.[130] This was certainly the case, yet emptying these barrels every single week would have required refilling them with water drawn from the river and then carried up hundreds of steps, or paying someone else an exorbitant fee to do this task, since the price of two buckets of water carried by shoulder pole immediately skyrocketed as soon as air raids and their resultant fires began.[131] And Chongqing may not have been any worse off if people refused to undergo this strain; in such a mountainous city with unpaved side streets, most dumped water would simply have turned the streets into a muddy mess before pooling down below, effectively moving the mosquito breeding pond to someone else's doorstep rather than removing it.

The water barrel ordinance followed the typical chain of command, instructive in and of itself. The Chongqing municipal government wrote the order (likely in response to a request from the Executive Yuan, though this time the record made no mention of it), asked the Bureau of Police to transmit it to the people via the *baojia* heads, then charged leaders of the CBPH cleaning team with the task of inspecting the water jugs—to ensure that they had in fact been emptied—throughout the city every three days.[132] Though it passed through multiple layers of bureaucracy, the actual order to the people came from their own neighbors—heads of the *baojia* neighborhood watch system—and low-level personnel within the CBPH enforced it. Thus, commoners experienced state health orders through people of more or less the same social status as themselves, who nonetheless carried a state mandate granting them power over their social peers. Given this situation, one can easily imagine scenarios between the two parties including everything from passive resistance and private resentments to outright shouting matches like that of Li Dianju with officers Chen and Xu.

CONCLUSION

A fascinating play unfolded on the stage of wartime Chongqing. A chain of command cascaded like a waterfall from central government officials down to *baojia* heads of neighborhood associations, while resistance rushed up like a geyser and created a documentary record of "hygiene criminals." These two forces intersected in the making of modern, hygienic citizens—a project that largely failed in the wartime capital because the logic of the masculinist state bred defiance rather than compliance. Many people disliked the imposition of a standard of cleanliness that only partly concerned their physical health and more directly concerned the Nationalist Party's political health. Their resistance ultimately left the showcase capital mired in filth; the Generalissimo's New Life Movement Demonstration District demonstrated nothing so much as the failures of the masculinist state to mandate hygienic behavior. Its health regulations proved to be paper tigers, notable more for the fact that so many people ignored them than for any dramatic change they instigated. Large portions of the health system functioned outside the state's grasp; despite a regulation mandating that all health personnel register for a government license, in 1944 fully half of the staff at the Chongqing Municipal Hospital—the city's largest hospital directly under CBPH administration—possessed no medical license whatsoever.[133] Ironically, the state had little control even over its NLM staff. When one foreign gentleman met a pretty Chinese lady and invited her to a restaurant, she arrived accompanied by a Chinese man who proceeded to proffer her sexual services in the manner of a pimp. Deeply offended, the foreigner made to leave, whereupon the Chinese men hollered after him, "You don't like her? If you want a nicer one I can help you. You can easily get ahold of me—I work at the New Life Movement Headquarters!"[134]

The dysfunction began with an overly dictatorial relationship between the central government and health officials. Although Chiang Kai-shek certainly cared about health principles and wanted results—as made manifestly evident in the multiple public health orders he authored each day—he placed far greater priority on his other duties. Minister of Health Jin Baoshan had to interpret every one of the Generalissimo's orders through intermediaries. CBPH Director Mei Yilin also encountered difficulties. Although he identified with the elite class and believed that instituting hygienic modernity required disciplining the bodies of the poor, as an educated health professional who cared about improving people's lives he chafed at the reduction of all health concerns into aesthetic showmanship. His resistance to this mode of public health prompted the NHA to cease paying his salary in January 1942, forcing the municipal bureau to assume the cost. He resigned that December, and Wang Zuxiang assumed the CBPH directorship in September 1943, stayed in this post through the end of the war, and ultimately followed the Nationalists to Taiwan.[135]

One key to understanding the New Life Movement and disciplinary public health comes from the study of Chinese death ritual—specifically, the distinction between orthodoxy (uniform belief) and orthopraxy (uniform practice). James Watson asserted that "the integration of Chinese culture was only possible because the state enforced orthopraxy and did not try to instill uniform beliefs among its citizens."[136] Evelyn Rawski posited that this dynamic held because Chinese rulers believed that adhering to prescribed behavior would in fact instill the prescribed thought; "proper action (behavior, or ritual) was an approved means of inculcating desired beliefs or values."[137] As long as people performed the requisite funerary rituals, prescribed by Confucian tradition and clearly explained in lineage manuals and ritual texts, they could adhere to a variety of beliefs about the rituals. This allowed religious and ethnic diversity to flourish within a unified empire. The design of the NLM suggests that Nationalist officials followed this logic, believing that inculcating certain behaviors would result in desired affects. Records from wartime Chongqing show that this logic failed them.

This is not just a story of failure, however. The government's retreat to Sichuan initiated a westward expansion of state health administration and brought profound transformation to the southwest. An admirable amount of public health work took place in a location previously out of reach of the Nationalist government: Chongqing, the bustling commercial center of Sichuan Province, previously the territory of Liu Xiang and other warlords. The Chongqing Bureau of Public Health existed only because of the city's designation as wartime capital. Likewise, the Chongqing branch of the Chinese Red Cross, first established in 1920 but dissolved soon thereafter due to lack of funds, was reestablished in November

1937 after having received an influx of cash when the city became the wartime capital.[138] The availability of funds from foreign charities allowed the CBPH and other health agencies partially to escape the privations of war and continue functioning, even as runaway inflation crippled the economy. This influx of donations, coupled with a diverse population of refugees and international sojourners, transformed Chongqing from a remote city in the hinterland into the heart of a cosmopolitan nation, a nation in which Sichuan—and the greater southwest—was an integral part.

Seen from this perspective, this is the story of Chongqing's growing pains. As it became a capital city of over a million people whose residents included high-status foreign diplomats, journalists, and military officials, Chongqing had to look a certain way, and this required that its people behave a certain way. The large town that had been seamlessly connected to its rural borderlands—with a smooth exchange of night soil for food, and pigs roaming freely on its streets—gave way to a cosmopolitan city whose streets were regularly cleaned and packed with police. These men, charged with disciplining the populace into the proper behavior, came face-to-face with people's insistence that they wished to continue living as they had done prior to the war, regardless of their city's changed status.

Gender analysis helps to clarify the apparent contradiction between health officials' failures in Chongqing and the successful expansion of state power across the southwest. Male state officials self-consciously accepted Chiang Kai-shek's militaristic style of governance in order to construct themselves as modern men. The targets of their reforms—garbage, beggars, mendicant *médecins*, cramped and muddy alleyways—manifested an unruly and "feminine" city with its overflowing piles of loose refuse, excessive tolerance toward vagrants and quacks, and secret doorways tucked behind yin shadows. Wartime health officials replaced these elements with their "masculine" counterparts of the Nationalist nation: tightly closed lids on hard-edged metal trash cans, zero tolerance for those who did not support themselves with "legitimate" employment within the orthodox economy, and wide, paved streets whose surfaces lay exposed to yang sunlight. An all-male force of uniform-clad policemen and *baojia* heads enforced the new order.[139] Just as in treaty-port Tianjin, in wartime Chongqing hygienic modernity did not naturally occur, but had to be "maintained through vigilant policing."[140] A select group of men used the power of the state to forcibly remove the city's shadowy, feminine elements in order to declare it hygienically modern and capable of representing a legitimate political party of men in charge of a sovereign nation. Men who worked on behalf of the state brusquely pushed aside the suffering poor—refugees living in "War of Resistance shacks," or beggars eking out a subsistence living—to protect the nation's reputation.

While their work of cleaning the capital largely failed, male public health officials succeeded in establishing new institutions and setting the parameters in which women worked. Lacking any claim to full political power, women freely assumed roles that allowed them to claim social power by caring for the needs of civilians and soldiers. Working as nurses, midwives, doctors, and volunteers, women and girls provided lifesaving services for otherwise neglected people across the country. Because they often labored under the aegis of the state, they represented it but worked in an entirely different fashion—one that cemented the affectionate bonds of citizenship and knit together the national community. The rest of this book tells this remarkable story.

2

Appearing in Public

The Relationships at the Heart of the Nation

We needed to find a way to construct happy homesteads in the wilderness, to be a ray of sunlight in the darkness!
—MAJOR GENERAL ZHOU MEIYU, DESCRIBING THE ATTITUDE OF A RURAL PUBLIC HEALTH NURSE

Wartime advances in healthcare could not have taken place without the work of thousands of women who administered to their patients on street corners and in living rooms, in converted temples and at roadside clinics, in military field hospitals and in air raid shelters. Working as doctors, nurses, midwives, and school administrators, these women transgressed gender norms to enter public spaces, touch the bodies of male strangers, and assume positions of authority over their patients' bodies. This required not only physical but also emotional labor. In the words of Zhou Meiyu, who created both the civilian and military nurse training programs, nurses must "construct happy homesteads" and lead people to healthier and more contented lives. As an upper-class woman educated in elite institutions both in China and abroad, Zhou interpreted poverty as a barrier to this happy life. Accordingly, she characterized her area of work as a "wilderness" where nurses could "be a ray of sunlight in the darkness" to illuminate the path to civilization for a benighted population. Many women shared this belief. When the state called upon women to contribute to the war as supporting caretakers, thousands answered that call with alacrity, partly out of eagerness to help their brethren in a time of dire need, partly to uplift themselves through work outside the home, and partly out of a conviction that they could make a difference.[1] Though they soon learned that impoverished communities were not simply devoid of culture, most nurses continued to believe in poverty as a force of "darkness" and their own work as a source of "light." Put simply, female medical professionals worked within the same structures and strictures of the masculinist state articulated in chapter 1, and quite frequently believed in them. Neither side could operate without the other, and both worked toward the mutual aim of teaching people to internalize state values and new hygiene practices, so as to save lives.

Yet women's work had a more powerful effect on wartime society. While men's work through overt discipline fostered resistance, women's work, at least when delivered with compassion and care, fostered compliance. Women therefore played the more important part in teaching people how to accept state regulations as standards for their own values and behavior, and extended state power further than did many men who represented that power more directly. This occurred because women performed their work in an entirely different manner—not as a result of any innate quality of the female sex, but because the gender expectations of the time cast them into a role distinct from that of men. Whereas men fulfilled the responsibilities of a disciplinary father, women who worked as nurses, midwives, doctors, and volunteers played the part of the nurturing, caring mother, delivering crucial services to people in need. Playing this role required women's "emotional labor"—work in which "the *emotional style of offering the service is part of the service itself.*"[2] Precisely because they performed this emotional work, modeled for them by none other than First Lady Song Meiling, women succeeded where men failed. The nature of women's work with civilian refugees, orphaned children, wounded soldiers, and general patients required that they communicate trustworthiness to their charges. Operating under the gendered assumption that, as women, they possessed a "natural" tenderness, women proved particularly adept at the emotional labor of healthcare.[3] They worked hard to earn their patients' trust and formed relationships with them. They served as representatives of state benevolence and thereby granted the masculinist state the necessary power to enter people's homes and affect individual bodies. Contemporary literature reflected women's power to transform their patients through emotional labor. One of the wartime novels by the famous author Ba Jin, *Ward Four (Disi bingshi)*, used the setting of a civilian hospital ward to reflect on this facet of wartime healthcare.[4]

This was not the first time that women had worked to soften the disciplinary power of a state, nor would it be the last. Women and girls who cared for suffering people in wartime China occupied a role that had long been established in colonial states. European women who worked as healers and teachers in colonies served as crucial conduits by which colonial states accessed indigenous peoples, precisely because their lower status and "inferior" gender placed them in a more intimate relationship thereto.[5] During the British colonial government's counterinsurgency against communist guerrillas in postwar Malaysia, colonial nurses played a key role in schooling the people in "cultural colonialism." As part of the Cold War politics of convincing people "to align with capitalist rather than communist countries," nurses served as a "tool in the propaganda war of the British government to demonstrate that it cared about the welfare of villagers."[6] Indeed throughout the British Empire, "medicine, public health, nursing and the clinic were themselves instruments and sites of colonial governance."[7] Though they worked for their own rather than a colonial state, women in wartime China played a very similar part in amplifying state power over the people.

It did matter that these women worked on behalf of an indigenous state. For one thing, this fact gave their work a dual purpose: it simultaneously rendered people's bodies available to the state for physical manipulation (e.g., to receive an immunization), and taught people what types of services they could demand from the state. Additionally, and more importantly, it taught people a new mode of relating to one another. This most crucial way that women's emotional labor in healing contributed to state power occurred at the level of interpersonal interaction. When thousands of women accepted the charge to heal soldiers and civilians, their work transgressed boundaries of gender, class, and region in a manner that shaped the national community. As healthcare workers they gained an unprecedented proximity to male bodies that profoundly challenged gender norms. Moreover, with less recourse to more-prestigious positions within the hierarchical health profession, women were much more likely than men to take on the less remunerative roles of the frontline responders, so people in need frequently encountered a woman at their moment of greatest vulnerability. Female healers' intimate contact with soldiers and refugees from all over the country fostered emotional bonds that bound the nation together through myriad quotidian medical encounters. Differences in sex, social class, occupation, level of education, and native region faded into the background in these moments when new relationships blossomed. Given the poignant needs of a nation under siege, the bonds that women built affected far more than two people; they formed the bedrock of a national community.

In defining the national community, this book affirms the emotional dimension of Benedict Anderson's classic work on nationalism.[8] It also parts from the emphasis of Anderson and subsequent scholars on print capitalism and the experience of simultaneous time through reading newspapers and novels. Though seductive to historians who work primarily with texts, this approach reveals precious little about the vast majority of Chinese of the time who could not read and had little to no experience with print culture. To be sure, illiterate people learned and shared information about their country through a variety of means. They attended performances of traveling drama troupes, requested the services of professional letter writers who set up shop outside post offices, listened to public speeches, shared rumors and news in market towns, and (especially in Sichuan) gathered in teahouses that served as sites of "neighborhood or community information center[s]."[9] They could certainly partake in public political culture, but direct attention to the written expressions of that culture teaches us little about how the illiterate majority understood it and their role therein, and much more about what the literate minority thought about their unlettered brethren. Analysis of how the latter fit into and gained membership in the national community therefore requires privileged attention to their emotional lives since, in the words of Haiyan Lee, "the modern subject is first and foremost a sentimental subject, and . . . the modern nation is first and foremost a community of sympathy."[10]

In China, this is poignantly expressed in the use of "a term of deepest emotion" to express patriotism, *aiguo* ("love of country"); the use of a familial term to delineate "country," *guojia* ("nation-family"); and the fact that leaders in both the Nationalist and Communist parties "sought to find a means of generating feeling among their supporters."[11] In their daily language, Chinese people continually affirm the centrality of emotions in nationalism. Therefore, in order to analyze the making of China's national community, the present work pays close attention to emotion—specifically, under what circumstances, with whom, and for what reasons people developed emotive relationships. Stories of healthcare during the War of Resistance demonstrate that medical exchanges fostered emotional bonds between civilians and soldiers and their female caretakers, in a manner much more pronounced than with male caretakers.

In order for women to perform the medical labor that saved lives, and the emotional labor that connected them in a communal narrative, they first had to normalize the public appearance of (particularly middle-class) women. Women had to transgress social norms in order to occupy public spaces, associate with men who were strangers, and assume positions of authority over others. Three factors made this transgression possible. First, these norms were not evenly distributed across the country. While inner provinces like Sichuan tended to have more-conservative gender norms, the arrival of refugees from eastern cities during the war created spaces in local culture for greater acceptance of women taking public roles.[12] Second, First Lady Song Meiling called for women to contribute to the war effort through public work, and frequently appeared in the press modeling just how to do it. Third, extraordinary times call for extraordinary measures. Just as the 1911 Revolution and the 1927 Northern Expedition had required the active—and often violent—participation of women, the War of Resistance required women to become highly visible medical authorities.[13] The demand was highest in professional nursing. While many women became doctors and midwives, the overall number of personnel in those professions remained fairly constant throughout the war. Nursing, on the other hand, experienced a dramatic increase in personnel. Between 1936 and 1937, the number of nurses registered with the National Health Administration increased from about 250 to over 4,500. By 1941 the number had increased again to over 5,500.[14] The relative ubiquity of female nurses during the war created social space in which women crafted a new role for themselves—not just as healers, but also as makers of the national community.

A BRIEF HISTORY OF NURSING IN CHINA

Although women had long taken care of the ill, they had generally done so in the confines of their own or their relatives' homes, and the care networks in which they operated overlapped with their family networks. The process of transforming nursing into a hospital-based profession took decades. It began in the late nineteenth century when foreign missionaries established training programs inside mission hospitals, first in the Margaret Williamson Hospital in Shanghai in 1887.[15] This was roughly two decades after the American Civil War in Williamson's home country had transformed nursing into a profession and granted middle-class women a space therein.[16] With the original goal of obtaining their own hospital personnel, the first missionary nursing schools accepted only male students because they were affiliated with men's hospitals, and missionaries chose to observe the strict gender segregation practices of Chinese elites. This worked until missionaries entered the field of women's medicine; by 1900 medical missionaries had succeeded in opening 12 women's hospitals of the country's grand total of 107. By the 1920s the missionaries celebrated their achievement in recruiting female nursing students to serve therein, which allowed them to proselytize not only their religion but also their gender ideology—specifically, their belief that nursing was an innately feminine venture and that female nurses in crisp white uniforms (the color of mourning garments in China) were an essential element of a modern hospital ward.[17] By 1934, 65 percent of all hospitals in China had female nurses attending to male patients, signaling a dramatic departure from previous policies of observing Chinese gender propriety.[18]

Foreign missionaries also played a significant role in standardizing nursing education. In 1908, the American Methodist missionary Cora E. Simpson founded the Nurses' Association of China (*Zhonghua hushi hui*). At its first general meeting in Shanghai in 1914, the association established curriculum standards and an annual exam that all nursing school graduates in China had to pass in order to receive a license to practice. The association also adopted the term *hushi* instead of *kanhu* to signify "nurse," at the suggestion of China's first woman to have studied overseas in England. The new term used the suffix -*shi*, meaning "scholar," adding a degree of professionalism to the role.[19] This work soon inspired local initiatives. In 1932, China's first government-run nursing school, the Central Nursing School, opened in Nanjing with a two-year course in nursing and a one-year course in public health and midwifery.[20]

As important as medical missionaries' work was, it did not take hold until Chinese women decided that professional, feminized nursing fulfilled their own goals of female emancipation. The shift began very gradually with two Christian converts, Kang Cheng (Ida Kahn) and Shi Meiyu (Mary Stone). In 1896 the two women returned to China with degrees from the University of Michigan Medical School and opened their own women's and children's hospital in Jiujiang, Jiangxi,

as missionaries of the Methodist Episcopal Church. In addition to treating hundreds of parturient women, Drs. Kang and Shi opened a new professional path for
their female compatriots. Like Chinese Florence Nightingales, they demonstrated
through their actions that respectable women could voluntarily choose the medical
profession and remain dignified.[21]

The radical feminist activist Qiu Jin (1875–1907) also played a key role in
promoting nursing. In 1904, Qiu left an unhappy marriage and two young
children to attend Shimoda Utako's Girls' Practical School in Tokyo. While there,
she encountered Japanese Red Cross nurses and became convinced that their
métier could also serve to liberate her own compatriots from their economic and
social oppression.[22] She translated a nursing manual, and she advocated nursing
as a suitable occupation for women in the feminist journal she founded, *Zhongguo
nübao* (Chinese women's journal), as well as in her public speeches. Qiu Jin had
left her family, lived alone overseas, joined Sun Yat-sen's Revolutionary Alliance
and other radical societies, dressed in men's attire, learned to make bombs,
conspired to assassinate the Manchu emperor, and would bravely face execution
at the tender age of thirty-two, yet she understood that most women would never
lead such radical lives.[23] She instead urged them to see professional employment
as a path to liberation and declared that women's feminine qualities made them
perfect candidates for nursing.

Through her advocacy of nursing, Qiu Jin inadvertently helped the missionaries
achieve one of their goals: promoting Chinese women to positions of leadership.
In 1921, Wu Zheying became the first Chinese woman to run a local nursing
school—in this case, the Shanghai Red Cross Nursing School, which had originally opened in 1909. In 1926, Wu became the first Chinese chairwoman of the
Nurses' Association of China. By 1935, the association boasted a majority Chinese
membership, and its 167 affiliated nursing schools (mostly missionary run) had
graduated nearly five thousand nurses.[24] As the number of professionally trained
Chinese nurses continued to grow, foreigners gradually yielded leadership positions
in accordance with their overall aim of promoting Chinese initiative in the nursing
profession, and the war spurred this process even further.

PUBLIC APPEARANCES: VISIBILITY, MEDICAL AU-
THORITY, AND CLASS POLITICS

Moving into public spaces was dangerous for women during the war, not least
because near-constant warfare made rape an omnipresent threat.[25] It also exposed
them to social ridicule and the risk of impugning their entire families.[26] Nonetheless, women frequently appeared on the streets of Chongqing as public health
providers and representatives of the state. Young women frequently worked on
vaccination teams that operated on busy street corners and in heavily trafficked

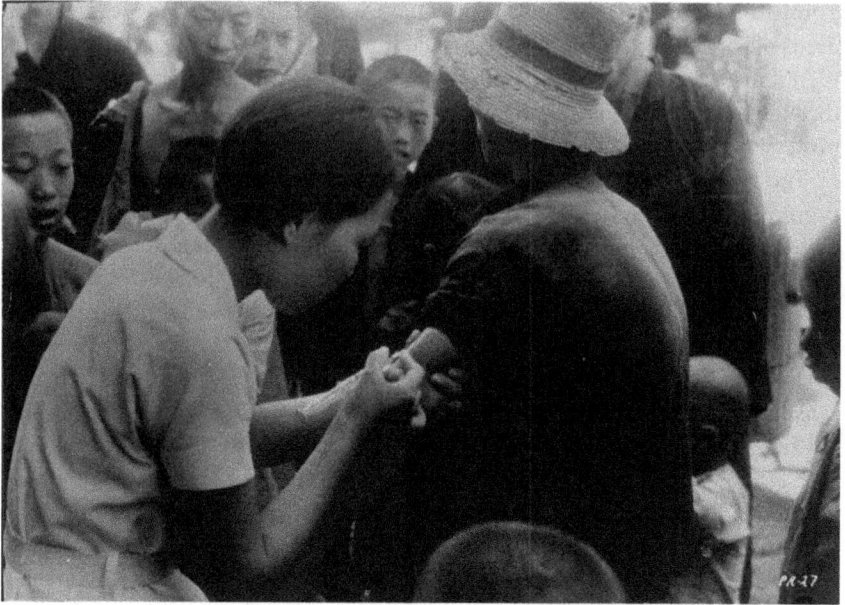

FIGURE 6. A young woman delivers vaccinations on Chongqing streets, ca. 1941. Box 86, folder "Vaccine Plant." ABMAC Records. Rare Book and Manuscript Library. Columbia University.

portions of town, such as bus stations, train stations, and wharves. During the vaccination campaigns that the Chongqing Bureau of Public Health sponsored every spring and fall, they worked long hours delivering free vaccinations. At a time when many Sichuan parents disallowed their daughters from traveling alone or even appearing in public, female vaccinators entered crowded spaces of largely male sociality armed with the tools of their trade—syringes, vaccine ampoules, and nurses' uniforms—that granted them medical authority over the recipients' bodies and a certain degree of protection. The woman shown in figure 6 appears not the least bit ruffled by the men and boys pressing in on her and operates her syringe with the steady hand of an expert. Her firm grasp on the recipient's arm displays an unprecedented intimacy between two strangers of opposite sex. Although curious onlookers congregate tightly around her, some of them scrutinizing her actions, her syringe and nurse's uniform, crisp and clean, set her apart from the crowd, granting her a distinguished singularity. Her hairstyle marks her as a "new woman," quite possibly a "downriver" refugee from a more cosmopolitan, coastal city.[27] She swiftly and effectively delivers the state's instrument of public health to people who welcome her service.

As a group, women possessed neither political nor military power, but this photograph demonstrates that as medical professionals, they did gain power over

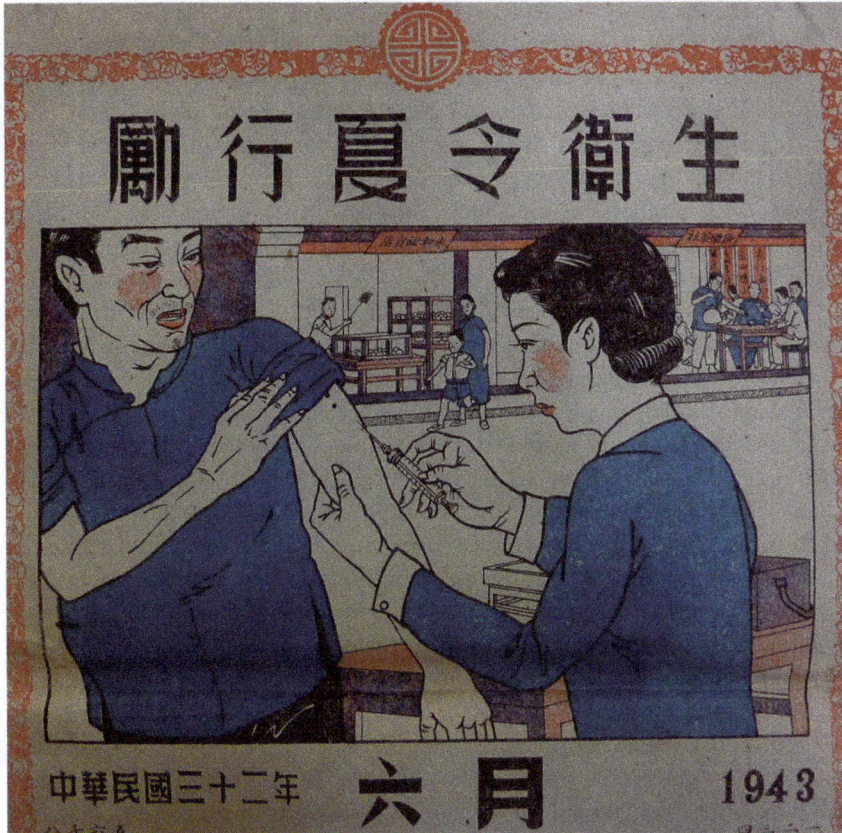

FIGURE 7. June 1943 page of the National Institute of Health public health calendar, labeled "Steadfastly Implement Summertime Health." NLM ID 101171294, History of Medicine Division Collection. Courtesy of the United States National Library of Medicine.

people's bodies. Women primarily exercised this power through delivering services that people wanted, so they encountered little resistance, but their actions served to legitimize masculine state power over people's individual bodies and the political collective. Recall that the June page in the 1943 public health calendar mentioned in chapter 1 claimed that, in order to prevent cholera, "it is imperative to mobilize the local troops immediately for earnest and strident prevention."[28] The placid picture accompanying this text employed the image of a caring woman to belie the violence of the claim that military intervention alone could protect the people from cholera. (See fig. 7.) The artistic double of the real woman in the photograph, this "new woman" with her stylishly short haircut and rosy cheeks gives a healthy-looking man a repeat cholera-typhoid vaccination with a sturdy syringe and a firm touch. She has placed her equipment right on the street and works out in the open. The artist who depicted a common scene in real-life Chongqing also employed artistic license to render it more civilized. The crowd has disappeared to reveal the owner of a sweets shop who diligently keeps flies away from his wares, and well-dressed citizens enjoying a civil cup of tea in a cleanly tea shop.[29] The viewer's eyes gravitate first to the woman's syringe in the middle foreground, then to the mother tending to her healthy son in the background. As I explain in chapter 5, the mother–son dyad indeed occupied the center of the Nationalist state's wartime politics, just as the mother and son occupy the center of this calendar page.

The regular appearance of female medical authorities on the streets of Chongqing announced a new era in local society as well as in the medical profession. Certified by the state and dressed in some form of recognizable uniform, such women were able to employ medical authority to supersede social norms that restricted women's appearance and movement in public. Women who regularly performed their professional labor in the streets defied the gendering of public space as masculine. They even challenged the domestication of public space that had occurred in the early Republican era in response to the more frequent appearance of middle-class women in public (with the opening of girls' schools, the establishment of new civic associations, etc.). In the eyes of male Republican officials, "a 'domesticated' public realm was an orderly, safe, and segregated zone where women could take part in public activities while being protected from physical contact with men."[30] Providing medical service, on the other hand, required not only physical proximity to men, but direct, skin-to-skin contact. If "limiting physical contact between the sexes was one crucial way to protect women" in the early twentieth century, "[b]y the 1940s, the cultural milieu had become more open in terms of accepting, and even encouraging, women to venture into the public sphere."[31] The war sparked the sea change that occurred between these two moments.

The primary factor fueling this change was need. Health officials in Chongqing needed women to be public and mobile in order to provide necessary healthcare. Accordingly, they ordered public health nurses to conduct biannual vaccination drives, as well as to carry the wounded to local and outlying hospitals for treatment after air raids. Panic-stricken and terrorized citizens repeatedly saw young women come to the rescue of the wounded. (See fig. 8.) In this photograph, the nurse in front wears a face mask to protect her lungs from post-air-raid dust, while the blown-out paper windows of the building and rubble on the street depict a beleaguered city desperately in need of the care that these women provide. They bear telltale signs of new womanhood; the woman in the face mask also wears a wristwatch, and all of the women have short, bobbed hair.[32] They carry a heavy load—a wounded man—but they provide the tender care of a mother figure. Therefore, although once in the hospital these women would touch the body of the man in order to tend to his wounds, their labor affirmed the domestication of public space.

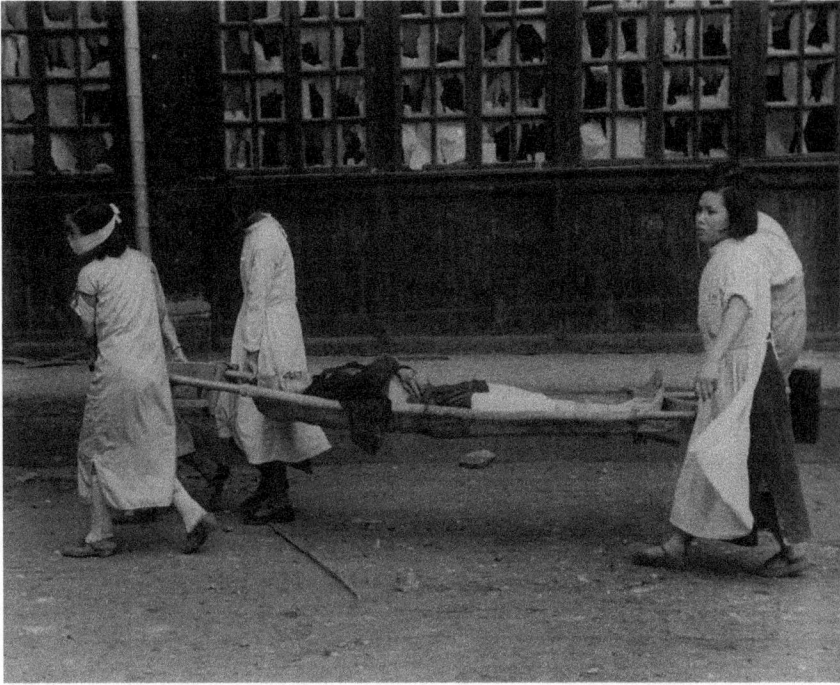

FIGURE 8. Young female nurses carrying a wounded man on a stretcher to their hospital for care after an air raid. LOT 11511–7, WAAMD #123, U.S. Library of Congress, Prints and Photographs Division.

Seen from this angle, women's wartime healthcare work marked the triumph of conservative gender politics. During the women's movement of the early Republic, women and their allies who took the radical position argued for immediate suffrage and legal guarantees of women's rights. On the other hand, women and men who adopted the conservative position "emphasized the need to rally to China's profound national needs even if that meant putting off suffrage."[33] During the War of Resistance women who challenged gender norms, gained personal autonomy, and achieved a new social position generally did so only because they willingly accepted difficult and risky work for relatively low pay. They furthermore had to follow Song Meiling's lead in playing the role of supportive caretaker *and* affirming a class politics of hygiene. The winning moment of moderate politics granted women some authority, but only if they worked on behalf of the nation in a caretaking role that supported the state's desire to universalize middle-class aesthetics.

Throughout the war, Song Meiling played the role of national mother and modeled the type of contributions women ought to make to the war effort. Hailed in the wartime press as "Madame Chiang" (*Jiang furen*) but granted her own full name in the present work, Song was highly visible to both domestic and foreign audiences; journalists and photographers recorded her every move in both the Chinese and international press. She held leadership roles in several local charitable organizations, and her open cooperation with known leftists further encouraged the remarkable nonpartisanship in women's wartime organizations, even as their husbands served political parties that remained bitterly divided. Song Meiling frequently appeared in the news, inspecting donations of medical equipment (see fig. 9), visiting wounded soldiers, sewing clothing for refugees, attending to children in orphanages, and giving stirring speeches to women's volunteer organizations (sometimes flanked by her two sisters of different political leanings, Song Ailing and Song Qingling).[34] As in this image, she almost always wore an elegant *qipao*, which marked her as a *taitai*—a married woman of the upper class who did not have to work outside the home and could therefore play a prominent role in philanthropy. While many upper-class wives had done philanthropic work prior to the war, Song galvanized them into even greater action during the crisis.[35] This photograph also clearly depicts another means by which Song gained international prestige as a woman: her physical beauty, a matter frequently remarked upon. To American audiences she appeared "gracious, beautiful, dignified, courageous," indubitably playing "the star role" and "captivat[ing] the hearts of the American people" by representing "the educated, the cultured, the beautiful, the tolerant, [and] the Christian in China."[36]

Song Meiling appeared in international media with much more frequency than her husband, Chiang Kai-shek, and definitively represented her country to foreign audiences. Yet in her fund-raising speeches in the United States, Song belied her powerful role in Chinese domestic politics and employed Orientalist notions of China as a defenseless country beset by rapacious Japanese and in need of protection from the progressive and powerful United States. She coined the English phrase "warphans" (war orphans) and made judicious use of these poster children for China's relief effort so as to raise the maximum amount of foreign charitable donations. Song's media presence informed the twentieth-century version of the so-called China mystique—an American version of gendered Orientalism that cast China as a nation of willing yet feminized and rather powerless modernizers, asking for help and guidance from Americans, who saw themselves as occupying the masculine role of chivalric saviors.[37] As a US-educated, Christian daughter of the prominent businessman Charlie Soong (Song Jiashu), Song Meiling capitalized on her ability to charm American audiences not only with her beauty and elegance, but also with her perfect English, spoken originally with the lilt of a southern belle and later with the studied affectation of a British accent.[38] Eloquent in both English and Chinese and ever the charming hostess, Song Meiling entertained foreign dignitaries long after her awkward and taciturn husband retreated to his bedroom, and actively participated in many foreign policy conversations.

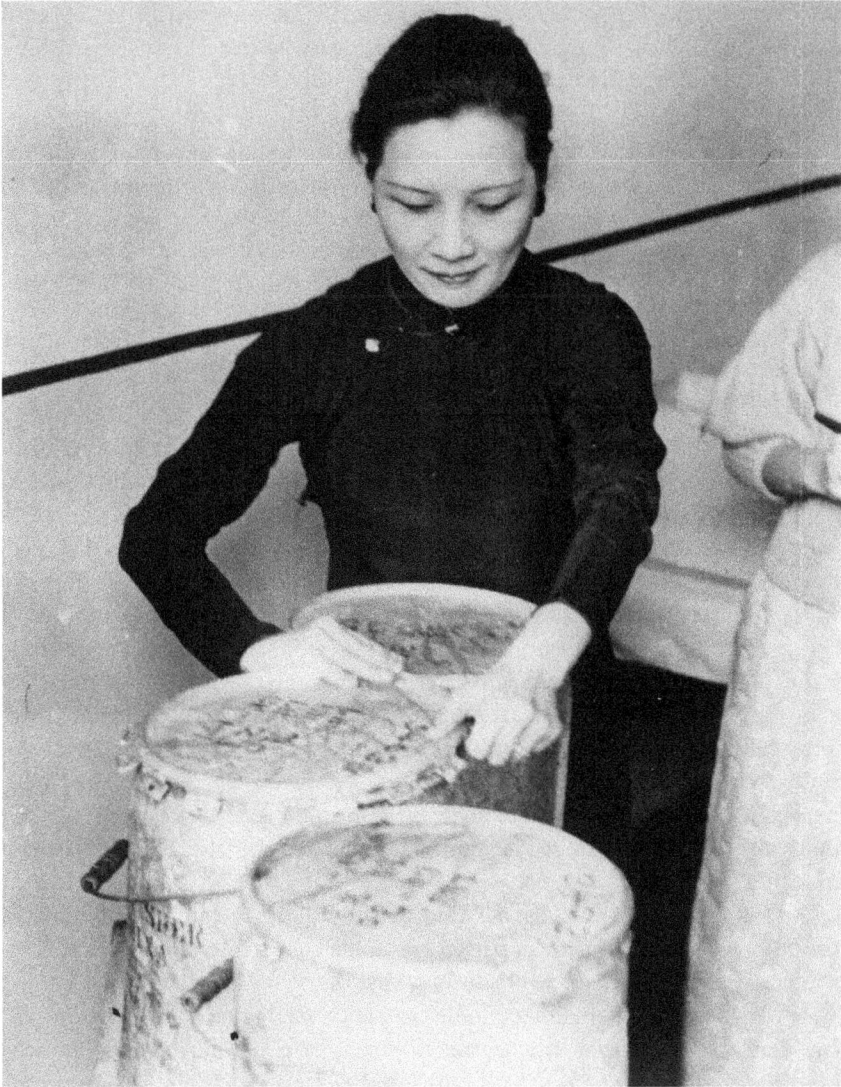

FIGURE 9. Song Meiling opens medical supplies donated from the United States. Box 85, folder "Surgical Relief Supplies." ABMAC Records. Rare Book and Manuscript Library. Columbia University.

Most Americans who dealt with the Nationalist regime during the war retained fond feelings for Song Meiling even as they began to disdain Chiang Kai-shek, and it was often Song rather than Chiang who represented China in American media.

Within China, Song Meiling represented the feminine side of the masculin-ist state, playing the part of the caring mother who tended to her flock but also held the responsibility of teaching them to follow the correct path. In a speech to delegates of women's organizations in Nanjing on August 1, 1937, Song Meiling delivered a rousing call to action:

> We must unhesitatingly and with courage throw the last ounce of strength and energy into an effort to secure national survival. . . . [E]very one of us Chinese must fight according to our ability . . . [and] we women are citizens just as much as are our men. . . . I hope each one of you will take a very enthusiastic part in this work and throw yourselves fully into it. While during war time the men are the fighters, it is the women who bear the brunt of carrying on at the rear. We must encourage the men and let them know that we are in our own way holding on and not letting them down; that we are just as ready to give up everything, even our lives, to support our fighters at the front . . . [because] the fighting morale of our men at the front depends on how much support the rear can give.[39]

While she underscored the equality of women's and men's labors, Song also designated women's role as supportive, self-sacrificing, and nurturing, while gendering militarism as exclusively masculine. Although in her speech Song asked that women commit themselves to the risk of death, she employed this as a rhetorical flourish. She knew her audience well and spoke primarily to women like her: the wives of government officials and businessmen who did not have to work for a living. Many of these women believed in an inherent superiority of middle-class values and behaviors and used activism to leverage their own political capital. By contributing to national defense through civilian relief projects that promoted loyalty to the Nationalist Party, these women demonstrated their usefulness to the state.[40] Others, like He Xiangning and Xie Bingying, who had organized military nurses in previous wars and did so again during the War of Resistance, posed more direct challenges to gender norms that defined the battlefield as a strictly masculine space.[41]

As with male discipline, female didacticism devoted the greatest attention to the poor. Song gave voice to her party's prevailing cultural attitudes about poverty and rural people when she wrote, in 1937, that the New Life Movement included "intensive course[s]" for rural Chinese "in public sanitation, rural economy, village industries, military discipline, and, most emphasized of all, methods of teaching the people to become *self-respecting and worthwhile citizens.*"[42] Her words betrayed her failure to recognize the fact that rural Chinese and the urban poor already were "worthwhile citizens" if one takes their contributions to the nation as primary barometer. Not only did they keep civilians and soldiers fed after the country lost nearly one-third of its territory; they also served as soldiers themselves and suffered the greatest number of casualties. Moreover, after migrating into the cities, the rural poor performed a variety of manual labors that kept those cities functioning: carrying water and other goods to householders, sweeping the streets, running the food markets, carting away dead bodies, and reconstructing buildings after air raids. Yet in the eyes of the NLM architects, rural Chinese would not become "worthwhile citizens" until they cast aside their own values in favor of those that government leaders deemed worthy of respect.

Song Meiling's words had political power not only because of her position as First Lady, but also because she served as Honorary Chairwoman of the Women's Advisory Council (WAC) of the NLM (*Xin shenghuo yundong cujin zonghui funü zhidao weiyuanhui*). Founded in the first provisional capital of Wuhan in March 1938, the WAC served as the clearinghouse for women's wartime mobilization and relief efforts. Its members helped the Nationalist state maintain social control during the war; their consistent work kept the NLM relevant to wartime society. The Association for the Promotion of the NLM (*Xin shenghuo yundong cujinhui*), with its main chapter in Chongqing, organized civilian relief projects that included orphanages, soup kitchens, refugee homes, services for wounded soldiers, war bond drives, and fund-raising events.[43] In both Wuhan and Chongqing, activism of upper- and middle-class women flourished; by 1941 over forty women's organizations had registered with the government in Chongqing. Women such as the feminist lawyer Shi Liang, Young Women's Christian Association leader and wife of a famous warlord Li Dequan, and communist activist Deng Yingchao all sat on the People's Political Council (*Guomin canzhenghui*) (PPC) and helped to found and run the most prominent female-led civilian relief organizations.[44]

Even these middle- and upper-class women could gain only indirect political power in the masculinist state, yet their work served to sustain its power. Women's relief organizations like the WAC relied on donations and a volunteer labor force comprising primarily women and girls. The PPC had a strictly advisory role, and state officials frequently ignored its recommendations. Nonetheless, women active within it promoted an image of the Nationalist state as caring and benevolent, and supported the state's aim to keep people healthy. Their medical and relief work therefore served simultaneously to obscure men's disciplinary power on the one hand, and to further its practice on the other. As the soft arm of the masculinist state, women's work—running soup kitchens, orphanages, services for wounded soldiers, and clothing drives for refugees—compelled people into compliance through both gentle persuasion and offering the services that people actually wanted. While the *direct* political power that women's leadership conferred had its limits, the *indirect* political power that women yielded as they regularly interacted with the recipients of their services rendered them indispensable servants of the state.

Women's success hinged on their emotional labor. Smiling and using kind words while they worked made the services that they offered much more accessible and desirable, and granted women access to docile rather than resistant bodies. In this way, women's work in civilian relief performed the most crucial step in helping the disciplinary power of the state get into people's homes and onto their bodies: that of instilling governmentality, or aligning citizens' desires with those of state officials. The recipients of women's work had the freedom to reject the services offered but seldom did so. Rather, they opened themselves to being schooled in a new behavior protocol and a new way of understanding the state as provider of services. They even began to understand themselves in a new light: as the deserving recipients of organized caretaking, performed with the aim of delivering them into citizenship all cleaned up and behaving properly.

Concrete examples of women's reforms in war orphanages and "family education zones" illustrate this point. Both locations took the family as the basic unit of social change, and women as the primary instigators of that change. They worked within a framework shaped by "Sick Woman of East Asia" discourse that had designated the home "a source of national pathology" and in desperate need of reform.[45] Three of the largest social reforms of the early twentieth century—the New Culture Movement, the New Life Movement, and the anti-tuberculosis movement—articulated the home in this manner. All three located dirt and vice within the Chinese family and created "a new technology of the individual," according to which citizens related more readily to the nation-state than to their own families and worked on behalf of the nation.[46] Working under Song Meiling's direction, female orphanage volunteers employed this "new technology of the individual" by inserting the party as the orphans' new parents and inculcating patriotic loyalty to the Nationalist state. They taught orphans to perform propaganda plays and sing patriotic songs. The lessons often rhymed, and some people could still recite them from memory as adults. In order to exploit the children's anti-Japanese sentiment, they decorated the walls of orphanages with drawings of Japanese soldiers slaying children, along with sketches of field artillery and airplanes. Images designed to teach the children personal hygiene hung alongside the war images, underscoring the profound connection between personal health and national salvation.[47]

Orphanage volunteers argued that orphans made excellent raw material for social transformation since they were free of the tainting influences of a bad family life.[48] Others worked to access families directly so as to transform them from within. In 1939, Minister of Education Chen Lifu declared that, of the three types of development that education fosters—intellectual, moral, and physical—only the first can occur in schools, while the latter two occur in the home. In an attempt to foster the type of moral and physical education that would support the civilizing mission that Song Meiling articulated and Minister Chen desired, in 1941 the Nationalist state established three "family education experimental zones," two near Chongqing and one in the northwest. Faculty and students of normal schools (teachers' colleges) located in these three zones performed a variety of tasks in nearby villages in order to "direct the improvement of women's life habits." They schooled rural "housewives" in their daily chores of running a household, took surveys, performed health checks, and delivered vaccinations.

They employed home visits, training classes, exhibitions, and various forms of entertainment in order to reach their target audience. The team of students in Beibei, just outside Chongqing, reached 256 households in its first two years of work (1940–42). Acting under the authority of Minister Chen, these women worked "to extend elite understandings of civilized child rearing and correct family behavior to the masses."[49]

These school programs in domestic reform trained young women to perform their work with a certain kind of affect designed to counteract the types of emotional resistance they might face. In compliance with this affect, articulated as "correct etiquette" or demeanor (*yitai*), they had to learn how to respond flexibly to people's "pride, humility, sincerity, arrogance, and modesty." This aspect of their training was crucial "because much of the power of the experiment [in reforming domestic life] relied on interpersonal connections and direct intervention."[50] As frontline troops in the civilizing mission of the New Life Movement, these women performed the emotional labor that had the power to transform poor and unhygienic Chinese from objects of pity and disgust into people worthy of direct contact. While the end goal of the masculinist state and women working within that state remained the same—to render middle-class hygiene norms a universal standard—their methods of delivery differed, and that difference determined their failure or success. Reformers who made an effort to account for the emotional states of the recipients of their reforms more readily entered into relationship with them.

The attempt to establish an emotional connection mattered a lot, regardless of the profundity or durability of the resulting relationships. Available records reveal very little about how people felt as they received instructions on how to sweep their floors and steps, keep flies away from their food, and teach their children to brush their teeth and wash their hands. Yet the women who reached toward them crossed a social chasm between the poor and the (relatively) wealthy in Chinese society. In describing poor people and their habits as unworthy of respect, NLM discourse gave voice to a widespread revulsion that had the power to cleave the country. In the words of political philosopher Martha Nussbaum, "[t]he need for emotions of loving concern becomes even more apparent . . . when we consider the threat posed to morality by disgust. Disgust jeopardizes national projects involving altruistic sacrifice for the common good, for it divides the nation into hierarchically organized groups that must not meet."[51] Disgust and feelings of (moral or physical) revulsion often keep people from sharing the same physical space. The mere meeting of people on both sides empowered the dream of making the nation whole. The war made this possible because it made the nightmare of its division more palpable. Indeed, "one way to overcome" the problem that disgust poses to a just society "is surely to link the narrative of the full humanity of the denigrated group to a story of national struggle and national commitment."[52] In daring to touch the bodies and hearts of orphans and poor farmers, women declared that they had an important role to play in the nation's present battle to survive, and in future dreams of continued strength. The next chapter demonstrates that one political party—the Communist Party—figured out precisely how to "link the narrative of the full humanity of the denigrated group to a story of national struggle," while the Nationalist Party utterly failed, with powerful consequences for modern China.

TRAINING FOR EMOTIONAL LABOR: ZHOU MEIYU AND THE PROFESSIONALIZATION OF NURSING

Nurses also received training in emotional labor that enabled them to form bonds with diseased refugees and soldiers, transcending conceptions of disgust to build an inclusive national community. Major General Zhou Meiyu (1910–2006), the person most responsible for professionalizing rural public health nurses and military nurses, explicitly trained them in this manner. One of the first women to attain the rank of major general in the National Revolutionary Army, Zhou correctly assumed that her country needed her expertise as a professional nurse trained at the Peking Union Medical College Nursing School (class of 1930), and later at the Massachusetts Institute of Technology (MS in Public Health) and Barnard College (MA in Education). While the next two chapters focus on Zhou's work in military nursing during the war, this section highlights her work to train rural public health nurses.

In 1931 Zhou went to Dingxian, a county in rural Hebei Province, in northern China, where she trained public health nurses for the Mass Education Movement (*Pingmin jiaoyu cujin hui*) (MEM) that had settled there. Much less an organization than a "loose coalition of reform-minded elites" working toward "rural reconstruction" (*xiangcun jianshe*), the MEM concentrated the energies of people interested in alleviating rural poverty through specific measures of community empowerment such as literacy campaigns, land reform, and public health services.[53] While many of her peers might have called this a hardship post, Zhou described it as a "great glory and honor," during which the lessons that she and her young colleagues learned from the villagers positively dwarfed their contributions.[54]

Zhou's own humility, and the humility she instilled in the nurses under her command and leadership, were not only a core attribute in Confucian culture but also an essential ingredient of the nurses' emotional labor. Zhou, a woman who had graduated from her country's preeminent nursing school and ultimately attained high rank within a male-dominated military system, had to convince other educated women to ignore the urge to climb higher on the social ladder, and instead descend it to live in an impoverished village among poor farmers who lacked even the most basic education. This in a country where many women attended nursing schools precisely so they could improve their social status. Zhou had to manufacture a social role for nurses that granted them moral prestige and personal satisfaction. To accomplish this task, she employed methods very similar to those Song Meiling used to convince upper-class wives to engage in charity work: she modeled moral rectitude in her every action, judiciously used titles and clothing to signal authority, and faced all obstacles in good cheer. In short, Major General Zhou Meiyu fully embodied the qualities that she wanted all nurses to cultivate, as is evident in figure 10.

Zhou Meiyu began this work in 1931 in Dingxian, where she developed a comprehensive training program for rural public health nurses who traveled to their patients. Trained in a rural setting for direct work among villagers, Zhou's nurses had an impact far beyond this single county. First, they constituted the largest workforce in a tiered medical system whose affordability and feasibility convinced the Nationalist state, after years of resistance, to support rural healthcare.[55] Moreover, precisely because of Dingxian's status as a model county under the close watch of Nationalist officials, the roving public health nurse became the lynchpin worker in the state model of rural public health, which Zhou's colleague Chen Zhiqian (1903–2000) spread across the entire province of Sichuan during the war in his capacity as Director of the newly established Sichuan Provincial Health Administration.[56] Furthermore, Dr. Chen intimated in his memoir that the Dingxian system served as a blueprint for the barefoot doctor program that the People's Republic of China implemented countrywide and that gained worldwide acclaim in the 1960s and '70s.[57]

In Zhou's model, traveling nurses took responsibility for all the villagers living within a twenty-*li* radius (about seven miles). This typically encompassed ten to fifteen villages with fifteen hundred to two thousand students. Focusing their work on local schools, the roving nurses performed health examinations of all schoolchildren every three months, looking in particular for signs of the common ailments of trachoma and scabies, and measuring all students' heights and weights to determine whether they had enough nutrition for proper development. Nurses also took responsibility for environmental health, ensuring that latrines and wells lay at least fifty feet from one another and that both had covers, disinfecting drinking water at schools that could not boil it, placing spittoons in each school, and providing students with personal teacups and washbasins to minimize contagion of the most common diseases, trachoma chief among them. To further prevent the spread of disease, they administered what preventive shots they had in the 1930s: vaccines for smallpox, cholera, and typhoid, and diphtheria antitoxin. They asked students to bring other family members and villagers to the schools on vaccination days, consciously making use of the youth to disseminate medical technologies and encourage other villagers to partake in this important preventive measure.

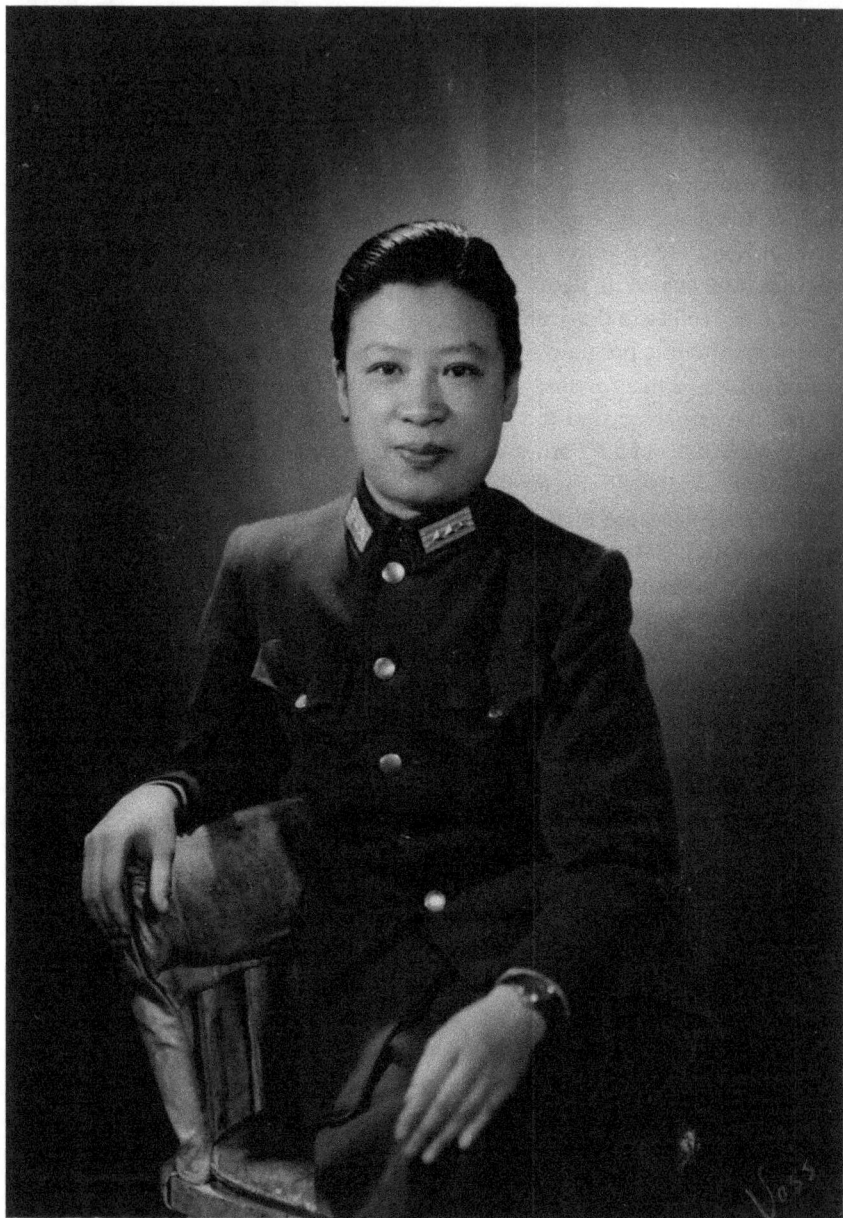

FIGURE 10. Major General Zhou Meiyu pictured in uniform, ca. 1940–1943. Box 75, folder "ABMAC no. 2." ABMAC Records. Rare Book and Manuscript Library. Columbia University.

Child delivery constituted another crucial part of nurses' work, and Zhou recalled that each nurse in Dingxian helped to deliver at least twenty babies, though at that time they lacked the cultural power to unseat elderly *chanpo* midwives.[58] (See chapter 5 for more on elderly midwives.) Most importantly, Zhou trained her nurses properly for the job. After working in Dingxian for two years, Chen Zhiqian concluded that "the modern urban-educated doctors and nurses do not fit the need of the rural villages."[59] For example, the PUMC offered little training in trachoma because the disease had largely disappeared from the United States, despite that fact that it was a nearly universal ailment of Chinese schoolchildren.[60] Though herself "modern [and] urban-educated," Zhou trained nurses to perform the care that rural villagers needed.

Beyond delivering crucial medical services to the people, Zhou had an explicit goal of professionalizing nursing and elevating its social prestige. Far from limited to China, this was a global problem that nurses faced around the world. Although simplistic narratives credit Florence Nightingale with single-handedly rendering nursing an acceptable and honorable activity for middle-class women, in actuality this process took many decades, hundreds of women, and the confluence of multiple social factors. Although her male contemporaries considered her "unfeminine and a nuisance," Nightingale during the mid-nineteenth-century Crimean War defied British cultural norms to enter the social space of unclean men and become the "Lady of the Lamp" and "ministering angel" in public media, even earning accolades from the British queen.[61] Nearly a century later, Chinese nurses needed their own Florence Nightingale to challenge the same social expectations of elite women: that they stay at home, never associate with men besides close family members, keep their distance from the poor, and by all means stay away from all sources of "filth."[62]

China was not singularly behind the times; nurses in other countries continued to struggle with these issues (and many still do today). In Argentina the Fundación Eva Perón (named after the First Lady of the populist government) throughout the 1940s and '50s "dignified the work of the nurse" through a rigorous education program whose curriculum focused on elevating the status of nursing to a respected profession.[63] In post–World War II Canada, where nurses' wartime contributions had earned them some measure of social status, nursing schools still struggled with middle-class women's "reticence to enter nursing," and the work to professionalize nursing continued well into the 1970s.[64] Indeed, the "quests for social, cultural, and professional authority" characterize the history of modern nursing across the globe.[65]

Sensibilities of social class and ideas about dirt constituted a staunch barrier to entry in Chinese nursing. Accordingly, Zhou trained rural public health nurses to make respect for the human dignity of their patients a central feature of their work. Nurses earned some social status by answering their country's desperate need for healthcare workers, but that status was immediately challenged because they worked among people whom so many of their compatriots considered uncultured, backward, and worthy of pity at best, disgust and revulsion at worst. The fact that their job required them to touch the bodies of the poor compounded nurses' struggle to claim professional dignity, all the more so because these bodies were often in states of decay and filth that triggered revulsion. Zhou Meiyu recalled:

> I've always been very interested in nursing and felt that the country needed that kind of work. At that time, everyone still looked down on nursing, believing that it was what a servant would do, and that cleaning a patient's body or taking care of their waste was dirty work. But from the perspective of the hospital, nursing service is performed for those who need assistance, and one must apply professional skills, experience, and knowledge in order to perform this service.[66]

Zhou's reflection underscores the fact that the professionalization of nursing in China entailed rendering the act of caring for poor people and unclean bodies a respectable enterprise. The enormity of this task can be appreciated through a juxtaposition with another Asian society that has as yet failed to achieve this goal. In Bangladesh, where the British colonial government introduced professionalized nursing in 1947, and most nurses are lower-class Hindu women living in a predominantly Muslim society, people currently "associate nursing activities with commercial sex work" and consider it "dirty." Although nurses do gain some measure of prestige for having access to education and a professional job, they are also "tainted" by their physical contact with strangers' bodies and suffer on the marriage market because "Bangladeshi Muslim culture prohibits physical touch between non-family females and males."[67] In a very similar cultural setting in the 1920s and '30s, Zhou Meiyu set out to challenge social norms and make the women she trained feel proud enough of their work that they could inure themselves to the criticism they would face.

Zhou fostered pride in nurses by tying their work to a grand narrative of national development. She called her students "future masters of our nation" and articulated the goal of their training as "seeking the welfare of our country and the world" (*wei guojia shijie mouqiu fuli*). In accordance with China's long-lived respect for learning, education was the primary vehicle for this work of national importance. Moreover, Rural Reconstruction activists, like public health nurses, understood that for maximum effect they had to encourage villagers to take charge of their own needs, so health education constituted an important aspect of the nurses' work. They delivered hygiene lectures to all teachers within their jurisdiction, held "hygiene chats" with the students each week, and conducted hygiene education in the villages. Nurses also organized students into cleaning teams to sweep out the schools and other public spaces, hoping that if students did the work themselves they would take pride in the results and continue it even after the activists had gone.[68]

Public health education was also a means of magnifying their labor. Roving nurses were keenly aware of the fact that they could work around the clock with no sleep and still feel that they had done little to satisfy actual demand for their services. Zhou described their workdays thus:

> We nurses worked tirelessly. We would often get up very early in the morning and together we would ride our bicycles several miles to a health center in a neighboring village, or directly to people's homes, or to a school to do health inspections. We would usually finish around 4 p.m. and then finally have lunch, so we ate just two meals a day. After eating, we would have a big meeting to discuss the day's work and stay in that particular village for the night before riding back in the morning. We worked together well and with delight.[69]

What motivated these women to do such demanding work?

Answering this question requires analysis of the dual effects of nurses' emotional labor. If Zhou's description is accurate, from the late afternoon onward each day the nurses had intimate experiences with the villagers, taking meals with them and sleeping in their homes. On the one hand, then, nurses' emotional labor of humbly submitting to hard physical work with little food served to make villagers feel close to the nurses, willing not only to submit to their care but also to feed and house them at night. On the other hand, this intimacy helped the nurses feel closer to the villagers and begin to understand the conditions of their lives from an embodied rather than a merely academic perspective.

The importance of health workers' embodied knowledge of village life is underscored in Chen Zhiqian's reflection on the successes of the village health workers—rural villagers who received remedial training before doing public health in their own communities. He noted, "I found the enthusiasm of the village workers really inspiring; they were always enthusiastic and eager to learn, they did not expect too much remuneration, and they were uniformly proud of their ability to assist their fellow villagers."[70] Public health workers who served their own communities established emotional closeness with the recipients of their care by knowing, intimately and personally, the struggles that they faced in ensuring their health and how they wished to overcome them. These villagers found their public health work sufficiently empowering that they willingly accepted low pay and eagerly sought new information. This, then, was the ultimate goal of public health workers who served strangers: to treat these strangers like their own kin, able to understand and address health problems *from their perspective.*

Writing of a similar situation in a very different place and time—Botswana's only public hospital cancer ward in the first decade of the twenty-first century—Julie Livingston describes the ability of the nurses she observed and worked with to create emotional closeness with their patients as founded on "moral sentiment." She argues that illness happens *between* people and is a "deeply social experience," and therefore "[c]are-giving is a moral endeavor. It is at once deeply personal and deeply social, and it is a vital practical matter, crucial to patient well-being and survival."[71] Because they understood this aspect of their work so well, the Batswana nurses always remembered patients' names (which the doctors seldom did), joked with them, cajoled them, put on smiles rather than faces of disgust when cleaning putrid wounds, prepared the patients' bodies for burial after their deaths, conducted the morning prayer service, and learned to love their patients and treat them like their own kin.[72] One nurse said, "We grow to love our patients only to watch them die. They become like our family. There are days when it is just so painful for us."[73] The intimacy of their labor explains why "more than doctoring, nursing is understood to require sentimental work."[74]

Nursing work in wartime China required a similar emotional labor. The combination of physical and emotional demands sometimes overwhelmed nurses. Zhou Meiyu recalled that riding their bicycles such distances left the nurses covered in dust head to toe and feeling utterly exhausted. They nonetheless continued to do their best in the face of unending work because they saw themselves as performing a unique and valuable service, which Zhou expressed in the phrase "[I]f we don't do it then who will?!"[75] A world of meaning lies in those words. Particularly in situations of resource scarcity—of both personnel and supplies—a healthcare provider must continually improvise and make do.[76] When the demands on one's time and attention never cease, that improvisation entails not only devising clever solutions with the materials on hand but also creating emotional states that have the power to supersede other emotional training, such as the disgust response, the desire for material comfort, or the acceptance of social norms about women's withdrawal from professional life after marriage. Emotional labor "requires one to induce or suppress feeling in order to sustain the outward countenance that produces the proper state of mind in others."[77] In order to "produc[e] the proper state of mind" in their patients, nurses had to continually perform confidence, love, and compassion, regardless of how filthy their patients' bodies or how hopeless their illness.

An essentialist analysis might posit that because nursing entails the physical care of others, performing these ministrations will "naturally" produce emotional care for others. Yet this argument ignores the fact that sometimes the opposite occurs, because emotional labor requires real work. Some nurses, unwilling to engage in challenging emotional labor, numb their hearts in an attempt to protect themselves from the death and decay in which their job immerses them. Some nurses feel revolted by the physical state of their patients. Some nurses get exasperated with patients who do not yield to their care or refuse treatment. Some nurses mistreat their patients; in another situation in which nurses cared for people of a lower social class than themselves—South Africa in the late twentieth century—middle-class nurses routinely abused their patients, both verbally and physically, as a means of asserting their social status and power over them.[78] Contrast this with the nurses in Botswana, who by nearly all measures faced a more difficult work environment but frequently sympathized with their poor patients and served as staunch advocates for them.[79] One Botswana nurse in the cancer ward explained her emotional labor this way:

> [N]urses of all people must have empathy. Not sympathy, not pity, but empathy. You have to really *feel* . . . that you want that patient to get better, to feel OK. With experience, you don't feel that sickness or disgust or fear from the wounds. You can't, if you are a nurse. You cannot let the patient feel that you are afraid of them or that you are disgusted by them. If nurses don't do this job, then who will? Who will?[80]

Nurses in wartime China and in twenty-first century Botswana came to the same conclusion: no matter how hard the job, we *must* continue to do our best because we are uniquely qualified for it. They judged themselves irreplaceable not only because of their professional training in the rigors of medical care, but more importantly, because of their profound understanding of how well they performed the emotional labor of nursing. Knowing that "part of the job is to disguise fatigue and irritation," nurses in both societies deemed themselves well trained for this work, and because they knew it to be real work, deemed others not (yet) capable of performing it.[81]

Zhou Meiyu understood the moral imperatives that nurses faced to calm, soothe, and indeed love their patients. She deliberately trained nurses to perform this emotional work, particularly in the military, and believed that women treated their patients more tenderly than did male nurses.[82] In discussing the work of military nurses she explained that sustaining a serious wound on the battlefield rattled a soldier's nerves, and claimed:

> It's better for a [female] nurse to deal with such a situation, mostly because female workers are of a gentle nature. Most of the wounded are men, but when they start to get angry and the nurse just stands by without saying a word, they dare not get too fierce.[83]

This gendered division of labor appears to have been widespread in military nursing; Yao Aihua recalled that the women in her unit cared for the gravely wounded, while the men cared for the lightly wounded.[84] In addition to increasing the chances that a wounded soldier would get emotional as well as physical care, it also reified gender roles. Zhou claimed that female nurses' ability to calm panicked soldiers stemmed from their "nature," when in fact she trained them to perform the proper behavior: to quietly stand by the soldier's bedside. This nonbehavior worked for two reasons. First, the refusal to engage with an angry soldier deprived him of fuel to keep the fight going. Second, a female nurse represented she who needed the soldier's protection, yet she stood by his bed ready to care for him. Her silence subtly reminded the soldier of this dynamic within the traditional gender system and exploited that system to make him ashamed of his outburst and ready to submit to the nurse.

Motivating soldiers to fight and to comply with orders was a significant problem for the National Revolutionary Army, partly because of widespread social disregard for soldiers, encapsulated in the phrase "a good man never joins the army" (*haonan bu dangbing*), and partly because conditions in the army were infuriating (as explained in chapter 3). Army Medical Administration medical officers, noting that a soldier's degree of despair frequently matched the severity of his wound, chalked it up to improper political indoctrination. They treated upset soldiers to motivating speeches, songs, and theatrical performances, and stirring testimonials from previously wounded soldiers who had decided to return to battle.[85] In characteristically disciplinary fashion, Nationalist officials passed a regulation in November 1938 stipulating the precise behaviors with which civilians must show respect to soldiers on their way to or from the front (stop all movement, remove hats, etc.), and in May 1940 mandated the use of the term "respected soldiers" (*rongyu junren*). Nonetheless, reports still circulated of civilians blatantly disregarding both the soldiers and the state's orders—by, for example, closing up their shops just before a trainload of soldiers rolled into town.[86] The disciplinary state failed again. In this context, the significance of military nurses' training to perform emotional labor that helped to calm a wounded soldier appears all the more powerful for its ability to communicate care and simultaneously shame men into complying with military medical authorities.

DIDACTICISM AND THE FAILURES OF EMOTIONAL LABOR

Not all nurses, or women in other healthcare positions, could complete the task of suppressing their disgust at or judgment of poor people. Some resorted to didacticism in an attempt to persuade people to adopt new mind-sets or behaviors. Precisely why they thought this might work remains unclear. Some had undoubtedly succumbed to the elitism that saturated Chinese culture and granted pride of place to the educated (an effect of centuries of scholar-officialdom). Some may have been responding to physical and emotional taxation in the face of seemingly insurmountable obstacles. In the 1930s and 1940s infectious disease, infant and child mortality, and malnutrition plagued the countryside. Few villagers had even basic literacy, people married very young, and childbirth could just as easily bring death as life.[87] Chronic poverty depressed peoples' spirits, and upstart urbanites with an elite education could make only so much headway, no matter how inspirational their politics or dedicated their hearts. In response to this grinding fatigue, many cloaked themselves in a veneer of self-righteousness. Their passionate desire to modernize China gave them courage to continue their hard work, but this very desire introduced another tension. Rural Reconstruction activists sometimes be-lieved themselves indispensable to reforming the countryside, which ran counter to their core mission of boosting villagers' own dignity and proud participation in rural activism. Chapter 5 demonstrates that this resulted in a notable failure in midwifery work.

Two short stories that Mass Education Movement volunteers wrote for use in hygiene education, *Gonggong weisheng* (Public health) and *Kepa de huoluan* (Scary cholera), also used in wartime Chongqing, illustrate the moralizing senti-ment that health workers often had as they worked to reform health behaviors.[88] MEM activists' "deep-seated belief in the positive potential of rural people" meant that much of their literature "extolled the benefits of rural living over urban," but according to many contemporary reports, their experiment with overt didacticism in theatrical dramas "did not appear to be making inroads into Dingxian's vil-lages."[89] Although villagers flocked to the performances, they appear to have done so only out of desperation for any kind of entertainment, for "local commentators noted that the spoken dramas did not outlast the reformers," and records of the Rural Reconstruction activists' interactions with villagers "showcase the cultural chasms that remained between even those reformers who had deep experience in the countryside and rural people."[90] Because its very tone implies disrespect for existing practices and beliefs, didacticism may temporarily entertain, but it rarely results in long-term change.

The MEM public health stories used in wartime Chongqing, all written in the vernacular and composed as colloquial conversations, follow a trite format juxta-posing an elderly and backward-looking character against a young and forward-thinking modernist who serves as the former's teacher and guide. Zhou Liaoxun's *Gonggong weisheng* (Public health) debuts with a scene of people gathered at Ti-ananmen Square in Beijing to hear a Public Security Bureau official deliver a pub-lic health talk. One individual, the foil of our story, gets up in the middle of the speech and stands on the sidelines, mumbling to himself, "What is this 'public health' he's talking about?" while rolling a cigarette from loose tobacco he keeps in a pouch. The old man's soliloquy continues:

> You can't drink, you can't smoke, you can't pee or poop where you want, when some-one at home dies of a contagious disease you gotta' burn 'em, you need to build some kinda' running water 'n' water pipes, 'n' places for butchering animals 'n' hospitals 'n' pharmacies. What a bunch o' rubbish! I don't understand this hygiene business and I've managed to eighty or ninety, hah! You want me to stop drinkin', stop smokin', well then I'll just die of boredom! And what if I have to piss really bad? If I don't go, then what? And I'm not supposed to take care of sick people at home? What? What? I can't even listen to this crap![91]

Hereupon the old curmudgeon runs into a young relative who takes it upon himself to educate his elder in the sagacious ways of an enlightened citizen who knows how to care for the public weal. The young man first explains the word *weisheng* not in the terms of individualized longevity practices long associated with Daoist meditation, but in the terms of hygienic modernity—of collectivized state medicine inextricably bound to national strength and political sovereignty.[92] He explains that "the logic of *weisheng*" is both passive (individuals protecting their health from illness) and active (individuals strengthening their bodies through exercise), and that since people "lead collective lives," collective health measures work only when everyone cooperates.[93]

The old man listens to the younger's diatribe on the benefits of public parks and disease prevention, but protests vociferously on the subject of sports, saying that when he was young his grandfather taught him martial arts (*wushu*) and it was tremendously beneficial to his health—so much so that he has reached a ripe old age in perfect shape without knowing anything of "public health." Here the younger interjects that martial arts, "which many people nowadays call 'national arts'" (*guoshu*), are also worthy, but since people have different tastes, a public park should make space for a variety of activities.[94] This passage shows the influence of the accumulated efforts of a community of martial arts practitioners based in Shanghai who transformed the martial arts into a modern sport by purifying them of religious and spiritual connotations and relating their practice to the pursuit of national strength, encapsulated in the new expression "national arts."[95]

The young man then launches into another diatribe, on the ill effects of tobacco and alcohol, punctuated with exaggerated claims such as that "the nicotine in a single cigarette can kill ten sparrows!" and "all cigarette smokers suffer from greatly diminished vitality." He also uses the timeworn and imprecise population count of four hundred million to calculate supposed losses of national wealth based on the improbable scenario of every single Chinese person smoking five coppers' worth of cigarettes per day. The story concludes with the old man, now thoroughly convinced by the young man's "amazing" words, denouncing himself and all cigarette smokers as "sinners."[96] The story leads readers to imagine that a pedantic lecture can transform a person's lifelong habits and beliefs in a single afternoon.

In *Kepa de huoluan* (Scary cholera), author Gu Qizhong employs an even more didactic style. The story opens with an old man, Wang Laosan, who contracts cholera from eating a cut melon on the street. Nationalist health officials did indeed outlaw cut melons for their propensity to attract flies and thereby spread disease; his experience fighting cholera in the 1920s gave Minister of Health Jin Baoshan a particular concern for this issue.[97] In the story, Wang goes to the hospital at the behest of his neighbor's son, Li Hua, who is a medical student. Here Gu Qizhong shows that Rural Reconstruction activists understood the necessity of trust to change local habits. Wang's choice to go to the hospital, a place that "rural folk don't know about," relies on his trust in two things: his personal relationship with Li Hua, and the power of institutionalized education. Wang stays for ten days and learns that, despite villagers' belief that hospitals employ "crude methods," the hospital is clean, the staff are friendly, and since they use needles their treatment is "no more painful than a mosquito bite," in stark contrast to his recollection of the village doctor's treatment of a wound on his hand, which "hurt to high heaven!" Wang emerges cured and with a newfound belief in hospitals, declaring to Li Hua, "Western medicine has saved my life!" (*gei xiyi jiule huilai*).[98]

Having thus set the stage, Gu then introduces a lecture posing as a short story. Wang Laosan admits that the hospital nurses were always too busy to tell him about his illness, so upon returning home he asks this information of Li Hua, who is only too happy to provide it. Li tells Wang that he contracted cholera, using the standard term from medical texts, *huoluan*. In order to teach Wang Laosan what "cholera" is, Li Hua tells him all the vernacular names for it, including *huliela* (a transliteration of "cholera" using the word for "tiger" and thus expressing its fierceness), *fasha* (eruption of granular-sand rashes), and three names that describe its symptoms: *jiaochang sha* (granular-sand rash that twists the intestines), *bieluosha* (granular-sand rash that produces sunken whorls [on the skin]), and *diaojiaosha* (granular-sand rash that makes your legs cramp and shake).[99]

The text simultaneously signals an openness to vernacular culture and a desire to school people in "proper" medical terminology. Meaning literally "sudden chaos," *huoluan* first appeared in print as a referent for cholera in the 1838 *Huoluan lun* (Treatise on sudden turmoil), by learned physician Wang Shixiong (1808–64). Writing after treating several patients during China's second cholera pandemic, Wang borrowed the term from the *Huangdi neijing* (Inner canon of the Yellow Emperor) of the first century BCE, wherein *huoluan* denotes "distinctive clinical cases characterized by their sudden onset and simultaneous vomiting and exhaustive diarrhea," though not to the exclusion of other acute gastrointestinal diseases with similar symptoms. Nor did Wang interpret it exclusively, though he voluntarily took the first step in solidifying *huoluan* as "cholera" by establishing a precedent for the association.[100] By the early twentieth century *huoluan* had shed all other meanings in the writings of health officials, but Gu's story confirms that among the people multiple names for cholera still circulated.

After his litany of terms, Li Hua speaks in rhyme of the symptoms of cholera, embedding a pedagogical mnemonic within the story to help readers (or listeners) learn how to distinguish cholera from less deadly gastrointestinal ailments. "You vomit and have diarrhea, your face narrows and your nose grows pointy, your skin dries up and your eyes sink in [to your skull], [and] your fingers and toes get all wrinkly [*you tu you xie, mian xia bi jian, pi gan yan xian, shouzhi jiaozhi quan fa zhouwen*]."[101] Both early-childhood Confucian classics and the primary MEM texts for adult literacy employed rhyme as a pedagogical method to render new concepts easy to remember.

Li Hua demeans another Asian culture, perhaps to make China appear more civilized. He explains that cholera originated in India where, in "ancient times," people drank the same water that they used for bathing and washing clothing, and though their behavior facilitated the transmission of cholera, they believed that it originated in miasma or from "people angering the gods," so they prayed and invited spirit mediums to intervene on their behalf—all of which Li declares "useless." Then (in 1884) a German doctor (Robert Koch) discovered the causative bacterium, *Vibrio cholerae,* and others subsequently discovered that sunlight, heat, steam, disinfectant, and acids all destroy this weak microbe. In fact, it dies within a few minutes in a 1 per cent solution of creolin (*chouyaoshui,* a disinfectant made from coal tar that kills bacteria and mites), or a few seconds in a diluted solution of hydrochloric acid, and even the stomach acids in healthy intestines can kill it. Nonetheless, Li explains, *Vibrio cholerae* is still very dangerous since it can live for several weeks in water, excreta, and gutters, or on wet clothing. Most frighteningly, "doctors say that twenty-five thousand microorganisms can stick to the legs of flies," and these insects love to rest on human food. Wang Laosan finally realizes that he got sick from the cut melon that he had eaten in the city, whose sweet scent must have attracted flies. After patiently listening to Li Hua's continued lecture on preventive measures (including both vaccines and staying warm while sleeping), proper identification, treatments to avoid (scraping, or *guasha,* and popular medicines such as *rendan* and *shaqiwan*), and the only treatment known to be effective (saline drip), Wang announces that he learned a lot and is looking forward to the next discussion with his learned neighbor.[102] Thus ends the long disquisition, just in time for the next story to introduce its two characters, "Mr. Today who breaks superstitions, and Mr. Ancient the stubborn old man."[103]

Collectively these stories suggest that no matter how hard they worked to empower villagers, Rural Reconstruction activists and other reform-minded intellectuals retained a sense of moral superiority, fully in keeping with NLM politics (whether or not they would have professed allegiance thereto). This stemmed primarily from their belief that as educated people they had something valuable that they must urgently impart to their rural beneficiaries. Chen Zhiqian expressed this sentiment well when he explained in his memoir that "scholars are a special class, but . . . with this respected status, went the responsibility, as educated men, of working for the good of the common people."[104] Although reformers like Chen and Zhou aimed to improve villagers' morale and self-respect, they in fact sometimes propagated a didacticism that disempowered rural Chinese for their lack of a specific kind of knowledge and value set. They had genuine sympathy and concern for the plight of their poor countrymen and women, but in their political naïveté they condensed the problems to poverty and ignorance, with little structural analysis of the root causes. It would be anachronistic to blame them for their innocence. Coming of age in the post–October Revolution era of global optimism about ending socioeconomic privations, when the fledgling Communist Party of China offered only one version of the story, most people in this generation lacked the political savvy to understand the structural inequality that poor farmers faced. Nor did they know what would occur during the Cold War, when capitalists took up the cause of rural development for their own, often with disastrous consequences for the communities ostensibly served.[105] Despite their shortcomings, the Mass Education and Rural Reconstruction movements created a cadre of highly educated young adults who had privilege but cared deeply about those who did not. That their genuine concern so readily mutated into pedantry may appear tragically naive today but made perfect sense in their own hour of national crisis. It also accorded with the political structure in which they worked. In the two model counties of Dingxian in Hebei and Zouping in Shandong Province, the Nationalist state mandated the transfer of power over "county government, including police and courts," to the Rural Reconstructionists.[106] Even the sincerest effort to empower villagers rooted itself in the politics of taking power.

ROMANCE OF THE NATION: NEW FORMS OF MALE–FEMALE INTIMACY

A sense of national urgency monopolized much of women's emotional labor, including that of the women who did not join the military as soldiers or nurses but worked in support positions. These women sewed and washed military uniforms, sent medical kits to soldiers, wrote letters to help illiterate soldiers communicate with their families, raised government bond monies to fund the military, and volunteered to comfort hospitalized soldiers with entertaining music and art performances. Women and girls performed this work by the thousands, often in prominent settings and with public recognition.[107] In so doing they followed Song Meiling's prominent modeling of such activities as a woman's proper wartime contribution that prioritized the needs of the nation. They also followed a script prevalent in romantic literature dating from the late 1920s, which "enacted [citizenship] again and again in the romantic motif of falling in love with and marrying *any* of one's fellow citizens regardless of genealogy or social station" and constructed love as "a linguistic and cultural resource mobilized and mobilizable by the project of modernity."[108] One way such literature mobilized love argued for "the postponement of love and the subordination of sexual relationships to the revolutionary agenda."[109] Operating between Song Meiling's model of national motherhood and literary models of deferred romance, young women could experience physical and emotional intimacy with male strangers without endangering their virtue; on the contrary, they demonstrated their profound love of nation through such closeness.

Thousands of educated young women who wrote letters for soldiers during the war adopted a powerful stance vis-à-vis the unlettered men and produced new intimacies between themselves and people previously deemed strangers. Literacy represented power in a society that considered writing (*wen*) the foundation of culture (*wenhua*) and civilization (*wenming*). The power to connect people separated by war had in fact been the foundation of the Mass Education Movement. When its founder, Yan Yangchu, interacted with Chinese laborers for the first time in his life while working in France as part of China's work-study movement in World War I, the largely illiterate workers begged this Yale University graduate to write letters home for them. Yan obliged, but then took the bolder move to teach them how to read and ultimately spearheaded the MEM in 1923.[110] As a measure of letters' importance during the War of Resistance, China maintained no less than three separate postal services during the war that fractured its territory.[111]

Beginning in December 1937, high school girl students in Hubei wrote letters for soldiers by decree of the provincial government.[112] Volunteering across the country from 1944 to 1946, women in the New Life Movement Friends to Wounded Soldiers Society wrote over sixty-five thousand letters for soldiers, and over twenty-two thousand letters for new recruits.[113] While we can only imagine the details that these letters contained, the emotional power that they possessed to connect people—soldiers to their distant family members, and volunteer letter writers to soldiers—is palpable. Qing, a young college student who in 1939 volunteered with several of her classmates to comfort soldiers in a village in Guangxi Province, told her story of the role that these letters played in fostering friendship between the soldiers and volunteers. Though her group had brought towels, needles, and thread, Qing reported that none of the soldiers had any torn clothing that needed mending, nor did they want the towels. Notwithstanding the students' missionary zeal, initially the soldiers also failed to respond to the daily propaganda plays and nightly meetings designed to incite anti-Japanese sentiment. The soldiers did make use of the four hundred mosquito nets, however, pleasing Qing, who ardently wanted the soldiers to know that people on the home front cared for them and wished to protect them from the predations of malaria-carrying mosquitoes.[114]

In contrast to the lukewarm or even cold reception of other offerings, many of the soldiers greatly treasured the letters that the college students wrote for them. Inside the third ward, which like the others held about a hundred patients, the soldiers surrounded Qing and her fellow volunteers each day, begging them to "write a letter for me too, teacher!"[115] The soldiers' common appellation for the students, *xiansheng,* literally means "first born" and at the time was an honorific title for a person with education or status. The "teacher/first born" title succinctly expressed the power of writing to connect these homesick soldiers to their loved ones back home, and the uneducated soldiers to the college students; were it not for the war, these soldiers and students would have had few opportunities to interact with and learn to respect one another. As the soldiers dictated their letters, the students learned intimate details of their lives and gained a new understanding of the heartbreak and hardships that the young men had to endure. Since most soldiers came from poor rural backgrounds, this understanding undoubtedly led to a greater appreciation for village culture and the hardiness of villagers among the children of the privileged urban class.

Scenes like the one depicted in figure 11 occurred around the country, tens of thousands of times each year throughout the war, and transcended social divides. Since girls of all but the most elite families had only recently gained access to formal education, the young women who could so deftly wield the brush on behalf of men were almost certainly of the urban middle class, while the vast majority of soldiers came from poor villages. While in normal circumstances members of these two populations would have had few occasions to meet and even fewer occasions in which to share intimate personal details, the war placed them in close quarters and made each dependent on the other: the soldiers for the volunteers' service, and the volunteers for a population to serve and thereby gain personal fulfillment and social recognition.

The photograph also clearly shows how new forms of male–female closeness in wartime settings allowed people momentarily to cross the artificial boundaries between certain social categories while simultaneously reifying heteronormative interpretations of gender. The union of the female volunteer and male soldier—two young, attractive people with no chaperone—in this small space speaks volumes about the social changes wrought by the war. Abandoning gender propriety in these extraordinary times, the two breach social code in order to strengthen their nation's ability to fight the enemy. Yet they remain unequal in their affection. The supine soldier stares directly into the camera lens in a moment of vulnerable exposure, his face fully recognizable and his identity laid bare. In contrast, the young woman's posture with her back to the camera affords her anonymity, while her bobbed hair, close-fitting cotton *qipao,* and ability to write mark her as a "new woman." Her willingness to volunteer in the hospital marks her a new woman of the war years, leveraging her social privilege on behalf of those less fortunate in service of a national cause. No bourgeois stain on her character, in this setting her privilege and education allow her to perform a sacred duty for the nation. She supplies the soldier with emotional relief—an afternoon with a pretty young woman who appears to care for him, and a letter to cherished family members that will ease their worries about his whereabouts and condition. Having received this relief, the soldier can more readily return to battle. The letter writer creates an intimacy with the convalescing soldier, not for the sake of romance itself, but for the romance of the nation.

Letter writing produced emotional intimacy, but medical care required physical intimacy as well. Medical work brought women into entirely new positions and unprecedented proximity with men to whom they bore no familial relations.

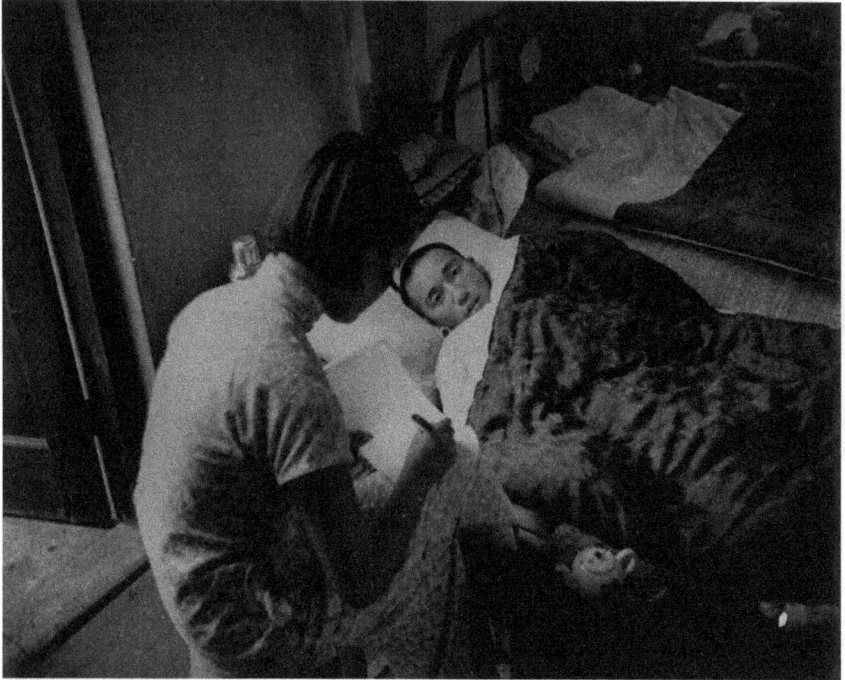

FIGURE 11. A young woman writing a letter for an illiterate soldier convalescing in hospital. LOT 11511-2, WAAMD #410, U.S. Library of Congress, Prints and Photographs Division.

Female nurses' and doctors' regular access to male bodies in mobile vaccination tents, medical wards, hospitals, and clinics changed the way that men and women interacted with one another in public and produced scenes in which onlookers witnessed new modes of performing gender. Figure 12 clearly demonstrates the singularity of such moments in wartime society. The patient's nervousness about the nurse's proximity to his naked chest reflects his anxiety that he could be perceived as improper if he shows any signs of enjoying or desiring the closeness. The nurse's poise and the precision of her movements show a contrasting calm that bespeaks pride in her own professional prestige, and confidence in her medical training. The nurse's stance indicates a status difference between the two that troubles traditional gender roles even as it affirms the woman as caretaker.

LITERARY REFLECTIONS OF GENDER TROUBLE: BA JIN'S *WARD FOUR*

Female nurses and one idealized female physician, Dr. Yang, feature centrally in famed author Ba Jin's (1904–2005) semiautobiographical novel *Ward Four* (*Disi*

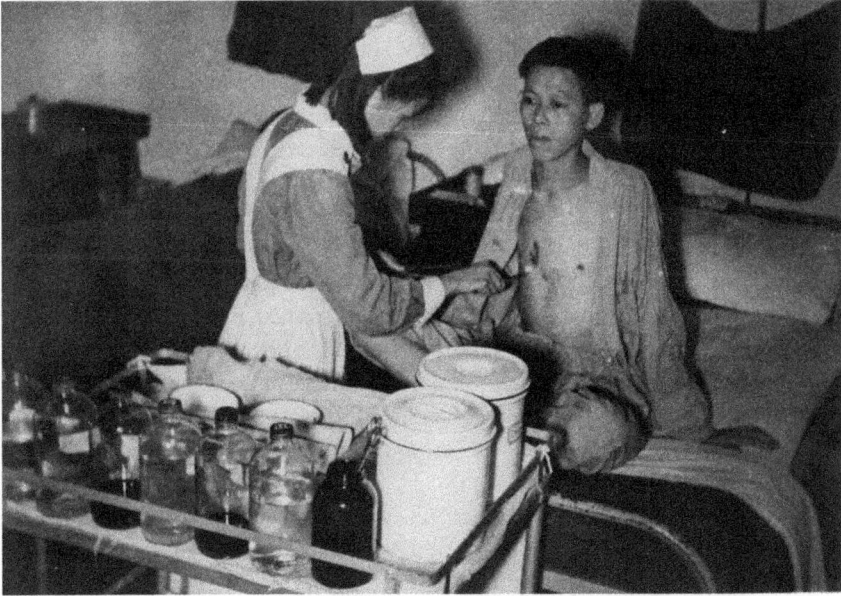

FIGURE 12. Nurse treating a man's bare chest. Box 75, folder "ABMAC no. 3." ABMAC Records. Rare Book and Manuscript Library. Columbia University.

bingshi), one of three novels that he wrote during the war and first published in 1946.[116] The book takes the form of a diary penned by a twenty-three-year-old man from June 1 to June 18, 1944, when he enters the third-class ward of a hospital with a gallbladder infection and encounters much more than physical suffering within its walls. Ba Jin depicts the callous hospital ward, whose name recalls death, as a microcosm of a society pushed to the very brink of survival. He underscores this vulnerability by refusing to name his main character and referring to other patients by bed number: "bed six woke up," "bed eight giggled."[117]

Dr. Yang serves as the diarist's angelic savior and "the only example of an idealistic doctor in the novel."[118] Her wisdom, kindness, and beauty give the young man hope in his darkest hour. Ba Jin self-reportedly created Dr. Yang as a combination of real and fictive components: "her charming smile and her dedication to her profession are based on two different doctors" he knew during his own hospitalization in Guiyang, but "her mind and spirit are totally made up." Nonetheless, the hospitalized Ba Jin "did consider the doctors as saviors," and the author notably selects the female rather than the male physician to embody this role.[119]

Dr. Yang also serves as the amanuensis of the anarchist Ba Jin, who, during his time in the lower-class hospital ward in Guiyang, felt appalled at the uneven distribution of medical services. The only chink in the armor of his idealized physician shows after one of her poor inpatients dies because he cannot afford full treatment. After this Dr. Yang admits, "[S]ometimes I feel like changing my profession and doing something else. I wish I'd never studied medicine." The main character tries to cheer her up by declaring, "Why? Isn't it a wonderful thing to be a doctor? A profession that saves lives and saves the world!" Dr. Yang responds, "You're looking at it like a child. . . . Even if I study medicine to the limits of my ability, that doesn't mean I can actually save people. I'm no match for money. People with no money can't benefit from my efforts."[120] This pessimistic view of wartime health services pointed to deep inequality in the social structure that permeated medical spaces. Within this context, it is all the more salient that Ba Jin selected a woman as heroine of his dark novel. Dr. Yang represented the thousands of women whose work partially alleviated this inequality not only because they were the most affordable and numerous staff members in health organizations, but also because they communicated a meaningful message of care through their emotional labor.

These factors made women's medical work quite memorable. Recalling his hospital experience seventeen years after the fact, Ba wrote, "I feel I could still see clearly even with my eyes closed the setting and the daily life of patients, as well as the facial expressions and language of several doctors and nurses."[121] As argued above, facial expressions, choice of words, and tone of voice are all central facets of emotional labor, and their memorability to patients—whether positive or negative—delineates the distinctive nature of work that entailed intimate exchanges between people living through their most vulnerable moments and the people trained to help them through the ordeal. Ba Jin's experience is likely to have been much less positive, since he continued this passage with the claim that he was "not willing to remember these people and my experiences there for long," even though "these impressions are too deeply left in my memories to be easily erased."[122] Ba had a profound and personal recognition of the value of genuine care in a hospital ward. Plagued by memories of his own painful experience, he gave his fictional self a savior—a woman who held fast to the emotional work of her profession and felt existential pain when that alone did not suffice to counteract social injustice.

Within the novel Dr. Yang exemplifies a woman whose mark of excellence lies primarily in the way she performs the emotional labor her job requires of her. Her advice to the hospitalized young man to "become kinder and purer" and "more useful to others" restores his hope in humanity after he has witnessed so many fellow patients die pitiful deaths, abandoned by their family members and forsaken by a society that granted the poor neither services nor sympathy.[123] The women who provide palpable care for their patients stand above the fray in this bleak setting. One patient underscores the view of nurses as embodiments of classic feminine virtue by declaring that "if you want a wife, get a nurse, if you ask me. They're caring and considerate . . . and nurses have an even temper."[124] All of the characteristics that make women good nurses, and good nurses desirable wives, have to do with emotional labor: being caring and considerate, and controlling one's temper.

Yet Dr. Yang also exhibits mannerisms that transcend traditional notions of femininity. Struggling to contain this powerful woman in a single figure, Ba Jin describes her as possessing both "masculine" and "feminine" qualities. His choice illuminates both the limitations of language to describe the shifts in gender roles that occurred in wartime medicine and the failure of imagination to comprehend the profundity of those changes. Dr. Yang's embodiment of the "feminine" qualities of magnanimous kindness and virtuous service recalls the role of Song Meiling in leading women's social activism. As if further mirroring the First Lady, Ba Jin crafts Dr. Yang as a strong leader who "walk[s] like a carefree man" and commands authority within the ward.[125] The author resorts to orthodox gender norms in an attempt to contain his own creation's transgression, delineating professional competence as masculine and self-effacing sacrifice as feminine.

Ba Jin's fixation on Dr. Yang's deft combination of seemingly dichotomous characteristics abandons his main character to a fantasy of self-improvement through adopting her gender-bending traits—a task that the patient dreams will allow him to escape the inhumanity of war. The book ends with the most direct expression of his obsessive fascination with his physician. When he describes his last encounter with Dr. Yang, he writes in his diary, "I could feel the blood drain from my face; my heart was beating wildly. . . . I looked up just as she reached the door. Her white hospital gown flickered briefly and was gone, gone forever."[126] The patient must now make his way alone in the world, without his angel.

Not all of the male patients in the story have the same response to female authority; most feel threatened rather than fascinated. Ba Jin sympathetically portrays the male patients' struggles to accept women's medical power and reflects men's anxiety about their uncontrollable vulnerability in the medical ward. Both male orderlies and female nurses attend daily to the physical needs of the all-male patients, including intimate procedures such as emptying bedpans and sponge-bathing the invalid. Most patients experience discomfort at losing their virile able-bodiedness and respond by attempting to regain authority. In order to ease their distress at their inability to perform the role of the dominant and capable man, they constantly tease and heckle the nurses to the extent that it becomes one of their only forms of entertainment. They try to resolve the ever-present tension between themselves as incapacitated patients and the young women as competent nurses through such statements as "Today I'm going to let Nurse Hu give me a shave"—a semantic overturning of the power dynamic that allows the disempowered man to imagine himself in charge of his own body.[127]

Constant though it is, their jovial banter can only momentarily reverse the gender inversion, and no one even attempts to perform it with doctors. To highlight this tension as a central feature of the ward, Ba Jin sets the first interaction between the main character and his savior Dr. Yang in a moment of extreme vulnerability: he has to bare his chest to his male doctor Feng in the presence of Dr. Yang during morning rounds.

> [Doctor Feng had] already "looked" in the clinic but he said he wanted to "look" again. This time there was a young (she couldn't have been more than twenty-five) woman doctor standing beside me, and I was embarrassed about exposing my abdomen in front of her. But I couldn't disobey my doctor's orders, so I reached down and lifted up my clothes (sweater, shirt, undershirt) for him. He leaned over and began to probe, thump, and listen.[128]

Dr. Yang's power to embarrass the main character is embedded in her gender and in the gender differential between herself and her charges. The need to expose their flesh in front of unfamiliar women rendered the male patients completely defenseless. Physical nudity underscored the social vulnerability that men, incapable of taking care of their own bodily needs, experienced when reliant on others.

At the same time, as if reflecting the image in figure 12, this first encounter hints at the productive tension born of social difference. Precisely because of their distinct identities as man and woman, patient and doctor, the two yearn to reach for each other across the social divides. Ba Jin makes this tension last. Immediately following the examination of the patient's bare chest, Dr. Yang and Dr. Feng speak to one another in English—a tactic that the physicians in the novel regularly use to exclude the patients from their dialogue and which reflects the class hierarchy of medical relationships. Ba Jin carefully presents these social distinctions between patient and physician, but their presence only increases the main character's ardor for Dr. Yang. For him, because her distinctiveness places her out of reach, it renders her wholly desirable, hinting at one possible reason for the compliance of lower-class men with caring women in wartime China.

CONCLUSION

China's geographic, religious, linguistic, cultural, class, and ethnic diversities had the power to put fellow Chinese at odds with each other, literally unable to comprehend one another's languages or enter each other's social worlds. Some women, in place to shape a new medical workforce, quickly learned that they could not let these barriers stand; they had to cultivate the trust of their charges in order to heal them. Accordingly, female nurses under Zhou Meiyu's leadership received specific training to communicate their trustworthiness by being the first to offer gendered intimacy. This emotional labor required that they communicate care through touch, facial expression, and tone of voice. Working at the front lines of demand to nurture refugees, orphans, and soldiers, women not only saved countless lives but also created the emotional ties that bound people together as members of a national collective. Their role as prominently visible representatives of humanitarian work made them not unlike today's female "etiquette volunteers" (*liyi zhiyuan*) who greet guests at major national events and represent China as a "civilized nation" through their docility, attractiveness, and modeling of Confucian virtue.[129] The role of women in anchoring national tradition and representing the nation long predated and long survives the war.[130]

Just as Florence Nightingale did not unseat British sociocultural norms in a single historical event, Zhou Meiyu and others only began their work in wartime China. She and her colleagues continued to train nurses and fight for their social recognition in postwar Taiwan for decades. Nonetheless, the War of Resistance created a variety of coalescing forces that allowed for rapid change in women's social roles. First, the war put so many people on the move, as both soldiers and refugees, that it produced new spaces for social encounters between strangers of different social status, region, and sex. The mobilization of the population also created an unprecedented concentration of highly educated individuals in the southwestern provinces, where they created medical institutions in which women of a lower social class could work. Second, women overwhelmingly occupied the lower rungs of these institutions and assumed roles that placed them on the front lines of medical response and squarely in the public eye. Third, prominent female leaders like Song Meiling, He Xiangning, and Xie Bingying called for women to contribute to the war effort through "feminine" caretaking work, modeled how to do it, and established the charitable organizations that provided the framework for its conduct. Fourth, unlike men, who authored and enforced punitive regulations that people resisted, women delivered services that people welcomed.

Most importantly, women learned how to perform the emotional labor that made them the most effective deliverers of state-sponsored medical work and granted them the power to fashion a national community out of docile bodies and to transform hearts. Throughout the war, many women played in public a role for which they had long received recognition in the private space of the home: that of the respected caregiver. As they worked in organizations designed to fulfill the mission of the state, these women leveraged their respectability to school people in "proper" modes of behavior that affirmed middle-class values. Best expressed in the New Life Movement, which took middle-class values as a universal standard against which to measure all Chinese, these hygienic behaviors became a marker of citizenship itself. Since they promoted better health, and therefore attracted the interest of well-meaning activists and public health workers, these behavioral standards gained sufficient momentum to become the means by which poor people could gain the status of "worthwhile citizen" in the eyes of their social superiors. Yet little progress could be made unless poor people reached for the services proffered, either in the manner of characters in didactic stories who proclaimed themselves saved by scientific medicine or asked their neighbors for long lectures, or in the manner of actual people who served dinner to public health nurses or willingly submitted to a vaccination shot. Through myriad interactions between and among health workers and patients, the war brought people of different sex, social status, and home province together in unprecedented encounters in which people reached for each other. This multitude of brief relationships, made all the more memorable for their birth at the razor's edge between life and death, wove delicate bonds that interlaced the eastern and western, northern and southern regions of a vast country into a new social fabric.

3

Healing to Kill the True Internal Enemy

We all thought: "We must work ourselves to the bone; saving one more
wounded soldier is like killing one more devil [i.e., Japanese soldier]!"
—YAO AIHUA, RECALLING HER WORK AS A VOLUNTEER MILITARY
NURSE DURING THE WAR

Though everyone assumed that war with Japan would eventually come, the actual moment caught the Nationalist government off guard and very nearly destroyed it. What came to be called the Marco Polo Bridge Incident (*Lugouqiao shibian*) took place just outside Beijing on July 7, 1937. Both sides' stubborn refusal to cooperate turned what might have been an isolated affair in the regional North China war that had begun soon after the Japanese colonized northeastern China (Manchukuo) in September 1931 into a full-blown war that engulfed the country and, a few years later, the entire Pacific.[1] During the first several months of fighting, Japanese soldiers tore through Chinese cities and villages, advancing like an uncontrollable forest fire and wreaking havoc on civilians and soldiers alike. Their rapid conquest of a vast territory, including the old imperial capital, Beiping (Beijing), and the actual capital, Nanjing, caused a health crisis that prompted the Nationalist state finally, belatedly, to fund and administer military medicine.[2] Though it grew as quickly as possible during the war, the underfunded and understaffed military medicine system could never catch up to the burning need, and young students like Yao Aihua, quoted in this chapter's epigraph, rushed in to fill the gap.[3]

Yao characterized her medical work in terms that simultaneously underscored its urgency and its role in supporting the Chinese military's aim to kill the enemy. She and her fellow nurses therefore supported the Nationalist state's ability to kill, by serving as the caring and benevolent face of a state that extended its reach into hearts and homes to save lives while simultaneously risking the lives of millions of men on the battlefields. Achille Mbembe argues that the political sovereignty of the modern state lies not only in its biopolitics—the structures it creates to affirm and protect life, such as schools and hospitals—but also in its necropolitics: its ability to determine who shall live and who must die.[4] The Nationalist state's killing machine—its organized military—placed at great risk not only the lives of Japanese enemy soldiers, but also the lives of its own soldiers, and women who worked in military medicine quite deliberately and consciously did the same. As Yao Aihua's words suggest, military nurses understood this direct connection between the work of healing and the burden of killing and in fact celebrated their ability to contribute to the war effort by nurturing the bodies of their own soldiers so that they could return to attacking the bodies of enemy soldiers.

Nurses could overlook their role in risking the lives of their own soldiers because they spent so much time and energy killing the soldiers' greatest enemy: disease microbes. Whereas in other belligerent nations battle had become the troops' most lethal threat (unlike during World War I), in China, with the exception of the first few months of the war, infectious disease and poor hygiene and nutrition still proved far more deadly than enemy soldiers.[5] Cholera, bacillary and amoebic dysenteries, typhoid, typhus, scabies, malaria, tuberculosis, tetanus, and relapsing fever all ravaged Chinese troops in an era when most of these diseases claimed easy victims. Among civilians, the burden of disease fell heaviest on the poor, and infantrymen—who often came from poor families and once in the army received insufficient food, clothing, and medical care—faced the greatest danger of all. Women who offered medical care formed a bulwark against these myriad threats and embodied the soldiers' hope of survival, even as they eagerly sent the soldiers back to the battlefield.

These women performed a crucial service for their country as well. Despite the rush of volunteers, staffing remained an intractable problem because China suffered a critical shortage of medical personnel. A 1937 survey of registered scientific-medicine professionals counted only 8,900 physicians, 2,740 pharmacists and druggists, 3,700 midwives, and 575 nurses nationwide.[6] In order to address this pressing problem, Major General Zhou Meiyu translated her training program for rural public health nurses into the military. Working with a man who had close ties to overseas funders, Dr. Lim Kho Seng (Robert Lim), and for a state that desperately needed her services, Zhou trained a large cadre of nurses more successfully in wartime than she could have done in peacetime since even as the Nationalist state's capacity shrank, the generosity of foreign donors grew.[7] Under the leadership of Lim and Zhou, the Chinese Red Cross Medical Relief Corps (*Zhongguo hongshizihui jiuhu zongdui*) (MRC) and the Emergency Medical Service Training School (*Zhanshi weisheng renyuan xunliansuo*) (EMSTS) trained frontline medics, stretcher bearers, and nurses as rapidly as possible. Working independently of but in cooperation with the government-run Army Medical Administration (AMA), the MRC and EMSTS formed the structure of a new military medical system.[8]

Ironically, the greatest peril to this system designed to protect soldiers' lives came from the Nationalist state itself. Many powerful state officials failed to recognize the terrible threat of disease and believed other entities more dangerous. According to Generalissimo Chiang Kai-shek, Communist "bandits" were the country's true "internal enemy" and deserved only death and suffering. Therefore, he and his allies grew suspicious of medical workers who treated all patients equally. They failed to understand the foundational role that emotional labor played in the provision of healthcare and decided that only Communists could feel genuine care for soldiers of the Communist armies. This emotional blind spot greatly strained China's military medicine system when Nationalist party rightists pushed Dr. Lim out of his leadership roles in the MRC and EMSTS, thereby threatening their smooth operation.

WHOSE "DISEASE OF THE HEART"? POLITICAL MYOPIA AND THE FATE OF THE NATION

The trouble began with defining the enemy. Three months before the war began Minister of Health Dr. Liu Ruiheng declared,

> China is on the eve of launching a great organized advance towards the elimination of preventable diseases. There are hordes of enemies which are destroying the national health and vigor, and until very recently no organized attempts have been made to retaliate.[9]

Depicting diseases as "hordes of enemies . . . destroying the national health and vigor," and fighting contagious disease as the foundational task of protecting national sovereignty, Minister Liu (and other health officials) attempted to coax the Nationalist government into committing precious resources to health programs. Although civilian and military healthcare gained substantial ground during the war, in many respects Minister Liu was shouting into the dark. When in 1941 *Time* magazine correspondent Theodore H. White interviewed General Chiang Kai-shek, the head of the Nationalist government famously stated, "[Y]ou think it is important that I have kept the Japanese from expanding. . . . I tell you it is more important that I have kept the Communists from spreading. The Japanese are a disease of the skin; the Communists are a disease of the heart."[10] While Chiang described the Communists as the country's true internal enemy, piercing the heart of the body politic, health officials more accurately described disease microbes—the internal enemy that penetrated a body's cells—as "hordes of enemies" that rendered soldiers unable to fight and civilians unable to rebuild the nation.

These definitions mattered. Because Generalissimo Chiang and other right-wing Nationalists treated Communists as sworn enemies, medical workers who treated them as fellow Chinese in need of care angered political leaders and faced personal danger. Right-wing Nationalists assumed that people who accepted the many privations of working in wartime healthcare must be devotees of Communist doctrine, for they could not conceive of another source of motivation. They understood only one of the two modes in which patriotism operates, for

> [p]atriotism is Janus-faced. It faces outward, calling the self, at times, to duties toward others, to the need to sacrifice for a common good. And yet, just as clearly, it also faces inward, inviting those who consider themselves "good" or "true" Americans [Chinese] to distinguish themselves from outsiders and subversives, and then excluding those outsiders.[11]

On the one hand, patriotism promotes philanthropic behavior toward people one considers part of one's community. On the other hand, it can promote social ostracism and mistreatment of those who are considered *not* part of this community. Precisely because Nationalist party rightists considered Communists and their political sympathizers a "disease of the heart," or outsiders inside the national community, they insisted that Communists receive no medical care when wounded. In other words, rightist ideologues had their own "disease of the heart"—the failure to understand that someone might wish to help *all* wounded compatriots out of simple patriotism, professional identity, or humanitarian impulse, rather than political alliance. This failure of imagination led them to decide that prominent military health leaders who followed the nonpartisan protocol of the International Committee of the Red Cross must be Communist, and therefore must be eliminated.

Dr. Lim Kho Seng (1897–1969), an overseas Chinese from Singapore, was the first to face this allegation. Dr. Lim exhibited the philanthropic form of patriotism from the beginning. On sabbatical in Europe when the war broke out, he gave up both his sabbatical leave and his appointment at the Peking Union Medical College (PUMC) to serve his ancestral homeland.[12] Once in China he established and ran the Chinese Red Cross Medical Relief Corps (MRC), which by November 1941 had trained nearly three hundred thousand medical personnel organized into 175 mobile medical teams.[13] Lim also established the Emergency Medical Service Training School (EMSTS), which by the spring of 1941 had trained nearly five thousand doctors, nurses, midwives, hygiene technicians, sanitation inspectors, and orderlies for both military and civilian services. Fully committed to serving anyone in need, Dr. Lim insisted that MRC units offer treatment not only to soldiers, but also to local farmers on the front lines.[14] He also assigned some of the MRC units to serve the Communist Eighth Route and New Fourth Armies, and he sent a division of the MRC to the Communist headquarters in Yan'an to treat people who had been wounded in guerrilla fighting in North China.[15] After facing pressure from multiple sides that left him in a constant state of fear, Lim resigned from the MRC in September 1942, and the organization entered a serious decline that lasted until December 1944, putting the country's military medical system at an extreme disadvantage precisely when the Imperial Japanese Army (IJA) launched Operation Ichigo (April–December 1944), the largest land offensive of the conflict, during which Japan nearly conquered China. Lim was also forced to abandon his position as head of the EMSTS in August 1943. Lim's colleagues kept the EMSTS in operation, however, and by late 1943 had trained over seven thousand medical officers and assistants, and over sixteen thousand by the war's end. Nonetheless, leading doctors in the EMSTS described Lim's departure as "an irreparable loss."[16]

This all occurred well after the New Fourth Army Incident of January 1941 spelled the death of the Second United Front and heightened mutual distrust between the two parties. In this same period, Chiang Kai-shek also disbanded Yao Aihua's medical service team on the suspicion that its members had Communist leanings since Mao Zedong and Zhou Enlai had publicly praised their service to wounded soldiers in the famous battle of Taierzhuang. (Yao's team soon regrouped.). Yao also recalled being transferred out of the 77th Regiment Hospital after half a year when the hospital administrators noticed how friendly she was with the New Fourth Army soldiers.[17] In a country with two fronts such friendships were politically suspect, but their interruption placed the nation at great peril.

Selfless service characterized not only Dr. Lim but the entire staff of both organizations he ran. To recruit personnel for the EMSTS, in October 1938 Dr. Lim visited Wuhan with Minister of Health Liu and delivered rousing speeches to educated refugees. In a short time the two men recruited over seven hundred doctors and nurses, with PUMC affiliates making up the majority.[18] Lim and Liu's success reflected the strength of their professional networks revolving around the PUMC, the emotive power of the war as a motivator to action, and the singularity of the war as a historical moment when a high concentration of educated people with fewer career options than in peacetime committed themselves to serving their country. Remarkably, Drs. Lim and Liu recruited so many people even though they offered such little compensation; MRC and EMSTS staff received a pay so low as to render their service virtually voluntary. This mattered little. Yang Wenda (PUMC, class of 1937), who as superintendent of the Chinese Red Cross Hospital supervised the training of hundreds of army doctors, so desired to serve his country that he declared himself willing even if he received no pay whatsoever. He noted that he and his colleagues worked alongside actual volunteers who included not only Chinese from within China and throughout the diaspora, but also non-Chinese from eleven countries around the world, including Romania, Poland, England, Germany, Spain, and India.[19] The presence of an international coterie of volunteers strengthened the employees' conviction that they worked toward a higher purpose.

Despite her distinction as one of the highest-ranked women in the National Revolutionary Army, Major General Zhou Meiyu also came under suspicion of being Communist and nearly lost her life when a Nationalist official sent someone to assassinate her. When the friend who had saved her told her of this plan, she merely scoffed and said, "That would be a waste of a gun. I'm not afraid!"[20] The mere idea that a member of her own political party might assassinate Zhou, who dedicated herself to saving soldiers' lives, seems absurd now but made sense amid the political paranoia that gripped the Nationalist Party during the war. In her oral history interviews in the 1980s Zhou felt compelled to explain: "At that time some people were very shortsighted and narrow minded; they always believed that if a person was doing something and asking nothing in return, they must be communist. This really was a big joke!"[21]

Though Zhou attempted to use laughter to dispel concern, this was not in fact a joke, or rather it was a big joke masterfully played on the Nationalists themselves. The emotional blind spot of radical Nationalists threatened the political stability of the country. Writing toward her own political goal (to promote the cause of cultivating certain emotions as the basis of liberal democracy), political philosopher Martha Nussbaum argues that "[c]eding the terrain of emotion-shaping to antiliberal [Communist] forces gives them a huge advantage in the people's hearts and risks making people think of liberal [Nationalist] values as tepid and boring."[22] Given that Mao Zedong famously declared to the Politburo during the Civil War, "[T]he battle for China is a battle for the hearts and minds of the peasants,"[23] the significance of the rightist ideologues' myopia is clear. They forgot that "patriotic emotion can be a necessary prop for valuable projects involving sacrifice for others."[24] They deliberately *discharged* nurses who befriended the soldiers to whom they provided medical care. This amnesia—or failure to understand in the first instance—ultimately cost them the country. During the Civil War, which bubbled beneath the surface of the War of Resistance and rolled into the open almost as soon as Japanese troops left, "the Communists proved far more effective than the Nationalists in mobilizing individuals and mass support by appealing to patriotism and anti-Japanese sentiment," and they won the war, and the country, in 1949.[25] The Communists understood how to build a national community on sympathy.

Nationalist leaders' paranoia did not secure their goal of uncontested power, but its exact opposite. All the midnight arrests and back-alley executions of Communists and suspected Communists proved again and again that Nationalist Party ideologues valued their own ideals more than human lives.[26] It also rendered the Nationalist Party ideologically empty, so the Communist Party could fully monopolize the spirit of service and personal sacrifice, even though in reality people across the political spectrum had this spirit, and both sides were simultaneously engaged in bloody conflict and suppression of "enemies." Extreme rightists relinquished the narrative of wartime patriotism because they failed to understand that the affective domain of healthcare existed within a politics of inclusion, rather than a politics of exclusion. General Chiang did understand the importance of caring emotionally as well as physically for soldiers, as demonstrated in the speech he delivered to military medical officers soon after the war erupted. Chiang told them,

> Our average soldier at the front, because he cannot rely on good military medicine and stretcher bearers, even as he fights bears the weight of worry over the fact that no one will be able to save him should he get wounded, and even should he be transported to the rear he still fears that he will not be healed, or even receive cruel and unfeeling [*lengku wuqing*] treatment in hospital. This decreases the soldier's courage in combat, and who can say how much it decreases our fighting strength?[27]

The key to Chiang's myopia lies in the first word, "our." He believed that care from "kindly doctors" (*cixiang de yisheng*) and "brave medics" should be limited to "our" people and denied to "theirs."[28] His virulent anticommunism left him unable to fathom that people who treated everyone equitably did not necessarily do so out of a commitment to communism. Nationalist ideologues who followed Chiang's lead consistently isolated and mistreated members of their own party who accepted personal discomfort to serve those less fortunate, and who performed this service in a spirit of equity.[29] Fortunately, Zhou Meiyu kept her calm and her life, and trained nurses to serve everyone who needed their care.

MICROBES: THE TRUE INTERNAL ENEMY

Chinese soldiers sorely needed people like Zhou Meiyu to accept personal sacrifices in order to help them, for their suffering knew no bounds. Soldiers faced hunger, exposure to extreme cold and extreme heat, and well-equipped enemies trained to treat them like animals. But their greatest enemies were invisible. After the first few months of blistering warfare far more Chinese soldiers died from the effects of pathogenic microbes than directly from wounds. Although the ratio of the total number of soldiers who succumbed to disease to the total number of wounded is fairly well matched—1.3 to 1.0—disease proved far deadlier than battle wounds. Whereas 44,847 soldiers perished of wounds in hospital, 405,753 perished of disease in hospital, a ratio of more than 9 to 1.[30] Just as Dr. Liu Ruiheng claimed, pathogens were "destroying the national health and vigor." Over the course of the eight years of warfare the National Revolutionary Army lost over half of its total fighting force to disease, wounds, and desertion.[31] This had devastating effects on units stationed throughout the country. For example, in a one-year period in which his nearly half a million troops saw no major battles, nine thousand of General Xue Yue's soldiers died from wounds and forty thousand of disease.[32]

Dreaded influenza—the same disease that sparked a global pandemic after World War I—earned pride of place on the list of lethal diseases, which also included tuberculosis, malaria, typhus, typhoid, and bacillary and amoebic dysenteries.[33]

In 1945, a professor of agricultural biology estimated that fecal-borne diseases caused fully one-quarter of China's annual deaths. These diseases included some of the soldiers' main scourges—cholera, amoebic and bacillary dysenteries, and typhoid—as well as the chronic complaints of rural farmers: schistosomiasis, hookworm, and parasitic roundworms. According to the professor's calculations, these fecal-borne diseases killed thirty to thirty-five million people during the eight years of the war, while the death toll of the war itself was fourteen to twenty million people.[34] Even accounting for the fact that soldiers did not suffer all of these deaths, adding vector-borne diseases—typhus, malaria, scabies, and relapsing fever—to this list affirms that minuscule microbes caused much more damage to China's fighting force than did Japanese bayonets and ordnance.[35]

One of the gravest dangers to Chinese soldiers, invisible to the naked eye, caused an insidious death: shigella, the rod-shaped bacterium that produces bacillary dysentery in the human digestive tract. The bacterium's namesake, Japanese physician Dr. Shiga Kiyoshi (1871–1957), had discovered the dysentery bacillus in 1897 while working at Japan's Institute for the Study of Infectious Diseases with its founder, Dr. Kitasato Shibasaburo (1853–1931), who himself had worked with Robert Koch.[36] Characterized by abdominal cramps, fever, and violent, unstoppable, bloody diarrhea, dysentery desiccates its victim to death in a matter of days.[37] Passed via fecal-oral transmission, shigella flourishes in the overcrowded, unsanitary conditions often present during war, even far away from the battlefield. Liu Feng, when recalling his experiences as an eleven-year-old apprentice in a Chongqing arsenal, said, "My greatest fear was diarrhea. In Chongqing I would shit until I got dizzy. It was so bad that by nighttime I couldn't see anything."[38] Currently treated with sulfa drugs, antibiotics, and the penicillin derivative ampicillin, created in 1961, bacillary dysentery was in the 1930s and 1940s often untreatable and frequently fatal.[39]

Cholera, another lethal disease that kills through chronic diarrhea and desiccation, also plagued Chinese soldiers during the war. Difficult to treat without antibiotics or immediate oral rehydration, it is caused by an agent, *vibrio cholerae,* that lives in water or food contaminated with human waste and can kill a person in a matter of hours. The victim first suffers nausea, vomiting, muscle cramps, and headache; impending death manifests itself in bluish skin and sunken eyes. Since the disease plagued both soldiers and civilians, military and civilian health organizations did joint prevention work. The NHA performed frequent cholera vaccination drives in which soldiers and prospective soldiers received priority, MRC hygiene engineering teams separated latrines from drinking water and disinfected wells, and military field medics learned how to devise a simple saline solution (or a sugar solution if no salt was available) for rehydration therapy. Yang Wenda recalled seeing the greatest number of corpses at any point of the war during a cholera epidemic in Nanchang. He and his MRC coworkers had to bury the bodies in mass graves of fifty to sixty corpses each, with a sprinkling of lime on top as a disinfectant.[40]

Recognizing that most field medics had undergone only brief training, the NHA produced portable, pocket-size pamphlets for military medics and emergency first aid nurses working on the front lines. Written in simple text without illustrations, these pamphlets provided detailed information on the prevention, identification, and treatment of all nine legally notifiable contagious diseases—typhoid fever, typhus, dysentery, smallpox, plague, cholera, diphtheria, contagious cerebral meningitis, and scarlet fever—as well as other common diseases such as scabies. The 1940 NHA pamphlet on cholera recommended traveling with a small quantity of bleach powder to disinfect drinking water, since soldiers routinely "drank from paddy fields."[41] The pamphlet also detailed proper management of a cholera patient's feces, though judging by the descriptions of military hospitals, sanitary feces management must have occurred rarely among sick soldiers.[42] Most of the suggested measures would have been impossible to follow in the field. For example, in many field hospitals the water supply barely sufficed for cooking and soldiers had to forgo bathing, so the medics certainly could not have washed the bedding each time it was soiled. Zhou Meiyu recalled that many a thousand-bed field hospital, unable to keep all thousand quilts clean, simply kept them in a closet and forced soldiers to sleep without bedding until an official came for an inspection.[43] A soldier suffering from cholera or dysentery would have soiled the straw or cot on which he lay multiple times a day, requiring the labor of many staff to maintain hygienic standards. Yang Wenda recalled addressing this problem by cutting holes in soldiers' cots and placing bedpans underneath so that sick soldiers unable to walk to the latrines could relieve themselves without soiling their bedding.[44]

By the spring of 1940, malaria and gastrointestinal diseases were demonstrably the primary killers of soldiers. Malaria had already proven its lethal might: in August 1938 "whole regiments were infected with malaria and an entire division stopped in its tracks." The MRC responded by distributing more than fifteen million quinine tablets in that single year of 1938. Nor did the danger diminish: a study conducted at the fourth EMSTS center in southeastern Sichuan from July 1943 to June 1944 recorded 10,760 cases of dysentery and 24,160 cases of malaria among troops in that area alone. Even partial data from the NHA showed a total of more than 1.7 million cases and nearly nine thousand malaria deaths between 1940 (the year data collection began) and 1945, as well as a huge spike in 1946, when the NHA recorded nearly a million cases and four thousand deaths. Nonetheless, the partiality of this data showed clearly when the United Nations Relief and Rehabilitation Association (UNRRA) produced its survey of annual communicable disease infection rates in China in July 1944, and estimated 21.3 million cases of malaria per year.[45]

Malaria illustrated the blurred lines between civilian and military health. With both mosquito nets and quinine in short supply, malaria spread even to the cold northern provinces when disease-ridden soldiers moved their battle lines there. Meanwhile in the southwestern province of Yunnan, where malaria was endemic, the disease incapacitated nearly 30 percent of the two hundred thousand laborers who built the Burma Road by hand; once again the civilian NHA and the military MRC collaborated to control it. In 1941 the National Institute of Health trained 138 male sanitary engineers in Chongqing, Guiyang, and Kunming in mosquito eradication techniques, which included draining ponds, covering standing water with kerosene to kill larvae, administering prophylactic drugs, and teaching people how to cover themselves while sleeping. Later, when the United States finally joined the war and had troops stationed in Yunnan, US Army personnel sprayed DDT across the area.[46]

The tiny louse joined the mosquito as a formidable foe. Typhus, relapsing fever, and other louse-borne diseases accumulated a tremendous death toll during the war, just as they had done across Europe during World War I.[47] Body lice wreaked havoc for the very simple reason that soldiers had little access to clean clothing and bedding; the NRA did not have the capacity to issue foot soldiers with more than one uniform. One soldier recalled that his single uniform "very quickly became infested with lice."[48] Staff in the MRC, NHA, and AMA recognized the severity of the situation and launched a war within a war against the minuscule and multitudinous louse. In September 1938 they began a delousing, bathing, and scabies (DBS) program to build mobile stations where soldiers could take baths, wash their clothes, and get haircuts. By June 1940 over two hundred such stations served soldiers around the country.[49] The showers had the added benefit of combatting scabies, another scourge of a dirty soldier and one that affected 70 percent of patients reporting to MRC health stations in 1938. In the ninth war area, by March 1943 bathing reduced the incidence of scabies from 90 to 10 percent. Proper cleaning of a soldier's lice-infested uniform required multiple steps. Liu Yongmao, the leader of the MRC environmental hygiene team, demonstrated to his staff that even when a soldier's winter jacket appeared clean after washing, thousands of lice still hid in the seams. Liu would run a hot clothes iron along the seams, then use a broom to sweep all the dead lice into a pile to show just how many more had been hiding inside. Zhou Meiyu and Yao Aihua both remembered that soldiers' body lice would attempt to crawl onto nurses while they tended to the wounded, so nurses tied the ends of their sleeves and covered their collars with bandages dipped in Vaseline to prevent the lice from getting traction. Nonetheless, "even with these kinds of careful protections, there were still incidents of contagion, so we did lose several nurses."[50] This gruesome reality underscores the fact that nurses not only accepted low pay and tough working conditions, but also risked their own lives to save the lives of others.

Because bacilli and bombs do not discriminate among their victims, the war created a certain degree of "social leveling" that opened the possibility for elites to empathize with their social inferiors through the common experience of suffering. Socioeconomic privilege could not entirely contain the traumas of war; even middle- and upper-class people lost their homes and family members to air raids and disease, especially as diseases expanded their temporal and spatial territory.[51] Refugees, enemy soldiers, and Chinese troops moved long distances, taking diseases with them.[52] Chiggers (trombiculid mites), for example, traveled with the Japanese army, expanding the range of scrub typhus all the way from Japan to China's Yangzi Valley and other regions of the Pacific War.[53] Epidemics began to follow new routes and timetables. In May 1941, Dr. H. W. Tseng of the Chongqing Methodist Union Hospital (*Chongqing Kuanren Yiyuan*) reported that he had seen "winter epidemics occurring in summertime," and that contagious diseases spread "far more easily than in peacetime."[54] Chongqing factory worker He Qiuping recalled that "cholera became rampant because of the Japanese bombings."[55]

Yet social leveling had its limits, and the poor undoubtedly paid the overwhelming cost of the war. Corruption in the military recruitment system placed the greatest burden of soldiering on poor families because the wealthy had many means of evasion: purchasing the services of a replacement; bribing someone to falsify census records (usually sons' ages); dividing family property prematurely to make all sons heads of household and thus ineligible for the draft; putting a son in school; sending a son to work in the city or a different village where he was not on the population rolls and could evade the local *baojia* head during conscription rounds; bribing recruitment officials; making one's son a recruitment official; or defending oneself with guns. Poor men were not entirely without means of defense: where the rich used guns, the poor used knives; and where the rich used bribes, the poor used their legs to run away from conscription gangs.[56]

Nonetheless, the majority of conscripted foot soldiers were poor and already in a state of compromised health before they even got to the battlefield (see figure 13). Sichuan supplied the greatest percentage of soldiers for the War of Resistance—giving a total of 3.4 million—and Chongqing shouldered a hefty share of this burden.[57] Rural Sichuan had very high rates of hookworm and schistosomiasis, and all of rural China had high rates of chronic gastrointestinal parasites, all of which compromise the body's ability to absorb nutrients from food.[58] In 1941, Minister of Health Jin Baoshan wrote that only 40 percent of four and a half million conscripts proved physically fit in a health examination, and 50 percent of these would likely develop an illness before getting to the front.[59] In one group of new conscripts bound for the ninth war area, 78 percent died in a dysentery outbreak due to malnutrition and lack of medicines.[60]

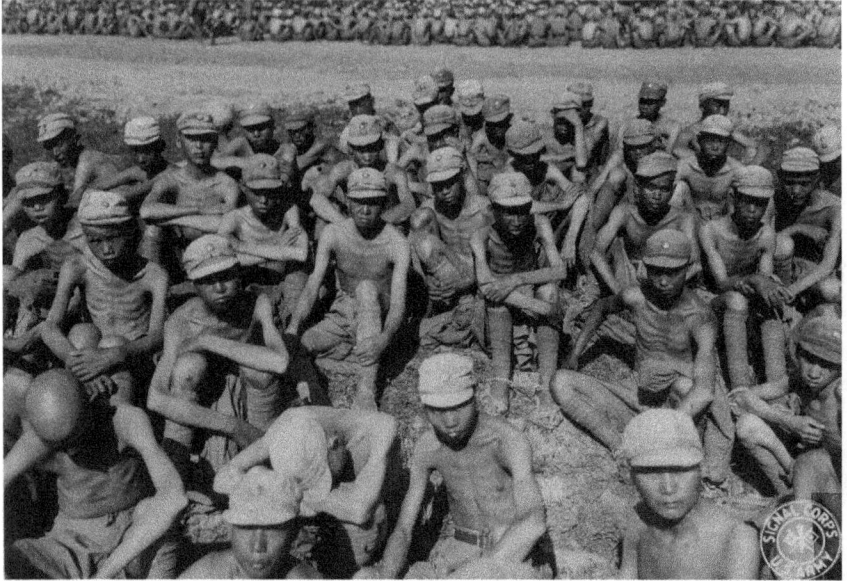

FIGURE 13. New soldier recruits already looking famished. Photo taken by the U.S. Army Signal Corps. Box 85, folder "Soldiers-Wounded." ABMAC Records. Rare Book and Manuscript Library. Columbia University.

New conscripts often had to march hundreds of miles just to get to their recruitment centers, then further to the battlefield. Traveling such distances often meant that soldiers arrived in a state of exhaustion in areas of the country where strange climates harbored diseases to which they had no acquired defense.[61] They might also lack proper clothing for the climate to which they marched; soldiers frequently wore threadbare uniforms and straw sandals that chaffed their feet, or no shoes at all. Superintendent Yang Wenda recalled treating many foot soldiers from Guangxi while supervising an MRC unit in Nanchang, Jiangxi. Yang stated that "these southern soldiers had no idea what winter was like in Beijing or Shanghai, so they traveled north in grass sandals and got frostbite. By the time they came back many of them had lost their toes and had to walk on the balls of their feet."[62]

LONELY SOULS AND WILD GHOSTS BURIED WITHOUT A COFFIN

The story of sixteen-year-old Pan Yintang illustrates how dangerous life in the Chinese army could be for the average foot soldier from a poor family—fourteen million of whom were conscripted throughout the war—as well as the suffering that ignoble death and improper mortuary treatment inflicted on soldiers.[63]

In 1938, Pan and 280 other young men fell victim to a conscription gang. The gang captured the men from Pan's home village of Shizi and nearby villages in Dazhu County, Sichuan. A farming boy accustomed to handling livestock, Pan likened their seizure to a farmer capturing pigs for slaughter.[64] This metaphor proved rather prescient, since most of his fellow captives never returned home.

The conscription gang threw Pan Yintang and the other captives into a desperate war. In raw numbers, the adversaries appeared to be evenly matched: by November 1937, China's NRA had 1.7 million troops in service but no reserves, while the IJA had six hundred thousand men in active service and nearly a million in reserve in the nearby Japanese colonies Manchuria and Korea. At its height the NRA fielded over four million soldiers, while the IJA eventually fielded 1.65 million troops in fifty-one divisions.[65] The NRA had to push more troops into battle because the Japanese had notable advantages in leadership, training, organization, munitions, and military hardware (chiefly tanks and planes), though China did receive crucial air assistance from the Soviet Union and later the United States.[66] The IJA therefore consistently inflicted greater casualties with fewer troops: in the Battle of Shanghai (August 13–November 12, 1937), Chinese casualties mounted to 187,200, while fewer than 10,000 Japanese soldiers died and a little over 30,000 sustained wounds. During Operation Ichigo, Japanese soldiers killed twenty to forty Chinese soldiers for every one loss of their own.[67] After conquering nearly all of China's coastal cities in the first few months of the war, including the capital, Nanjing, the Japanese Army had logged only 100,000 casualties. Meanwhile, China had suffered so many fierce defeats that reporters elided details in order to sustain morale.[68]

NRA leaders, unable to avoid the facts, began to make rash decisions that actually increased Chinese civilians' suffering. In December 1937 Chiang Kai-shek abandoned Nanjing rather than defend it, and then General Tang Shengzhi did the same rather than fulfill his sworn promise to Chiang to defend the capital to his death. This dual abandonment left civilians defenseless and at the mercy of an angered and rapacious enemy in an event that has been memorialized as the "Nanjing Massacre" or "Rape of Nanjing."[69] In November 1938 General Xue Yue, fearing a Japanese invasion of Changsha, preemptively burned the city to the ground rather than yield it to his enemy, thus becoming the city's destroyer rather than its protector.[70] Wishing to stall the Japanese advance on the first provisional capital of Wuhan, Chiang Kai-shek ordered the destruction of the dikes holding back the mighty Yellow River at Huayuankou in June 1938, killing half a million people and rendering another 4.8 million refugees. This disastrous act delayed the Japanese advance by only five months, and Wuhan fell in October 1938.[71] It also characterized the Nationalist state's extractive relationship with the natural environment, which led to immense ecological devastation throughout the war.[72] Though trading space for time came at such a great cost, space was indeed China's major advantage. Continually moving his troops and his administration across vast distances, Chiang trapped his Japanese adversaries in the "China quagmire" and bought himself some time to revitalize his armed forces.

The NRA sorely needed a revitalization. The losses at Shanghai alone had included over 70 percent (thirty thousand) of the German-trained and highly loyal officers in Chiang's army.[73] The remaining disloyal officers could cause serious problems. In the famous battle of Taierzhuang (March 24–April 7, 1938), General Li Zongren expressed his Janus-faced patriotism by refusing hospital access to soldiers from his commander Chiang Kai-shek's Central Army and offering treatment only to soldiers from his own power base of Guangxi Province.[74] Although feted for bringing his countrymen their first major victory in the war, General Li confirmed Chiang's suspicion that divisions within his own command could fracture the power of his army and directly endanger soldiers' lives.

Soldiers of course already faced myriad dangers, one of which is well reflected in Pan Yintang's story: their utter lack of training and preparation. Pan and his fellow conscripts first traveled to Guizhou, then to Kunming, where they received an extremely rudimentary training. He recalled that "each man was given a gun and three bullets, and we tried out the guns a bit, then we were considered ready to go to the battlefield." From there they went to Burma, where Pan and his fellow troops faced starvation. He recalled that they received no pay and meager rations, so they stole pumpkins, cucumbers, and beans from the farming fields and ate them raw. Still, they were frequently dizzy and nearly blind with hunger.[75] Napoleon Bonaparte is credited to have said, "An army marches on its stomach." As Pan Yintang's experience demonstrates, China's army had very little to march on. Though a particular problem in the Burma campaign, chronic malnutrition plagued all Chinese troops. While on paper a soldier had adequate rations—twenty-four ounces of rice per day, a sufficient amount of salt, and one pound of pork per month—in reality many officers resorted to corrupt practices to squeeze these rations out of their men and take the lion's share for themselves. Soldiers who did receive field rations often had little but uncooked rice kernels, so they frequently stole food from civilians as they passed through villages.[76] In 1945 US General Albert C. Wedemeyer wrote in a report to Chiang Kai-shek that "as [Chinese soldiers] march along they turn into skeletons; they develop signs of beriberi, their legs swell, and their bellies protrude."[77] Wedemeyer ended his report with a reference to the profound corruption within the Nationalist military—a severe problem that made Chiang Kai-shek irate. Ultimately, Chiang ordered an extensive investigation and the executions of the head of the conscription service, Lieutenant General Cheng Zerun, as well as the commanding officer of a particularly egregious recruitment camp. However, Chiang acted too late to save soldiers from abuse—in July 1945, one month before the war's end.[78]

Pan and his companions had been conscripted into the Chinese Expeditionary Force that fought with US General Joseph Stilwell in the disastrous 1942 Burma campaign. Despite General Stilwell's ability to spin the story to his advantage such that most English-language histories to this day paint him a hero, the campaign ended with the defeated Stilwell abandoning the Chinese troops in the Burmese jungle, where most died of starvation and disease.[79] Even during the second Burma expedition in 1944—Stilwell's attempt to massage his bruised ego—four out of five Chinese soldiers sustained combat wounds or died. Fortunately for these wounded men, substantial medical aid from the US military provided sufficient medical care for 60 to 70 percent of the wounded to return to battle (where they once again risked their lives in combat).[80]

In 1942, Pan Yintang and his fellows in arms could not rely on such aid. Their death toll mounted; of the 280 men taken from Pan's county in Sichuan, 178 (64 percent) perished of starvation, disease, or battle wounds. In the end only 35 made it out alive and well, while another 67 returned home disabled. Pan ultimately decided that in war most of the conscripted men "became lonely souls and wild ghosts" who died far away from home and received but a summary burial.[81] Soldiers frequently suffered this fate, even if they died on the Chinese side of the Himalayas. Yao Aihua recalled that "at first when the wounded started to die they would get a coffin of thick wood; later on as the death toll began to mount, the coffins grew thinner and thinner, until in the end they received no coffin at all."[82]

The pain of witnessing improper treatment after death is quite close to universal in human societies, but it had particular poignancy for Chinese soldiers.[83] In traditional Confucian culture, the idea of *luan*, or "internal confusion and chaos," was "feared more perhaps than the external invading army," and *luan* is exactly what death produces—a tear in the fabric of the social, an unstable (if temporary) proximity of this world to the afterworld, an opportunity for the dead to seek vengeance against the still living if they are improperly guided to safe harbor in the hereafter.[84] Funerary ritual, properly performed by the right people in the proper space and time, fulfilled the immensely important job of safely guiding the dead to a settled life-in-death in a parallel universe.[85] Those who died away from their families and communities, for whom no one could perform the requisite rituals, suffered not only an ignominious death but the existential angst of an uncertain postmortem existence.

Properly speaking, the dead themselves did not feel this after their passing, for as corpses they could feel nothing, but the soldiers who witnessed so many of their comrades' bodies treated like so much detritus likely dreaded that such a fate might befall them as well. Soldiers who survived also might easily have feared the power of the "wild ghosts" that their fallen comrades had likely become. Such wild ghosts—people who died at the wrong time or in a manner that superseded normalcy, such as during warfare—had the potential to disrupt the safety of the living. At least in northern China through 1945, "[t]here was generally a pervasive concern with the dangerous power of the spirits of those who had died by violence." Such individuals could easily feel wronged by the unnatural circumstances of their deaths, remain unsettled by the lack of proper funerary ritual, and use their powers as "unhappy spirits" to disrupt the lives of those who remained on earth.[86] Particularly those whose bodies suffered significant trauma in death, and therefore lacked a complete body with which to enter the afterlife, became "demons" for whom "even access to hell was denied."[87] The living therefore felt a profound responsibility to honor the dead with proper mortuary ritual and burial, and suffered when circumstances prevented this. During the war they also suffered in the absence of secure knowledge of their relatives' whereabouts; the NRA had not systematized its tracking and sometimes recorded soldiers as "without a trace" (shizong)—a word whose simplicity belies the torture that this lack of closure entailed for family members. Famous author Lao She passed devastating months wondering about his mother's whereabouts, of which he wrote, "[P]eople whose mothers are alive have secure hearts. I feared, feared, feared that a letter from home would tell me that I was now a plant without roots."[88] For some of the people who died while sojourning in Chongqing, neighborhood associations and charitable organizations stored their coffins throughout the war and worked to return them to the deceased's hometowns after victory. For the soldiers and others who followed the Nationalists to Taiwan, repatriation of remains to the mainland became impossible, and banishment to "a land where none of your relatives are buried" caused psychological torment that set their very identity on edge.[89] During the Cultural Revolution (1966–76), when all forms of traditional culture in mainland China were under siege, "one of the most intense anxieties experienced by survivors of the dead was their inability to attend properly to the traditional rituals of death and dying."[90] The same situation pertained during the War of Resistance. So profound was this pain for Pan Yintang that many decades after the war ended, he encapsulated his experience as bearing witness to the men around him as they "became lonely souls and wild ghosts."

ZHOU MEIYU AND THE ROLE OF WOMEN IN MILITARY MEDICINE

As with civilian nursing, military nursing expanded more dramatically than any other sector of military medicine during the war. Extrapolating from May 1948 data, at the end of the war China had 10 dentistry schools, 25 pharmacy schools, 91 medical schools, and 171 nursing schools.[91] The dramatic expansion in nursing could be described as an "intentional accident" in that it arose from a confluence of factors both planned and unplanned. The Nationalist government had devoted inadequate funding and preparation to its military medicine system prior to the war's outbreak but had also instituted mandatory nursing training for high school girl students that, sure enough, provided a pool of cheap labor when the crisis hit. No one could have predicted exactly how many hospitals would fall into Japanese hands, but once they did the AMA called in civilian help and authorized the creation of two additional military medicine organizations under independent leadership: Dr. Lim Kho Seng's Chinese Red Cross Medical Relief Corps (MRC), founded in August 1937 to create a mobile medical service to staff the more than two hundred AMA hospitals spread along the front lines, and the Emergency Medical Service Training School (EMSTS), founded in May 1938 to provide short-term, intensive training in medicine and epidemic prevention to fulfill personnel needs within the rapidly expanding civilian and military medicine systems.[92] Female nurses worked in all of these organizations, as well as in a variety of civilian volunteer groups, and did the most work to care for civilians and soldiers amid the trauma of war.

The rapid and, to civilians, rather unexpected advance of Japanese troops created an immediate crisis in the medical system, made all the more urgent due to the Nationalist government's poor preparation. At the beginning of the war, the AMA had only one doctor per seventeen hundred soldiers, and thousands of inadequately trained medical personnel. The total of three and a half million soldiers who served during the duration of the war could count on only 1,922 military doctors.[93] Although war began in July 1937, there were no regulations governing the transport, treatment, or reenlistment of wounded and ill soldiers until September, and field hospitals and triage centers could not be established throughout the war zones until the founding of the Central Management Office for Wounded Soldiers (*Zhongyang shangbing guanlichu*) in October.[94]

The wounded therefore quickly overwhelmed all available facilities. Famous author Xie Bingying, who organized women's volunteer medical corps in 1927 for the Northern Expedition and in 1937 for the War of Resistance, recalled of the wounded soldiers streaming in from the Battle of Shanghai (August–November 1937):

> [T]hey were lying crowded together in every room and even on the steps in the central courtyard. . . . Some had legs or arms severed by explosions. Others had lost half their brains in bomb blasts. Some had been hit in the stomach by machine guns and their small intestines were spilling out. Some had bullets still lodged in their flesh, and they cried out day and night from the pain. Some were missing two-thirds of the skin and flesh on their thighs. Some had wounds in which multitudes of maggots grew. Some had only a single tendon left in their hands.[95]

Wounded soldiers and the nurses who tended to them confronted gruesome scenes like this one throughout the country. Such experiences were common in military nursing; during World War I, Russian military nurses "were bombarded with numerous dramatic, indeed traumatic, sensory perceptions" and often felt "immediately and strongly repelled" by the sights and smells of wounded bodies.[96] Yet military nurses were trained not to make the "disgust face" that psychologists claim to be universal; they posit that humans in all societies and animals alike exhibit scrunched eyebrows, a curled upper lip, and a physical jerk away from the offending item.[97] In China as in Russia, this telltale sign would have affirmed the soldiers' physical repulsiveness, but as chapter 2 explains, nurses were expected to perform the emotional labor of smiling through difficult work in order to communicate care.

Japanese troops advanced far more rapidly than new personnel could be trained, so the government sought another source of medical personnel: female students. In December 1937, the Hubei provincial government required high school girls to undergo nursing training and contribute an eight-hour workday per month in a local hospital. In 1934 the Ministry of Education made nursing a mandatory class for female high school students, added three months of summertime training in 1936, and in 1940 mandated three hours a week of civilian and military nursing training for female students of high school age and up. Also in 1940, Hunan and Sichuan required young women who graduated from high school to work either as rural public health nurses or as military nurses, all the while promoting nationalism and organizing local women for similar work. Between 1934 and 1935, the provincial ministries of education in Jiangxi, Jiangsu, and Anhui provinces duplicated the central Ministry of Education regulation and required female students to study military nursing. Given the limited strength of the Nationalist state, it is likely that many provinces did not follow this regulation to the letter, but some clearly did.[98]

By providing the labor force that the state desperately needed to care for its soldiers, (young) women proved their indispensability to the nation and attained a position of power in constructing it. In late imperial China daughters in elite families were often educated so that they could teach their own children (with a focus on grooming sons for the civil service examination). In the Republic advocates of girls' education leveraged its benefit to the nation to argue their position, claiming that uneducated and bound-footed girls (the "Sick Women of East Asia") made the whole nation weak.[99] Whether for the patriarchal family or the patriarchal nation, women gained access to education not because it directly benefited them but because it benefited a larger social collective. This simultaneously put women at a disadvantage—always required to put others before themselves—but also placed them at the fulcrum of constructing this collective. During the War of Resistance women became conduits of state power, even as young students.

High school students clearly had some agency in how they answered this government mandate. For example, when students in Zhejiang found their nursing courses boring and irrelevant, their principal changed their program to include three hours per week of practicum in a local hospital, which they reportedly enjoyed. Beginning in North China in late 1936, students from Taiyuan (Shanxi Province), Beijing, and Shanghai all organized their own relief teams and went to the front to treat wounded soldiers.[100] In volunteering to nurse soldiers, these high school students were in good company. Prominent women such as Hu Lan-qi (1901–94), Xie Bingying (1906–2000), He Xiangning (1878–1972), Jiang Jian (1902–40), and Wu Jufang (1911–99) volunteered across China to care for soldiers and raise funds for the wounded.[101]

These women responded to an acute crisis in military and civilian hospitals in the first months of the war, where the AMA's lack of preparation left wounded soldiers in the lurch. Yao Aihua recalled that in the first few months of her work as a volunteer military nurse, wounded soldiers poured in from the fronts at Shanghai and Nanjing when her volunteer medical team was stationed in Zhengzhou (the capital of Henan Province). The wounded filled all available hospital spaces, and "some soldiers were just out on the streets. Some of them had their intestines hanging out, all bloody and indistinguishable from their other flesh. It was so pitiful!" A lack of ambulances meant that wounded soldiers often traveled by stretcher, rail, or river.[102] (See fig. 14.) Since the army itself did not always manage the transfer to hospital, troop commanders frequently lost track of their wounded, making it impossible to deliver a soldier's stipend for hospital fees and food and often difficult to redeploy a healed soldier to his original unit.[103] The sheer number of soldiers moving between hospital and field quickly exceeded the organizational capacity of the military's belatedly established transit system.[104]

The stretcher bearers in figure 14 appear to be civilians. Their clothing bears no mark of medical personnel, and the sparse attire of the man in front indicates a likely status of poor farmer. They may have received payment for their arduous labor, but the mountain's steep decline challenges even the surest-footed among them. A wounded soldier, pressing part of his weight onto a handmade cane and still carrying his rifle, follows closely behind. He may have witnessed his fellow soldier's first moment of agony; if they make it to the hospital, he will hear many more soldiers moan and cry. Someone with a full belly, a whole body, and a camera captured this image, freezing the moment when this limping soldier might have been worrying about whether his buddy would make it, whether he would be able to walk down this mountain, how far they would have to go to get medical care. No field hospital appears anywhere in this wide lens; these farmers are rescuing the two soldiers from certain death. In the absence of a functional state system, they have stepped in to suture the ruptured social contract.

Figure 14 captures a common reality of the war: soldiers often had to travel a long way to get medical care. A military officer explained that even if a medic was stationed nearby, the requisite medical supplies frequently lay at a distance of several hundred *li*, making even the slightest wound quite lethal.[105] Wounded soldiers therefore frequently arrived at a hospital in a terribly compromised state. Yao Aihua remembered,

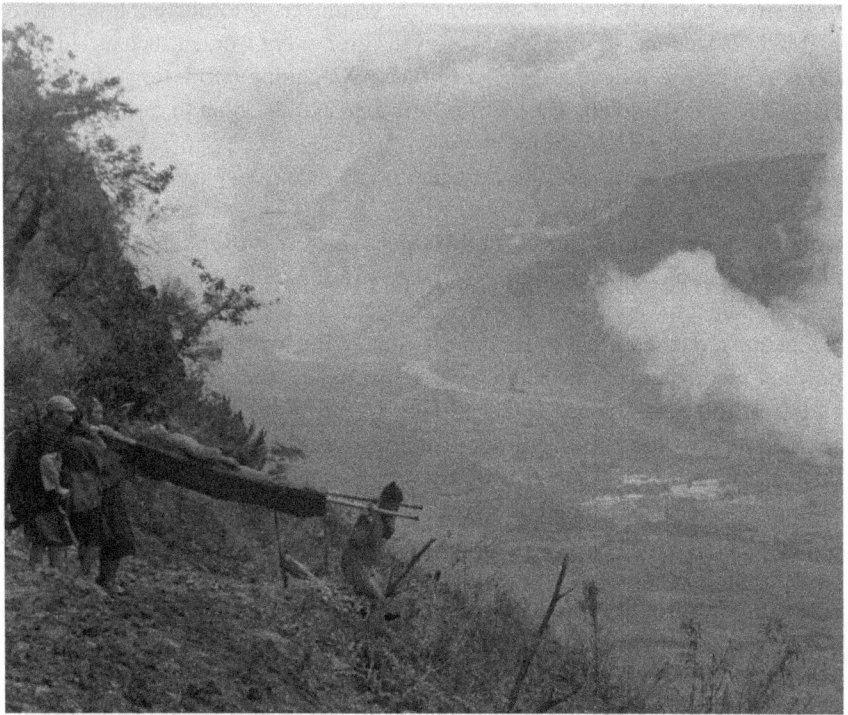

FIGURE 14. Civilians carrying a soldier down a mountain on a stretcher. Box 85, folder "Soldiers-Wounded." ABMAC Records. Rare Book and Manuscript Library. Columbia University.

> Because of the sweltering heat, by the time they got to [the provincial hospital in] Baoding most of the soldiers' wounds were filled with pus and maggots and stank to high heaven. With so many wounded close together they gave each other tetanus, and the death rate was very high. . . . The soldiers' bodies were full of lice, and as we changed their bandages the lice climbed onto us.[106]

The paucity of medical personnel made Yao Aihua's story more common than unique: at the age of sixteen she and all of her middle school classmates answered the call for volunteers from the local Baoding YMCA and Chinese Red Cross and followed their principal to the front after a single week of training in basic first aid. The unending strain of their work, which often began at daybreak and ended after midnight, left Yao so fatigued that at one point she slept through an air raid; her fellow volunteers thought she had died. She also recalled that the shortage of nurses in Zhengzhou meant that they could change a soldier's dressing only

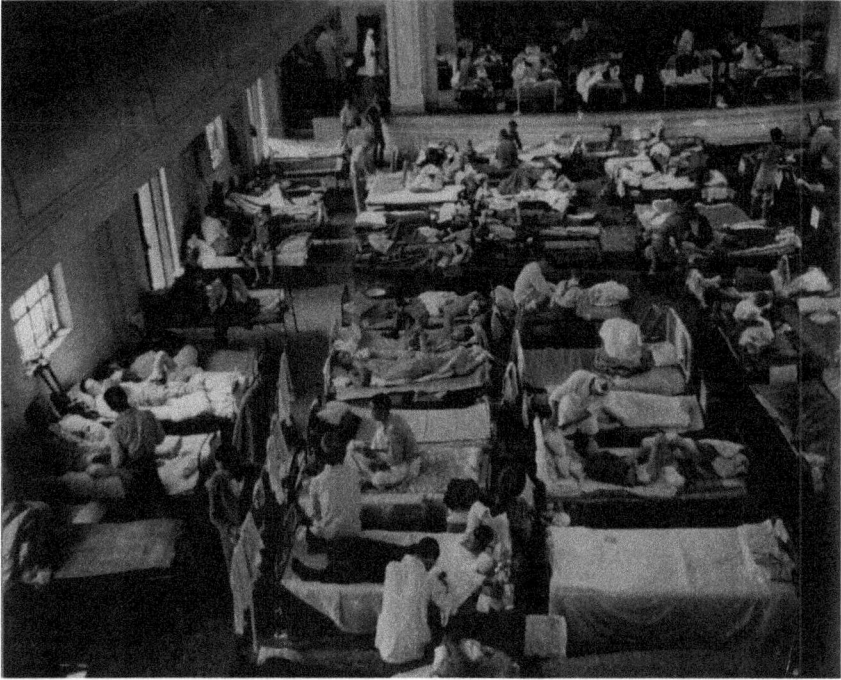

FIGURE 15. As battle lines advanced, hospital staff and patients repeatedly had to flee, and makeshift hospitals were built to accommodate wounded soldiers. This photo depicts one such temporary hospital in a school gymnasium. LOT 11511–7, WAAMD No. 411, U.S. Library of Congress, Prints and Photographs Division.

once every three days, making it difficult to stave off infection, particularly in the summer heat.[107]

Another problem joined the shortage of medical personnel to exacerbate the crisis: insufficient hospital facilities. The Central Hospital of the Chinese Red Cross in Nanjing, which boasted three thousand beds, seven operating rooms, and over three hundred medical staff, fell to the Japanese just one month after it opened.[108] Medical personnel had difficulty tending to refugees when they had to join them in flight. A great number of hospitals and clinics operated out of temporary quarters originally built for other purposes, and many soldiers ended up in such makeshift hospitals, where they often received inadequate treatment. The temporary hospital pictured in figure 15 had a handful of open beds and housed at least one profoundly emaciated patient (front right).

Demoralized staff who paid little attention to basic hygiene compounded all of these problems. A 1938 Red Cross report stated that "most hospital wards are untidy and the floors messy. Patients' clothes appear pathetic and uncared for.

Their bodies are unwashed, their hair long and nails uncut, and their quilts covered with lice. The dysentery or diarrhea cases lie in beddings soaked with excreta. . . . Many are infected with scabies."[109] Other reports from field hospitals around the country showed that such conditions were far from anomalous, and this posed a serious danger to soldiers. Battle wounds that began as minor injuries could easily turn lethally gangrenous or infectious due to lack of medical attention or supplies, improper antisepsis procedures, or poor hygiene in a field hospital. Hospitals in recruitment camps had the barest of supplies. Colonel Lyle Stephenson Powell, a US Army medical officer stationed in Guiyang in 1944–45, described one such facility:

> I have seen a good many ghastly sights, but I have never seen anything that gave me such a complete turn as did this "hospital." The building consisted of a long, earthen-floored, thatched-roof hut, the sides of which had practically all disappeared, presumably as firewood. Two or three [patients] had old overcoats of some sort pulled up over them; the rest had only shirt, trousers, and either bare feet or straw sandals. For warmth they were lying as close together as possible and were too sick to get up to answer the calls of nature; as a consequence the foulness of the place was beyond belief. As I went along looking at these people I counted several that were dead, some already as stiff as the boards they were lying on.[110]

The destitute conditions of Chinese field hospitals illustrate what a ghastly war can do to an impoverished country. Facing the prospect of improper medical care and callous treatment after risking their lives on the battlefield, many soldiers grew angry. Newspapers reported fights between medical staff and soldiers, and usually blamed the latter. Some hospitals refused service to wounded soldiers. One sympathetic reporter, Ji Hong, told the story of an injured soldier who, having had to hop a railcar by himself to get to an unoccupied city for treatment, was refused aid at all five hospitals he found. Ji also said that hospitals often failed to give soldiers proper food, and that he had met a soldier from Sichuan who had received a meager $1.50 in pay after four months of fighting. At one hospital that Ji visited to report on soldiers who had been waiting for three days without treatment, a wounded officer told him that while he could withstand his physical pain, the civilian doctors' brash disregard for his troops' suffering had gravely wounded his heart.[111]

These stories underscore the difference that a caring doctor or nurse could make at a time of vulnerability in a soldier's life. Particularly in the later years of the war, many of the soldiers were teenage boys, often far from home when they sustained a life-threatening battle wound or caught a deadly disease. In face of mortal danger and strident social prejudice, soldiers greatly appreciated and respected nurses who treated them with dignity and kindness. Medical personnel who treated poor men with decency communicated a rare message: your life is valuable, and you are worthy of care.

TRANSFORMING "BAD ATTITUDES":
EMOTIONAL LABOR AND NECROPOLITICS

Female nurses' first message to convalescing soldiers communicated valorization and care. The assumption that men must fight held strong even though the country they defended so often failed to acknowledge their basic human dignity. At least, this held for poor men; many a rich man thought nothing of dodging his responsibility. Nurses could therefore make a tremendous difference in the lives of poor soldiers by giving them both medical care and human caring. They worked within a system directed mostly by men, and among some male military nurses and men in other medical roles (frontline medic, stretcher bearer, physician), but women did the most to provide the emotional labor that helped soldiers to heal.

At the same time, analysis of women's emotional labor helps to explain a remarkable aspect of the War of Resistance, which it shares with other "great wars" of the twentieth century: "the colossal numbers [of people] persuaded to lay down their lives."[112] Women simultaneously provided affective care that encouraged soldiers to feel bonded to the nurses, and employed that bond to send them out into battle once more. In this manner they supported the nation as a "community of death."[113] Nurses frequently employed didacticism to play their role in affirming the supremacy of the nation's needs over the needs and desires of individual soldiers. They looked to upper-class women's groups for models, and to media representations of Song Meiling as their leader. A heavy class politics saturated these media and taught a generation of women to treat male soldiers as their students and as objects of reform.

The communion of female providers and male recipients of care placed women in positions of authority and power. One young nurse's impassioned speech beautifully illustrates the power differential, deriving from her social class, that existed between herself and the soldiers under her care. Her choice of words also illustrates how much her own sense of fulfillment stemmed from her belief that she had the power and responsibility to educate the soldiers to behave differently—precisely what Song Meiling instructed women to do in their volunteer work.

> At the time most wounded soldiers had a poor understanding of the war, so very few of them wished to return to the front lines after they healed. This was a very dangerous situation, since if they returned they would undoubtedly be more experienced than fresh recruits. So we used every opportunity to turn their hearts, talking with them, doing propaganda work, singing war songs, and we would slowly transform their bad attitudes into resolve; they would eventually tell us that once they got better they'd go back to fight the enemy.[114]

As much as nurses' medical treatments crossed class lines to create emotional intimacy, their attitudes and language could redraw those lines in stark terms.

This nurse's words clearly delineated her belief in her power to "transform bad attitudes," "turn hearts," and educate soldiers out of their "poor understanding of the war."

In reality, convalescing soldiers wished to return home precisely because they understood the conditions of war better than did the nurses stationed at hospitals in the rear, though nurses stationed at the front of course witnessed and sometimes personally experienced its horrors. Dreams of desertion rather than of battlefield victory occupied the mind of many a soldier. Poorly trained, ill equipped, underfed, and frequently underage, the average Chinese soldier had little chance of surviving combat against the troops of one of the world's most powerful armies. Particularly in the later years of the war, when press gangs rather than recruiters delivered most of China's troops to the front lines, they also had little ideological attachment to the role and looked upon military service as a death sentence.[115]

Male military nurses exacerbated the problem because they tended to browbeat convalescing soldiers, and this mistreatment made their patients feel uncared for and less willing to risk life and limb once more by reporting back to their units. Major General Zhou Meiyu discerned both the problem and how to solve it. She sent *female* nurses to the hospitals housing soldiers who had a chance of recovery and returning to duty. She instructed these women to treat the soldiers with tenderness and use their attentive care and encouraging words as a means of shaming the men back into uniform. In her oral history interviews, Zhou explained that every time some soldiers had healed and were soon to be sent back to the front, the hospital would ask Zhou to send in some of her female nurses, because there would always be a few soldiers who would get angry and start to fight, arguing that they were not fully cured. The nurses who followed Zhou's training spoke encouraging words to these angry soldiers, which helped to calm them down.[116]

Zhou's astute use of women's emotional labor to increase the fighting power of the NRA accords with the fact that "reciprocal injuring is the obsessive content of war . . . [but] its centrality often slips from view."[117] Not merely "angels of mercy" who soothe and console, female nurses also play a central role in the system of mutual injury, for an "effective medical system . . . contribute[s] to war precisely by contributing to one side's ability to out-injure the other side."[118] In wartime China, female nurses repeatedly sent their own healed patients back to face Japanese soldiers who had been schooled in anti-Chinese racism and trained to treat their adversaries like beasts.[119]

Despite their work in exposing their own soldiers to harm, female nurses celebrated their healed charges' decision to return to battle with send-off parties. In one such case at a bus station, the nurses overheard a soldier saying, "Those girls treated us extremely well. If we don't return to the front to kill the enemy we're not doing right by our country." This comment led one nurse to declare, "Once we heard this, how happy we were! We redoubled our efforts, and we learned a valuable lesson: *the work of educating soldiers was just as important as the work of healing their wounds.*"[120] This "education" consisted of self-conscious performance of heteronormative femininity—the embodiment of tender care—so as to shame men into accepting the duty of heteronormative masculinity: sacrificing one's own life for that of the nation.

This report therefore confirms that many women accepted their role in supporting the Nationalist state's exercise of necropolitics. In other words, they saw one important aspect of wartime womanhood as the ability to prop up the nation's fighting men and urge them to sacrifice themselves in military service. Yao Aihua articulated this even more pithily (as quoted in this chapter's epigraph): "We all thought, 'We must work ourselves to the bone; saving one more wounded soldier is like killing one more devil [Japanese soldier]!'"[121] Yao may have learned such words to describe her experience as a military nurse in part by reading the autobiography of Xie Bingying, in which Xie declared that their motto for relief work was "Saving one soldier is like killing one enemy."[122] Regardless, a female nurse's necropolitical power stemmed not from her ability to effect death for members of the invading army (politics as usual), but rather from her power to send her own country's soldiers back to the front lines, where they once again stared into the yawning mouths of early graves.

Her power relied on heteronormative gender roles that posited heterosexual attraction as the basis for male–female relationships and therefore placed women in a position of seductive power over men. The centrality of this relationship in Chinese gender roles dates to the early twentieth century, when the social space for male–male bonds shrank after the 1905 abolition of the civil service examination—the chief means for elite men to form all-male social networks—and globally circulating theories about evolution and human social organization assigned primary importance to the male–female procreative bond. Chinese theories of modern personhood formed at this time, leading people to "rethink gendered social relations as heterosexuality." The normalization of the male–female sexual bond, signaled in the language of pursuing women's education and "natural feet" for the sake of healthy progeny—that is, in the language of the "Sick (Wo)Man of East Asia"—eclipsed the social visibility and permissibility of nonheterosexual relations. In other words, "social theories of eugenic heterosexuality sought to reorder organic life around the procreative couple at the expense of the bond of filial father and son and brothers."[123] For both men and women, then, innate sexual difference and heterosexual identity based on the presumption of that difference lay at the foundation of modern selfhood.

As the new standard presumed to be universal, heteronormativity served as the fulcrum around which ideas about producing life (strengthening the "Sick Woman" to bear strong children) and about taking life (strengthening "our" soldiers so that they can kill more "enemy" soldiers) danced around and transformed into one another. The Nationalist state's necropolitics mobilized men and women into distinct and directly contrasting social roles that nonetheless worked toward the same goal of building a strong nation and defeating the Japanese army. Just as a great part of the power of modern warfare lies in people's ability to obfuscate its violence, heteronormativity in the medical workforce posited women as the caring, nurturing, supporting partners in the creation of mass-scale death who could coerce, cajole, and shame men into killing more ruthlessly. This system presumed that heterosexual identity—which placed primacy on maintaining one's attraction and attractiveness to members of the opposite sex—would secure women's psychological effect on men. Therefore, the more a woman embraced her role of strengthening the nation through nurturing its progeny (i.e., nursing, but also midwifery and childbirth), the more a fighting man felt compelled to embrace his work of killing on behalf of the nation. Military medical infrastructure extended the caring arm of the state, which in turn supported its killing arm: the exercise of necropolitics relied on women's healing as surely as it relied on men's murder.

Nurses may not have fully understood their role in obscuring the bald facts of military violence—that war's purpose is "to alter (to burn, to blast, to shell, to cut) human tissue"—because direct recognition of this fact requires a certain measure of fortitude. They nonetheless played a most essential role, for "the perpetuation of war would be impossible without the disowning of injuring."[124] While ample evidence suggests that many women yearned for the chance to prove their mettle in military nursing, their primary motivation could just as easily have been to provide succor to their own as any explicit desire to harm the enemy. Regardless, many women celebrated their ability to employ what they believed to be their uniquely feminine attributes: the caring touch of gentle nursing; a patient ear to quell a soldier's anger; rousing words to encourage a frightened boy to resume his manly duty on the battlefield. One nurse worked for two years without a single day of rest while she moved with the battalion she served, from Zhejiang to Jiangxi to Hunan to Guangxi provinces. She believed that the most crucial lesson these two years taught her was how to have patience with the soldiers so as to understand their "hardened hearts," gain their trust, and boost their morale. She wished to publicize the fact that "now no one dares refuse to return to the front," and clearly felt proud of her ability as a military nurse to populate her country's battle lines.[125] Another nurse revealed how attractive military nursing appeared vis-à-vis civilian nursing. She said that she had come from a missionary hospital in Shanghai, where she and her coworkers "were all depressed" because they wanted to come to the interior to serve in Free China but had family obligations, economic limitations, and no contacts to help them along the way. She stated, "If the government could establish networking organizations and escort them into the interior, I'm willing to bet that many nurses would come."[126]

She may have been right, since the famous authors Ding Ling and Xie Bingying, acting on their own and without government aegis, had little trouble recruiting women to go to the front as volunteer nurses. Ding Ling organized a group of women from Beijing who went to Baoding when soldiers wounded in nearby fighting filled all the local hospitals.[127] Xie Bingying claimed that she could have brought more to the front had she not had to leave in haste. As Xie recalled, "My program was no sooner announced than many nurses and female students got in touch with me—and thus the Hunan Women's War Zone Service Corps was established in four days flat."[128] As educated urban women and published authors, both Ding Ling and Xie Bingying could draw on a wide network of like-minded women who wanted the adventure of serving at the battlefront. Xie described it in this way:

> We received no official support for this project because some people said women should work only behind the lines, at home. We, on the contrary, seized the opportunity to rush to the front lines. In fact, everywhere in China women were beginning to mobilize.[129]

Working at their nation's front lines, women mobilized themselves to heal and soldiers to kill.

CONCLUSION

All available information confirms that, despite the brutality of the fighting, disease constituted the Chinese soldiers' greatest killer during the War of Resistance. This yields a heartbreaking picture of a conflict that China did not choose, that came too soon, and that thoroughly exacerbated all the extant problems in the country's healthcare system. The Nationalist government's failure to prioritize and sufficiently fund civilian health systems before the war ensured that most new soldier recruits hailed from villages and cities with minimal health services, while the chaos and disruption of the war itself often left them malnourished and overworked. Soldiers frequently began their military experience already in a poor physical state, and the deplorable conditions of recruitment camps and medical facilities both behind and at the front lines, coupled with the stressors of military life, ensured a low survival rate for the average NRA soldier. Soldiers suffered unduly from diseases, untreated wounds, poor sanitation, lack of clean drinking water, and insufficient food and clothing to such a degree that they themselves constituted an abused social group, asked to sacrifice their lives for the very state that failed to protect their bodies. Being a poor man of military age during the war considerably decreased one's life expectancy.

A handful of well-trained and dedicated medical professionals aligned their work against two formidable enemies: soldiers of the Imperial Japanese Army, and disease microbes. Nonetheless, their due diligence could not solve the underlying problem of deep ideological divides that made sympathy for soldiers appear morally and politically suspect to certain Nationalist authorities. The two most competent leaders in military medicine during the war came under suspicion of being Communist, and only one managed to avoid damage to her career. Most egregiously, Nationalist Party rightists got in the way of soldiers' lifesaving health services on the battlefields where they spilled their blood on behalf of a state that prioritized politics over human lives. While no one can prove that the Nationalist Party would have been more open to compromise had the war not pushed it to near extinction, there is ample evidence that the war escalated tensions both within the Nationalist Party and between it and the Communist Party. Over and over again, people who possessed a spirit of service, who willingly underwent personal privations in order to help others, who treated the poor as worthy human beings, were suspected of being Communists and persecuted. Those who made it to the top of the Nationalist Party power structure, with the dogmatic ideologue Chiang Kai-shek in charge, had no means of understanding such a commitment, feared its ardor, and treated its proponents like political enemies. Lim Kho Seng and Zhou Meiyu proved unstoppable, as did their institutions, but the rift between the Communists and the Nationalists continued to grow until it eventually tore the country apart. In a broader sense, the War of Resistance pushed both the Nationalist and Communist parties to the edge and exacerbated their mistrust of one another despite the renewed United Front agreement. It also gave members of each party a distinct experience of the war, in two very different regions of the country, that could be told as an exclusive narrative, and each has been told in this way for decades.[130]

One way to interpret the competing visions of military medicine is as two distinct "emotional communities." Historian of emotions Barbara Rosenwein created this concept to describe groups of people who may or may not share social communities such as neighborhoods, temples, and native place associations, but who do share normative values about the expression (or suppression) of certain emotions. Multiple emotional communities exist in any time and place, but people can move between different emotional communities only if they overlap significantly.[131] Interpreting rightist Nationalists' disdain for Communists and medical workers' insistence that Communists be given equal treatment as reflections of distinctive emotional communities suggests that China's civil war between the two parties had an important emotional component. The War of Resistance sponsored the creation of two ultimately incommensurable emotional communities. In the end, the fissure that tore the country in two appeared along a political *and emotional* fault line and drove members of the two communities to two distinct territories: mainland China and island Taiwan. Thinking in terms of emotional communities further shows just how deeply "nested" the War of Resistance and Civil War were within one another, since the process of the two communities moving apart began in the former but crystalized in the latter.[132] Viewed through the lens of the history of emotions, the gendered analysis of military medicine helps to explain why the Nationalists won the war against Japan but eventually lost to the Communists in a civil war during which entire battalions switched sides.

Necropolitics and the logic of war as organized injury help to explain the apparent contradiction in the fact that nurses' emotional labor to *save* the lives of soldiers was simultaneously a labor to *endanger* their lives yet again. While female medical workers challenged patriarchal gender norms that would have them stay indoors, they also extended the power of the patriarchal state by embodying its control of citizens' and soldiers' bodies. Because they worked during a war, female nurses were trained to employ their gender to shame men into performing their obligatory masculine role by returning to the terrifying battlefield to risk their lives once more in defense of the nation. Battlefield conditions and Japanese soldiers' ferocity suffice to explain why a healed soldier would resist returning to the front, but in the hands of Zhou Meiyu, China's military medicine system accounted for this reticence and mobilized women to police the men's gender performance through conformance to their own prescribed gender roles as gentle caretakers. Military nurses worked within a structure tightly defined by gender, but also exercised their own agency to bring death and destruction to the enemy. Female nurses proved so useful to the military that the Army Medical Administration stopped accepting male nursing students in 1947. Though the exigencies of the Civil War soon forced them to accept men who already had nursing training, the message was loud and clear.[133] Women had proven themselves of utmost utility to the masculinist state. The "Sick Woman of East Asia" had become her country's best healer.

4

Authority in the Halls of Science

Women of the Wards

Of course the material conditions [in the hospital where I worked] were very bitter; for example, I remember when two male volunteer orderlies worked for less than a day before they tried to run away, and when they were caught and brought back they spent the entire day crying in the hospital. This story illustrates just how hard the life was. Yet we women were willing to eat some bitterness for the war effort, and we've never cried or run away.

—ANONYMOUS FEMALE NURSE, NOVEMBER 1939

As the epigraph to this chapter suggests, women who entered the previously masculine spaces of the hospital and the battlefield worked hard to challenge expectations that they would fail and did so by calling attention to the ways in which they proved more capable than men. In openly speaking about this, as did this woman in a nurses' discussion group reported in the pages of the magazine *Funü shenghuo* (Women's lives), such women claimed authority not only over the bodies of the people they treated, but also over definitions of womanhood itself. Nursing "offered [women of] the new generation a route to emancipation."[1] Many of the women who volunteered to provide medical care for soldiers did so in part to escape arranged marriages and the control of their families.[2] Women who studied in state-run and missionary nursing schools lived in dormitories and gained professional skills that allowed them financial independence. This gave them the necessary autonomy to redefine women's role in public life, most explicitly in specific spaces of medical work: hospitals, clinics, and nursing schools. In these spaces infused with the authority of science, women expanded their own powers to heal and to make themselves anew. Through calling attention to the distinctive work that they did as healers who dared to look death in the eye and accept personal suffering in order to help others, these women claimed superiority over men whose courage faltered.

While the development of public and military health infrastructures gave women the *physical* space in which to perform new professions, restrictive social rules still prevailed. Women had to work within the patriarchal structure of the masculinist, necropolitical state. Previous chapters showed how this structure often worked to reify certain forms of femininity; this chapter analyzes the means that women employed to affirm their own rights and freedoms within this restrictive environment. The figure of the woman who used her power to heal bodies to support the state's power to kill and to build the relationships that comprised the national community did not just emerge whole cloth when the war changed social conditions. Actual women had to work very hard to change their own and others' perceptions of women's position in public life, in the nation, and in medicine in order to create and occupy this role.

The authority of science proved to be one of the most useful tools to expand cultural assumptions about what women could and should do. In China's encounter with western medicine—first as a distinctly foreign import in the early nineteenth century, then as an indigenized system of healing by the mid–twentieth century—scientific medicine "became symbolic of a shared striving towards the ideals of modernity."[3] Especially because Japanese pretense to medical superiority played a central role in Japan's imperial expansion, the translation of scientific medicine into China had tremendous significance for the country during the war.[4] It was also a matter of great consequence for women, for whom the growth of institutions of scientific medicine meant greater access to careers outside the home. The authority of science also helped women to challenge the cultural disdain for "manual operations" in medical care, rooted in the tradition of literate Chinese-medicine physicians who limited their physical contact with patients to pulse diagnosis and demonstrated their "skills in managing patients through words." In contrast, medical missionaries had distinguished themselves from this tradition and presented touch as a skill rooted in "the superior, advanced Western culture of medicine," not the "plebeian technique" as elite Chinese physicians would have it.[5] This granted women trained in mission institutions the ability to claim authority even though their close contact with patients' decaying, damaged, and putrid bodies could just as easily suggest otherwise. Yet merely occupying the spaces of scientific medicine—hospitals, clinics, laboratories, medical and nursing schools, and so on—did not automatically guarantee women respect therein, as the story of PUMC School of Nursing dean Vera Y. C. Nieh illustrates. Dean Nieh received steadfast support from her female colleagues, and interminable challenges to her authority from male colleagues.[6]

Most nurses assumed the normative gender role of the female caretaker, but also hitched their emotional labor to the creation of a national community as a means of escaping the alienation inherent to selling that labor. Just as with physical labor the worker can become alienated from the product of her labor, in emotional labor "the worker can become estranged or alienated from an aspect of self . . . that is *used* to do the work."[7] Even if the move were unconscious, the realization that they were producing something important for the whole country allowed at least some women to feel that their work mattered. In other words, even when they were paid low wages, worked near the bottom of a hierarchical profession, suffered through difficult working conditions, risked their reputations as "proper" women, and even risked their lives to help others, nurses got an emotional payback through asserting that their work had a high moral value. This, too, is encapsulated in the statement "We women were willing to eat some bitterness for the war effort, and we've never cried or run away." This nurse, who claimed to speak for her female coworkers, asserted that she and they had the necessary stamina and fortitude to perform lifesaving work that the nation desperately needed. In contradistinction to the assumption that women have less control over their emotions, these women performed the emotional labor of *not* crying even while working under extreme duress so as to demonstrate their fitness for the task.

Women also performed the emotional labor of making a new emotional community, which male leftist intellectuals, who decried their compatriots' inability to sever their emotional ties to their families in favor of the national family, failed to interpret as the potential backbone of patriotism.[8] The famous writer and mobilizer of volunteer military nurses Xie Bingying wrote in her memoir, "[W]e looked upon the battlefield as if it were our own home."[9] One of Xie's friends took to calling her "uncle," employing a gender-bending kinship term of endearment to manufacture a sense of home in the alien space of the front lines.[10] Zhou Meiyu likened the camaraderie within the Chinese Red Cross to the warmth of a family.[11] Yao Aihua recalled that the volunteer nurses she worked with during both the War of Resistance and the Civil War came from all over the country, but they all became close friends. Nurses and soldiers also crossed regional and ethnic differences in order to build trust with one another, and sometimes even behaved like kin. Yao Aihua got along very well with a group of wounded soldiers from Guangxi, in southern China. Even though they could not understand one another's dialects when they first met (Yao was from Hubei Province, in northern China), Yao tenderly changed the soldiers' dressings each day, and the soldiers took to playing with her son Fuxing while she worked.[12] Yao served as a surrogate mother/wife for lonely men who suffered the pain of being ill while away from home, and they in turn served as surrogate fathers to the young son of an overworked woman whose husband's unit was often stationed elsewhere. In a similar fashion, female military nurses in the American Civil War justified their public role on the battlefield by referring to the soldiers in kinship terms.[13] This phenomenon suggests that the making of a new form of womanhood rested in part on the construction of a new emotional community whose members employed the language of family to define themselves as a group adhering "to the same norms of emotional expression and value."[14]

Nurses also transformed local conceptions of the female gender through performing actions, in public and on behalf of the state, typically reserved for men. Even as military nurses described their work as innately feminine caregiving and fulfilled the heteronormative role of the seductress who manipulated men into returning to battle, their actual duties required performing tasks conceived as men's work. Nurses put themselves in the line of fire, rode on horseback into the battlefield, inured themselves to blood and gore, carried wounded soldiers on stretchers, worked endless hours with no rest, and developed emotional resistance to the constant strains of warfare.[15] Just as public health nurses in Chongqing regularly transgressed gender norms, working on the streets during vaccination drives and after air raids, female military nurses also occupied spaces of male sociality and learned to interpret this not so much as transgression, but as transformation. The ability of wartime nurses to invoke "a concept of the woman on other than normative terms" alerts us to the potential analytical limitations of the gender category as currently employed.[16] While female military nurses described their work as entering into the masculine space of army life, they also learned how to make it their own while celebrating rather than retreating from their female gender.

Words can deceive and obfuscate as surely as they can clarify. Women whose behavior simultaneously reified and transcended the heteronormative system of the war years defied language itself, forcing people to resort to linguistic play. Journalists, authors, and fellow colleagues described female doctors and military nurses as "manly" in order to convey what they felt about their behavior and bravery. Their semantic inventiveness exposed the gap between practice and prescription. Histories that include "women's own view of their worlds" demonstrate the ways in which, for centuries, Chinese women maneuvered around social limitations and arranged their lives to include unorthodox actions, even if speaking about them in orthodox terminology.[17] Chinese women's actions in war, often articulated in masculine terms, challenged the idea that femininity equated docility, helplessness, and passivity. Rather than wait for men to save them, these women went out of their way to save men. They donned soldiers' uniforms and worked day and night in blood-spattered hospital gowns.

These actions placed women in a new relationship to their gender identity, one in which they both accepted and challenged its strictures. It may therefore be possible to consider that the "historical site of [female] heterosexual subject formation" in wartime China was a "site of contestation . . . [of] binary analytics itself."[18] Women who took up the mantle of medical service during the war accepted that as women they had a distinct role to play, and even frequently defined it in gendered terms, but they rejected the idea that their femininity rendered their contributions any less important than or distinct from the fundamental goal of men: to serve the country. That the moment of stretching the boundaries of gender occurred in an era of heightened nationalism and militarism when most aspects of civilian life were hitched to the nation produced a flavor of modern womanhood quite specific to China. Questioning the applicability of the gender binary as currently applied in scholarship to the Chinese experience pushes analysis outside the dominant paradigms built by generations of scholars whose primary examples came from modern Europe, and even more specifically from modern France (scholars such as Simone de Beauvoir, Michel Foucault, Julia Kristeva, and Joan Wallach Scott). Such a move could inform an understanding of non-European gender systems on their own terms; call it a means of provincializing Europe in gender studies.[19]

For centuries, late imperial Chinese gender ideology characterized a stable empire as one in which "men plow and women weave" (*nangeng nüzhi*)—that is, both men and women performed productive labor that anchored family income year-round. Once women achieved access to institutionalized education in the early twentieth century and, as school graduates, developed specialized professions, they employed this logic to link their respective métiers to the urgent task of building the modern nation-state. They characterized social stability as the joint product of men's and women's productive work and asserted that women's domestic labors were neither confined to domestic space nor solely important to their own families.[20] As explained in the preceding two chapters, this expansion of the *physical* space and ideological significance of women's work predated the war and was furthered by it when the country experienced a sudden, dire need for medical workers that women were poised to fill. As they fulfilled their duties, these women expanded the *cultural* space of medicine to include women as authoritative figures within its ranks.

In so doing they both operated within and challenged the logic of the "Sick Woman of East Asia"—the idea that women's weakness was the primary source of national weakness, and therefore all work that empowered women both physically and socially should be done for the nation. Many women accepted that their work had national importance, but also insisted that it have personal value to them. Taken together, the rapid changes in women's professional opportunities and social perceptions of women in medicine set the stage for greater cultural change in the 1950s and 1960s. When peace finally returned to China, and the new Communist government had an ideological commitment to gender equality as well as an economic imperative to mobilize women for agricultural and industrial production, phenomena such as the "Iron Women" (*Tienü*) built upon the legacy that had begun in the making of the Republic and become a widely recognized norm during the War of Resistance: women working as equal partners with men to serve the nation.[21] Slogans about women "holding up half the sky" (*funü neng ding banbiantian*) and contributing to national reconstruction described not what the new government wished would come to pass, but what had already existed for decades. During the war, millions of civilians and soldiers received medical care from trained and competent women who bore the mark of their education and

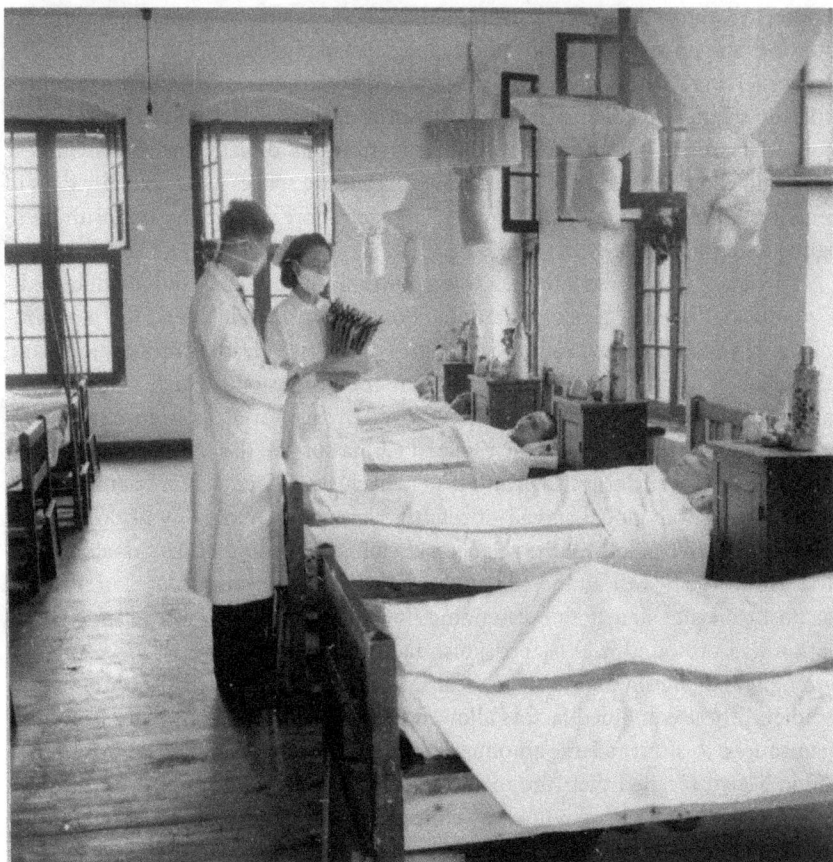

FIGURE 16. Doctor and nurse in a Chongqing Mission Hospital ward. The nurse's pristine white uniform, face mask, nurse's cap, and stack of patient records all indicate her status as a medical authority. 2000.017P/120 N, United Church of Canada Archives, Toronto, Ontario.

status as representatives of scientific medicine in their clothing, medical equipment, and posture.[22] (See figure 16.) In numerous encounters between patient and professional, Chinese people learned to recognize women as leaders in the spaces of scientific authority.

WOMEN AND SCIENTIFIC MEDICINE

Analysis of women's medical work during the war draws attention to a pivotal era in the history of indigenizing scientific medicine in China. Both the rise of the female nurse and the social phenomenon of the woman empowered with medical authority originated in the growing emphasis on scientific medicine during the war. Although women had long played key roles in medical care in China—chiefly in home-based care and midwifery—the most lucrative and socially prominent roles in Chinese medicine remained the near-exclusive domain of men.[23] Therefore, the growth of scientific-medicine institutions directly benefited Chinese women, who had been encouraged to work in these spaces from the early days of mission hospitals and during the war had even more reason and opportunity to study and practice scientific medicine.

Three factors spurred a tremendous growth in the influence of scientific medicine during the war: foreign charitable donations and volunteers, the predominance of Chinese with scientific-medicine education in leadership positions, and the labor of women, principally in the nursing profession—which both military and civilian medical organizations prioritized.[24] The War of Resistance inspired a global philanthropic network that helped China survive the war's predations, but also steered it ever closer to a health system exclusively founded on scientific medicine. During the global spread of total warfare, "the technology of destruction moved decisively ahead of the science of healing."[25] Medical professionals around the world watched thousands die and worked under a constant pressure to race against time and stanch a never-ending flow of blood. China, whose large population had profound health needs, also faced a formidable foe whose combined strength and determination struck fear into the hearts of all who encountered its soldiers. These combined factors allowed Chinese civilian and military health organizations to attract a large amount of foreign aid from many different countries. Zhou Meiyu recalled that "the medical supplies donated from overseas piled up like a mountain in our warehouse; we measured our quinine pills in tonnage."[26]

This aid could not have come at a better time. Just prior to the war the Nationalist state had expressed interest in developing a nationwide state medicine system, but the war threw the state into disarray and robbed it of a large amount of its tax income, curtailing plans that would have been lofty even in peacetime.[27] It fell to individuals working in a now skeletal health structure to carry the torch forward, and they faced crushing financial stress.[28] Luckily, they could call on foreign friends for help. In Nationalist-controlled areas the most active organizations included the Rockefeller Foundation's China Medical Board (CMB), the Chinese-American-founded American Bureau for Medical Aid to China (ABMAC), the American Red Cross (ARC), United China Relief (UCR, a conglomeration of seven American charitable organizations), the British United Aid to China Fund (BUAC), and the Friends Ambulance Unit (FAU). The China Defence League (CDL) and the China Aid Council (CAC) focused on Communist-controlled areas in North China.

This funding connected China to the world, largely through the networks of the Chinese diaspora. Prior to Japan's conquests in Southeast Asia, which blocked donations from overseas Chinese communities in the region, Chinese in Java supplied nearly the entire budget of the Chinese Red Cross (CRC). Dr. Lim Kho Seng then asked the American Red Cross to support his military medical services, responsible for the care of roughly three million soldiers at the time.[29] After this point the American Red Cross accounted for 70 percent of all foreign donations to the CRC.[30] The CRC used ambulances donated from India, Java, Sumatra, the Philippines, England, and the United States, the funds for most of which came from overseas Chinese fund-raising events.[31] In its five years of operation, the Friends Ambulance Unit China Convoy (*Gongyi jiuhudui* in Chinese) attracted two hundred foreign volunteers—hailing primarily from England but also the United States, Canada, New Zealand, and elsewhere—as well as sixty Chinese, mostly Christian students from WCUU.[32] In the Communist guerilla base in Yan'an, foreign volunteers including Drs. Norman Bethune (Bai Qiu'en), Shafick George Hatem (Ma Haide), Dwarkanath Shantaram Kotnis (Ke Dihua), Bang Wooyong (Fang Yuyong), Andrei Orlov (Aluofu), and Hans Müller (Mile) helped to build a military medicine system anchored by the Norman Bethune International Peace Hospital (IPH). Hailing from Canada, the United States, India, Korea, the Soviet Union, and Germany, this international group saved thousands of soldiers' and civilians' lives across North China.[33]

American dollars dominated. Over the course of the eight-year war, ABMAC gave nearly $10 million in medical aid and supplies to all the major institutions of both civilian and military health, while only 1 percent of total donations went to overhead.[34] Having originally aimed to raise $5 million, eventually UCR contributed more than $36 million in aid to China between its founding in early 1941 and late 1945. (This included over $70,000 from the personal fortune of Henry R. Luce, the publisher of *Time, Life,* and *Fortune* magazines.) Medical aid for both civilian and military organizations accounted for over $12.5 million of this sum. Though the bulk of UCR funds supported refugees and war orphans, by 1945 it had sponsored surgeries, hospitalizations, and other medical care for well over thirteen million soldiers and three million civilians.[35]

ABMAC, the sole organization founded by Chinese-Americans, funded virtually every medical project, civilian or military. For example, in 1941 ABMAC supported two first aid stations in Chongqing that serviced 120,000 air raid wounded; an NHA program that provided epidemic prevention services to over two million people; and the vaccine production plant of the Chinese Red Cross in Guiyang, which supplied cholera vaccine to ten million people—yielding an annual total of three million soldiers and well over twelve million civilians served.[36] ABMAC also created a penicillin project in late 1943 to develop penicillin within China as soon as facilities and supplies could be secured, sent many ambulances and automobile chassis into China, sponsored the evacuation of medical school faculty and students from occupied territories, and shipped medical textbooks and journals to schools taking refuge in the interior.[37]

ABMAC's gender politics reflected contemporary culture. As with other organizations, in its promotional materials women served to sanitize the violence from military medicine but could play that role only by embodying essentialist narratives. Figure 17 illustrates this very well. Only women appear in this promotional photograph created to advertise American medical donations to China and incite others to donate. Clearly instructed to smile either openly or subtly, the women all wear placid expressions that belie the bloodshed that the donation in fact represents: according to the photo's caption, these supplies will be smuggled at night across enemy lines into "Free China" and used to treat wounded soldiers, who will then return to killing. The two Chinese women legitimize the kindly American donation by sartorially representing their country in a dress—the modern, close-fitting adaptation of the high-necked Manchu *qipao*—notable for its attractiveness to "foreign friends" well into the 1950s.[38] The women were selected for their good looks and infantilized in the caption, which began, "Under the inquisitive eyes of two pretty Chinese *girls,* a group of nurses sort and catalog surgical instruments collected by the Medical and Surgical Relief Committee of America for rush shipment today from New York to Hong Kong."[39]

As noted below, ABMAC had progressive racial politics and accepted blood donations from African-Americans. It also included ethnic Chinese in its leadership structure. Yet even this racially integrated organization harbored Orientalists. Cofounder Dr. Frank Co Tui applied Hegelian notions of Oriental time to understand the country of his birth, writing in 1943:

> To understand the reason for China's technological backwardness, of which her medical backwardness is but one aspect, one has to remember that up to 1912 China was almost hermetically sealed to outside influences. . . . But while she remained in this stage of frozen culture, of "splendid isolation," the western world had experienced the industrial revolution and discovered scientific medicine.[40]

Falsely depicting Chinese culture as "frozen" in time and existing in "splendid isolation," Tui painted previous practices as thoroughly antimodern and antiscientific, and therefore denied their legitimacy so as to highlight his own role as heroic savior.

This illustration of the attitude of a hygienic modernist serves less to impugn the staff and volunteers of ABMAC than to illustrate the ardent love affair with science that gripped many health professionals in the war years. In the era of sulfa drugs and penicillin, many people engaged in saving lives had an unchallenged faith in scientific medicine. Many Chinese nationals applied the aid that they received from abroad to the project of promoting scientific medicine in their country. Indeed, they did much more than did or could foreigners to promote scientific medicine over and above indigenous medical practices.[41] According to ABMAC

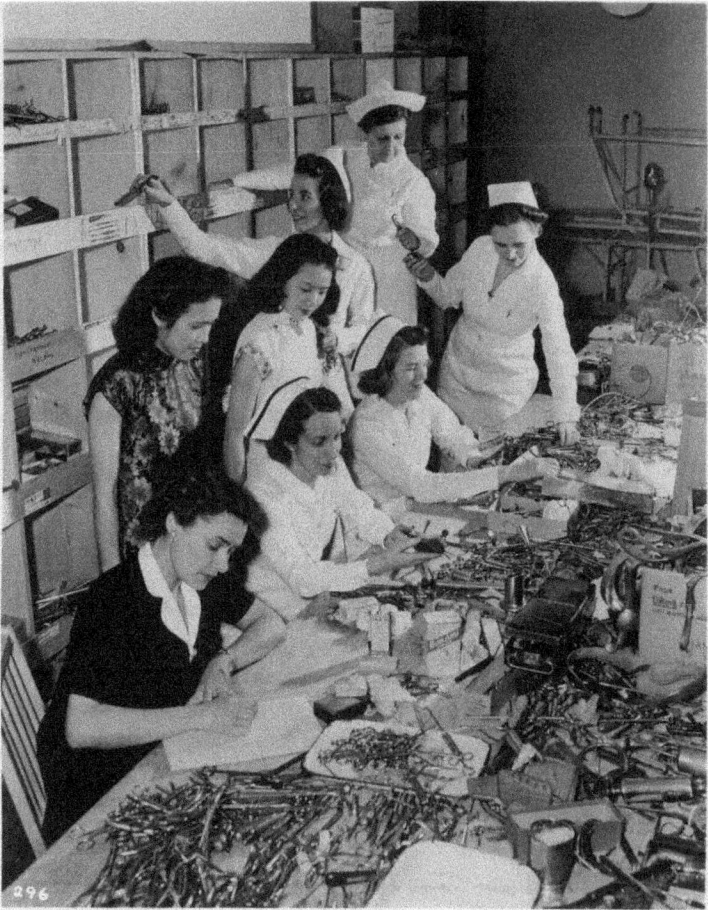

FIGURE 17. Six Caucasian women sort donated medical supplies for shipment to China while two Chinese women supervise. Dressed in *qipao*, they represent Chinese tradition, ca. 1938–1939. Box 85, folder "Surgical Relief Supplies." ABMAC Records. Rare Book and Manuscript Library. Columbia University.

president Dr. Donald Van Slyke, "complete and frank cooperation" characterized all dealings with China.[42] While foreign donations provided a crucial source of funding, it was the efforts of Chinese health workers that augmented the institutional and cultural power of scientific medicine and promoted its indigenization in China.

Among American donors, none had more power than the Rockefeller Foundation, whose total donations to China topped $44 million from 1914 to 1951, with nearly $33 million going to medical projects.[43] Much of this money supported the PUMC and the PUMC School of Nursing, whose graduates had the most power to spread scientific medicine. Virtually everyone who occupied a position of authority in wartime medicine and public health had either been trained at PUMC or served on its faculty.[44] Countless other graduates worked in health organizations in nonleadership positions. One alumnus estimated that roughly 80 percent of his fellow students went into public service or health education.[45]

The PUMC trained generations of Chinese who promoted scientific medicine in their own country as recipients of a benevolent imperialism. Indeed, "no other American institution's intellectual reach better exemplifies 'cultural imperialism' than that of the Rockefeller Foundation," which utilized "the ideologies of American science and medicine as a template" for its global philanthropy.[46] The Rockefeller patriarchs, from the ardent Baptist JDR Sr. through JDR III, all fashioned themselves as "missionaries of science."[47] In this role, the Rockefellers extended the influence of scientific medicine beyond missionary institutions and into secular life through an imposition of soft power, backed with millions of dollars. Their money disseminated the American model of nursing and public health around the world.[48] Within China, they had a deep impact on wartime Sichuan when a star PUMC graduate, Chen Zhiqian, served as director of the newly established Sichuan Provincial Health Administration (*Sichuan sheng weishengchu*) (SPHA) from May 1939 to November 1945. Headquartered in Chengdu, the SPHA gathered enough staff and money (principally from the Rockefellers) to establish county health centers (*xian weishengyuan*), based on the Dingxian model, in 131 of the province's 139 counties.[49] With this rate of activity, Sichuan alone accounted for nearly 19 percent of the total wartime growth in county health centers (from 242 centers countrywide to 938).[50]

Chinese students at PUMC had to adapt to multiple foreign cultures. Students who came from southern provinces had first to adapt to northern Chinese culture, including a distinctive cuisine and more-brusque mannerisms. Both Yang Wenda, from Jiangsu, and Chen Zhiqian, from Sichuan, had strong memories of this culture shock when they composed their memoirs many years later.[51] In the case of Lei Ting On, from Guangdong, he felt such pressure to conform to the intense nationalism of Beijing that he adopted the Mandarin pronunciation of his Cantonese name and became Li Ting'an for the rest of his life.[52] The use of English as the exclusive language of instruction and administration, coupled with the luxurious facilities, made PUMC feel like "a foreign country" to many students. It also made the school very elite; a 1935 survey revealed that every single PUMC student had come from a private university or mission college, since no others could pass the English-language portion of the entrance exam. Even then, roughly one-third of the students failed each year.[53] This new field of study—which included courses in anatomy, physiology, histology, biochemistry, and parasitology—not only constituted just one part of the foreign environment to which students had to adapt but was also the least shocking aspect of PUMC life for the students, who had deliberately chosen to study medicine. In other words, to these students, scientific medicine seemed less foreign than the English language used to describe it, the direct speech of northerners, the crisp new uniforms they wore each day of the week, and their two-person dorm rooms that were professionally cleaned each morning.

Having adapted to this environment, alumni of PUMC and mission colleges enjoyed two crucial assets: fluency in English, and the ability to develop personal relations with overseas funders. They signaled their cultural and linguistic competence by writing English-language letters in gorgeous calligraphy, signed with westernized sobriquets (such as P. Z. King, C. C. Chen, and C. K. Chu) or Anglicized names (such as Vera Nieh, Marion Yang, and James Yen; Yen had received a large personal donation from J. D. Rockefeller in 1928 after spending a week with the family in their summer home).[54] Other influential leaders such as Robert Lim (Lim Kho Seng) came from overseas Chinese communities and, as colonial subjects, spoke a non-Chinese tongue (in this case, English) as a native language; Lim had to brush up on Chinese in order to work in his ancestral homeland.[55] Once these individuals occupied positions of power within the Nationalist state, their comfort with foreign cultures became a crucial asset at a moment when China teetered on the brink of disaster.

This framework of mutual benefits contextualizes Chinese people's agency in their reception of the Rockefeller Foundation's cultural imperialism. With the conscious motive of using the medical technologies of the Western and Japanese imperial powers to resist these very nations' political and economic dominance, Chinese who indigenized biomedicine, as well as those who reformed Chinese medicine to conform to European scientific principles, carefully considered which aspects to accept, which to translate, and which to reject. As human beings they could believe in the therapeutic superiority of biomedicine, but as Chinese they could never forget its embeddedness in the cultures of white Western Europe and North America. Rather than adopt a "faith in science as the unmediated discovery of reality," Chinese adopters in this period knew that they must figure out how to effectively blend biomedicine with their own cultures of healing.[56] At the same time, all of the people involved in this project, both Chinese and foreign, deemed biomedicine a necessary component of modernity, public health, and political sovereignty. PUMC advisers wanted Chinese in positions of power, but they wanted those influential Chinese to eschew folk medicine practices in favor of biomedicine. This is somewhat ironic given that JDR Sr. himself preferred homeopathic to scientific medicine.[57] Nonetheless, PUMC graduates and their colleagues ultimately transformed scientific biomedicine into a central component of Chinese medical practice.

This transformation under conditions of war put high-quality education at the disposal of those who may never have had such an opportunity in peacetime. Yao Aihua, who at age sixteen had volunteered to serve soldiers on the front, had received only a single week of first aid training until her military hospital was stationed near the third Emergency Medical Service Training School (EMSTS) training center in northwestern Hubei. Despite the fact that the war had interrupted her middle school education, in 1943 she passed the EMSTS entrance exam, which trainers had repeatedly adjusted in order to accommodate students' low education levels.[58] Yao recalled that "because the principal of the school, Ma Ji [sic, Ma Jiaji], was a doctor from PUMC, and all the teachers were from PUMC, the quality of teaching was very high. The main class had over one hundred students."[59] Although Yao had the unique opportunity to learn from these faculty in her native language, she did not enjoy the luxurious PUMC facilities at its Beijing campus, but rather the inventive tactics with which people worked around the privations of war: "We had no desks or textbooks, but just took notes on our laps. The male students would go out to find corpses; we would cook off the flesh for our osteology classes. For clinical training we would study classic cases of wounded soldiers in the hospital."[60]

Nursing students in wartime Chongqing had access to better equipment. In 1937 the Canadian Mission Hospital Nursing School completed construction of a new, four-story building that could accommodate 120 nursing students, just in time for the spike in demand for its graduates. (See figure 21 later in the chapter.) Its students learned anatomy with the aid of posters displaying the anatomical body—the foundation of scientific biomedicine and a force for displacing "[t]raditional views of the body."[61] Anatomy and physiology occupied the greatest number of hours in the nursing curriculum—sixty classroom hours and sixty laboratory hours.[62] By the war years, Chinese women had come to occupy positions of power in settings legitimated by anatomical knowledge, and had therefore adopted a measure of its authority. As seen in figure 18, nursing students in the Canadian Mission Hospital Nursing School learned from Chinese women, not Canadians, and they all wore the white nurse's gown and hat that distinguished them from other women and marked them as possessing—or on their way to possessing—the authority of medical knowledge.

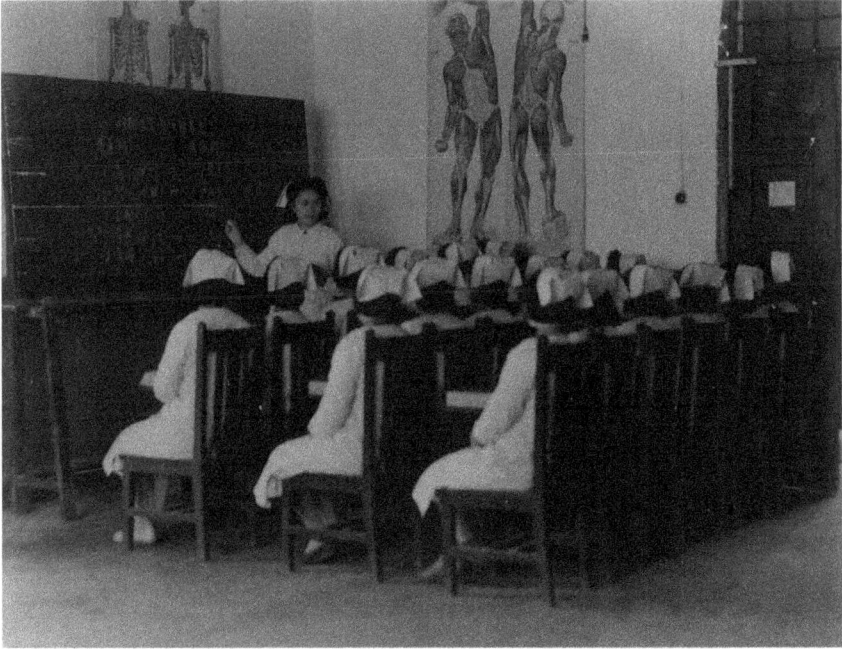

FIGURE 18. Classroom of the Chongqing Canadian Mission Hospital Nursing School, 1941. Box 77, folder "AMA no. 3." ABMAC Records. Rare Book and Manuscript Library. Columbia University.

Nursing students also studied chemistry, spending, in schools that followed the Nurses' Association of China (NAC) guidelines, twenty classroom hours studying the subject and forty hours in the laboratory.[63] (See figure 19). Other scientific subjects that the NAC required of nursing students included bacteriology and parasitology, *materia medica,* surgery, medicine, pathology, psychology, first aid, pediatrics, gynecology, obstetrics, nutritional sciences, communicable diseases, "mental nursing," physiotherapy, otolaryngology, advanced nursing arts, and public health nursing. Social studies rounded out the curriculum, with course work including nursing history and ethics, sociology, home economics, personal hygiene, Chinese, English, and citizenship. This curriculum, which combined the traditionally masculine subjects of laboratory sciences with the traditionally feminine subjects of social studies, reflected the way that nursing simultaneously reified traditional gender roles for women and granted them access to scientific authority. Yet nursing education was foremost a practical degree; the curriculum included over twenty-six hundred hours of clinical practice in the wards.[64]

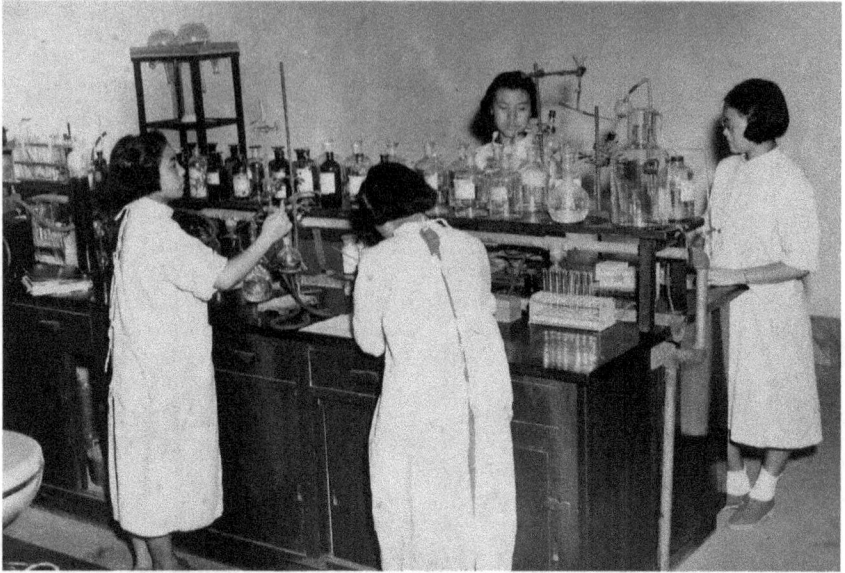

FIGURE 19. Nursing students studying chemistry. Box 83, folder "NHA and Nursing." ABMAC Records. Rare Book and Manuscript Library. Columbia University.

Clinical practice could also be an arena in which women occupied positions of authority, as seen in figure 20, a photograph of a woman demonstrating clinical techniques of bedside care in a classroom. With the exception of one male student, women occupy the front-row seats and appear to have equal status in this mixed-gender classroom. All of the students, male and female, are learning not only the content of the day's lesson but also to recognize women as medical authorities. The instructor employs the method of establishing her scientific authority that medical missionaries had created to propagate their teachings among women: the embodied knowledge of "concrete daily practice, [expressed] in observing, diagnosing, and treating patients."[65] The war helped to create such scenes of women in the spaces of scientific authority, not only by heightening the demand for their labor, but also by enhancing the social power of scientific medicine through increased availability of foreign funding and the movement of elite medical school graduates into wartime health institutions. Many people celebrated these accomplishments, not least the foreign missionary community that had first initiated embodied clinical practice as the foundation of women's medical expertise. A pamphlet promoting the work of West China Union University (a mission college in Chengdu) proclaimed, "[S]cience may be said to have permeated the world when it has become an integral part of higher learning in as remote a spot as Chengdu, Sichuan."[66]

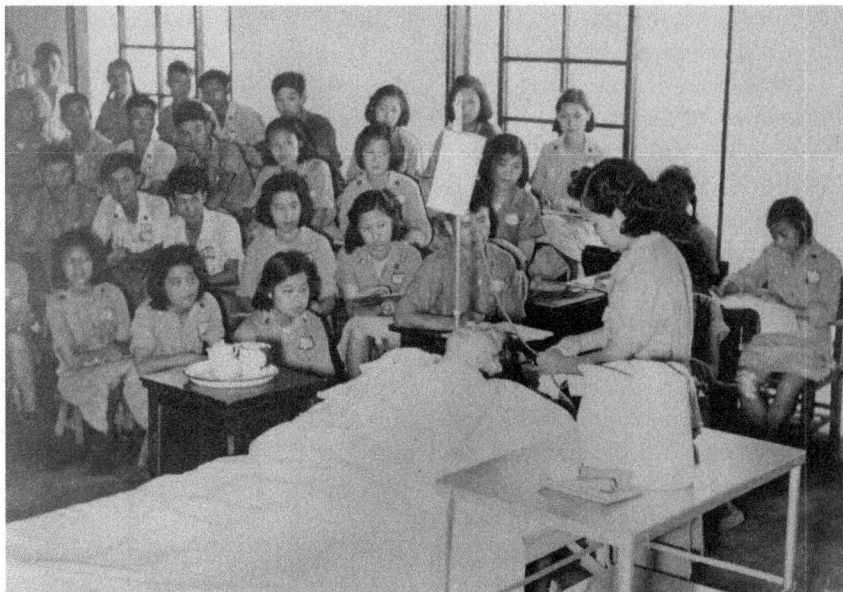

FIGURE 20. Woman demonstrating medical techniques to a mixed-gender classroom. Box 82, folder 2. ABMAC Records. Rare Book and Manuscript Library. Columbia University.

WOMEN AT THE FOREFRONT:
NURSES IN THE SICHUAN HOMELAND

One of the most challenging social norms that remained even after women gained access to nursing education was the idea that once a woman married, regardless of her level of education or previous career, she should stay at home to take care of the children and clean the house. In 1937, only 575 nurses were registered with the government, even though thousands had graduated from accredited nursing schools.[67] Though insufficient government registration certainly accounted for some of the discrepancy, the first major drop-off occurred when nursing school graduates faced pressure from their husbands and in-laws to become housewives and mothers rather than pursue a career in nursing. Even graduates of the country's best nursing school, the PUMC School of Nursing, faced tremendous pressure to abandon their professional ambitions. The school's dean, Nieh Yuchan, wrote a report claiming that the school's graduates not working professional jobs in the field were "rendering invaluable service in their homes, and are to be credited for the successes of their husbands." Nieh included a quote from one of the graduate's husbands to reinforce this claim—to wit: "I will always strongly support the PUMC Nursing School, because she produces good house-wives."[68] As further evidence that this attitude enjoyed cultural currency, it also emerged from the mouth of a hospitalized male character in Ba Jin's novel *Ward Four*.

As had been the case for Florence Nightingale during the Crimean War, for white nurses during the American Civil War, and for Japanese Red Cross nurses during Japan's early-twentieth-century wars in Asia, the War of Resistance gave Chinese women an opportunity to challenge the belief that nursing education found its best outlet in homemaking rather than in professional work.[69] The war therefore also gave women the *cultural* space in which to create a new definition of femininity. In a time of national emergency, this new womanhood hinged on national contributions as before, but now required that women perform physically strenuous and dangerous work in public spaces. No longer a mere extension of domestic duties and demure demeanor, nursing became a valiant and honorable means of contributing to the war effort. This shift occurred when many female nurses willingly accepted personal sacrifice and crafted a self-image centered on their ability to shoulder a *greater* burden than men in the same role, refusing to cry or "run away."[70]

The country in wartime required many more nurses than in peacetime. A 1942 report estimated the need for civilian public health nurses at twenty thousand and noted that the country had only twenty nursing schools capable of graduating more than one hundred nurses per year, suggesting an annual graduation rate of roughly one-tenth the actual need. Members of the NAC leadership committee, which included Zhou Meiyu, recommended the provision of scholarships that would cover "board, uniforms, books, and even pocket money" to increase the number of students.[71] Nursing schools in Chongqing worked to increase their capacity and establish agreements with nearby clinics and hospitals to secure clinical training spaces for a larger number of students. The concentration of refugees in the southwest gave them a much larger pool of potential students. At the same time, recognizing that China needed to increase its medical capacity, many missionaries renewed their commitment to putting Chinese staff in charge. By the war years, foreign staff constituted a decided minority in missionary institutions, and many Chinese occupied positions of authority. For example, by the end of the war in 1945 Chongqing's Canadian Mission Hospital (*Kuanren yiyuan*) had an entirely Chinese staff (see figure 21) supervised by a single Canadian working as superintendent and chief physician: Dr. Alexander Stewart Allen.

The transition to Chinese staff had a gendered component. Whereas foreign male doctors consistently complained in letters and reports to the mission board about their male Chinese colleagues' incompetence and unsuitability for leadership positions, foreign women generally celebrated their Chinese nursing colleagues' assumption of leadership roles and lauded their professional competence. Canadian missionary nurse Irene Harris wrote from Chongqing that, between returning from furlough in 1941 and 1943, "I have filled a more or less nonentity

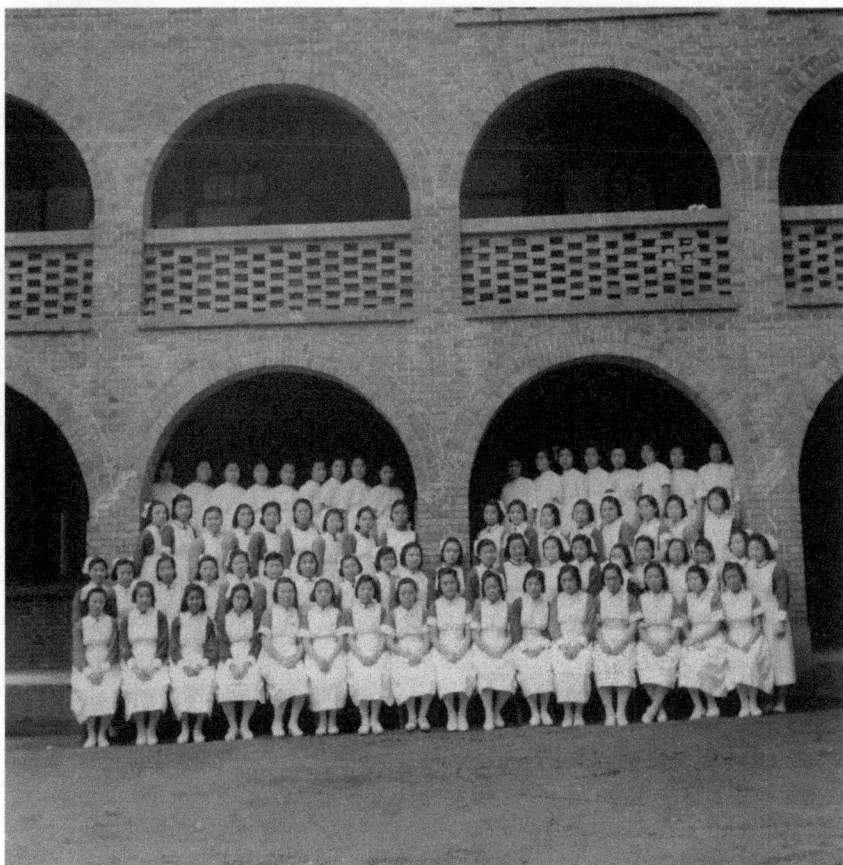

FIGURE 21. Chongqing Canadian Mission Hospital nursing staff, ca. 1930s. 2000.017P/96, United Church of Canada Archives, Toronto, Ontario.

position, the Chinese nurses having risen to the place where they can be heads of departments, Superintendent of Nurses, Principal, Dean of School of Nursing, etc., etc., and . . . I have simply filled in, acting in an advisory capacity, standing behind them, making suggestions but letting them carry through."[72] In October 1937 the Canadian Mission Hospital hired its first Chinese superintendent of nurses, Tang Chi Yuan.[73] In 1950, Gladys Cunningham wrote from Chengdu's West China Union University Women's Hospital:

> Later this month my senior Chinese colleague, Dr. Helen Yoh, will be back from London England. She will then assume Leadership of the Department. With another senior woman and two who will come back next year (all Sichuanese, I am glad to

say, so they will stay in this country) this department is in good shape. My work is really done. I can leave in peace. Not only for these am I thankful but for all OB-Gyn women all over this land, in whose training we have had a hand.[74]

A 1942–43 report from the China Inland Mission in Baoning, in northeastern Sichuan, stated that "the happy time has come when Chinese nurses are entirely responsible for that important department, the Operating Theatre."[75] All of these foreign nurses celebrated the creation of competence in their Chinese colleagues and eagerly handed control to them. By contrast, when Dr. Alexander Stuart Allen reviewed current medical facilities around the country in 1946, he wrote that one mission hospital in Changde, Hunan, had sufficient staff to open a nursing school "as soon as a missionary nurse arrives," evincing lack of confidence in Chinese leadership.[76] It makes little sense to assume that in every case male missionaries knew only incompetent Chinese medical workers, so it appears that women, unaccustomed to holding unchallenged authority, were more willing to share professional responsibilities with their Chinese colleagues.

Irene Harris's 1943 report also included a description of the work of then-current graduates of the Canadian Mission Hospital Nursing School that affirmed her opinion about her Chinese colleagues' abilities. Twenty-eight graduates served on the three-hundred-bed hospital's staff, and three were in charge of the nursing school. Three worked full-time in the mission's outpatient clinic in downtown Chongqing, including one woman who also took charge of home-based obstetrical care and childbirth. One of the graduates directed the health center for a local cement factory with three hundred employees. One had launched an entrepreneurial public health organization that employed student nurses to conduct immunizations in twenty-six firms as well as in two nearby schools with a combined total of twelve hundred students, for each of whom the nurses had also compiled complete physical examination and vaccination records.[77] Harris mentioned a total of thirty-eight nurses conducting their profession in industrial, educational, and medical facilities throughout the city as highly visible authorities.

These nurses did so much work partly because there was so much that needed doing. Hsu Ai-chu (A. C. Chu) (PUMC School of Nursing, class of 1930) keenly felt this need. Hsu had supervised public health nursing at PUMC's Beijing demonstration center before the war and in 1940 moved to Chongqing, where she became head of nursing at the National Institute of Health in Geleshan. In 1942 she became president of the Nurses' Association of China, and in that capacity established three new nursing schools—one each in Chongqing, Lanzhou, and Guiyang.[78] Like Zhou Meiyu, Hsu later led nursing work in postwar Taiwan.

This gave Chongqing four nursing schools: two mission establishments, one private school originally established by German physicians with cooperation from the German government in Shanghai, and the central government school. All of these schools worked to increase their student capacity and competed with one another for students. The four nursing schools in Chongqing had a minimum annual capacity of four hundred students. Posting successive ads in 1942 in the major local newspaper, the *Dagongbao,* they all solicited applications from young, unmarried women between the ages of seventeen and twenty-five who had a middle school education. The Canadian Mission Hospital Nursing School had openings for forty students; the National Central Hospital Nursing School also sought forty students; the American-run Methodist Union Hospital Nursing School sought twenty-five students; and the National Tongji Medical College Nursing School, which had moved from Shanghai in 1940, sought twenty students.[79] These schools jockeyed with one another for students; they ran their newspaper ads contiguously and sweetened their offerings. The National Central Hospital Nursing School in Geleshan, the sole government institution, offered discounted tuition for students who agreed to work for a state-run health organization after graduation. Not to be outdone, the American Methodists offered free tuition for the top five examinees in a test that covered the Chinese and English languages, mathematics, and a physical examination.[80]

With the near certainty of obtaining a job after graduation, and the promise of social approval for contributing to the nation in its time of need, young women had great incentive to attend nursing school during the war, particularly if they received financial assistance. On the other hand, they had no access to some of the more lucrative options. Only men between the ages of fifteen and twenty could apply to pharmacy schools, where they received a monthly stipend of 120 yuan in the first year of study, 160 yuan in the second, and a monthly salary of 200 yuan in their third year of apprenticeship, with promise of full employment and a salary increase upon completion. Moreover, pharmacy students did not have to remain unmarried, and had only to be free of "bad habits" (a euphemism for gambling, excessive drinking, using opium, and visiting prostitutes) in order to be eligible for the examination.[81] In other words, a male pharmacy student in Chongqing faced fewer bars to entry than an employed female nurse and received twice the pay, and a pharmacy apprentice received nearly six times the pay that Major General Zhou Meiyu received when she directed the entire nursing program of the Chinese Red Cross.[82]

Gender undoubtedly determined the hierarchy of the medical system. Women overwhelmingly occupied low-rank positions and received less pay than men and were expected not only to express deference to their senior male colleagues but also to view the inferior rank as their "natural" calling. Nursing schools looked for young, unmarried women who would not challenge authority. Likewise, young, unmarried, and obedient women much more readily accepted training in aseptic midwifery than did older midwives, who had long practiced their craft and gained some authority through their expertise.[83] Nursing nonetheless constituted a new career opportunity for most. Training in nursing school helped them to develop a professional identity in which they created feelings of solidarity with women from around the country; in 1943, fifty of the Canadian Mission Hospital Nursing School students hailed from other provinces.[84]

This growth in the nursing profession extended beyond Sichuan. In March 1944, the Nationalist government reported a count of 5,799 licensed nurses in Free China.[85] While this number does not necessarily imply an increase in trained nurses, it does illustrate an increase in government registration thereof—itself a clear indication of more nurses working in the profession. The NAC kept statistics on the number of nursing schools that operated in the occupied areas throughout the war, as well as the number of male and female students who graduated from these schools and passed the annual NAC exam. From 1937 to 1946, a total of 3,941 students passed the exam, thus becoming eligible to receive their degrees and licenses.[86] In the same time period, the number of licensed nurses across the country rose to 5,972.[87] Considering that all of the nursing schools that registered with the NAC had managed to train a grand total of 4,805 nurses from the time of the first school's opening in 1900 until the eve of the war in 1937, these numbers show a marked increase during the war, even though they do not include military nurses.[88]

These statistics illustrate another important aspect of wartime nursing: its transition from a mixed-gender to a solely feminine undertaking. Of the 3,941 passing students in occupied China, 3,506 were women and only 435 were men. Only four male students graduated from nursing school in 1945, and not a single one graduated in 1946.[89] In 1947, the Army Medical Administration ceased accepting male nursing students altogether.[90] Nursing had become an entirely female profession, primarily because of changes taking place in military nursing.

WOMEN AT THE BATTLEFRONT: NURSING THE MILITARY

Women's work to challenge gender norms did not end once they entered the battlefield. The transformation of femininity required that women not only perform their gender differently, but also believe new things about themselves, their abilities, and what constituted "appropriate" behavior for a woman. The new settings in which women found themselves in wartime allowed this dramatic shift to take place in a short period of time. Xie Bingying articulated just such a rapid transformation in her description of working at the front with fellow volunteer military nurses:

> At first we felt very uncomfortable when our hands were stained with blood, so we washed whenever it was time to eat. Later, with the blood of more and more injured soldiers dripping on our shoes and our clothes, and smeared all over our hands, we not only were unafraid of blood but *regarded it as a badge of honor.* Sometimes in

slapdash fashion we used only a little cotton soaked in alcohol to wipe our blood-dripping hands before we held up our rice bowls to eat.[91]

Taking pride in rather than shrinking from hardship emerged as a central feature in many memoirs and oral histories of female nurses. Willing to wear white nursing gowns (the color of mourning garments), work outside the home, and touch the bloody bodies of unknown men, Chinese nurses bravely executed a triple transgression of gender, class, and station. War produced the circumstances that allowed them to defy social norms and seek the extraordinary.

Judith Butler theorizes that gender is not a concrete reality but the product of re-iterative social performance. It can therefore be rewritten and reinvented through performance of new modes of being, as Xie Bingying and her comrades showed.[92] Women who thus redefined femininity during the war had many models to draw on. They may have read fictional stories that began to circulate in the late 1920s coupling revolution with romance and articulating a new heroine, "the modern *ernü yingxiong*" or "heroic daughter," who grounded her revolutionary spirit in a passionately expressed love.[93] Wartime drama troupes delighted audiences with reenactments of the story of Hua Mulan, who had joined the military on behalf of her father.[94] The close friends of famous anarchist Qiu Jin, who had been beheaded in 1907 for her plot to assassinate the Qing emperor, were busy memorializing her within the tradition of the female knight-errant (*xianü*).[95] Shi Jianqiao, who had famously killed a man in 1935 to avenge her father's murder, also led a highly publicized campaign to raise money to purchase three airplanes for the Nationalist military at a time when "public patriotism was gendered feminine."[96] Women in medicine, through repeatedly acting with confidence and assuming authority over their patients both male and female, crafted a new womanhood that the conditions of war made possible and their collective actions solidified. All performance requires an audience, and witnesses to this drama did not always accept it as fact, but many women fought back.

Perhaps the need to engage in this battle for recognition explains the rather dramatic format of Xie's autobiography. Her tone underscores the degree to which embodying the wartime version of "new womanhood" entailed the self-conscious formation of a new personality. Her story also suggests that, to a certain extent, performing new womanhood at the front required adherence to the rules of an equally constructed and circumscribed manhood. According to Xie, she and her fellow volunteer nurses cemented their performance by "sacrific[ing] individual freedoms and submitt[ing] [them]selves to strict military regulations, written in iron:

1. Sacrifice all; fight to the finish.
2. Work with dedication and energy.
3. Live and die with our soldiers, sharing their sweetness and pain."[97]

Although Xie's words may seem melodramatic, nurses did indeed live and die with soldiers. Chinese military nurses often served close to the battlefront and followed troops as they moved. They suffered through many of the same conditions that soldiers faced, including overwork, malnutrition, poor living conditions, disease, and even death. Government statistics counted over 320,000 military medical professionals who lost life or limb during their wartime service.[98] In this regard their experience was quite distinct from that of Japanese Red Cross nurses, who worked on ships stationed in safe harbors and at home-front hospitals during the Russo-Japanese War, but very similar to that of Russian military nurses of World War I, who also moved with the troops and worked at the front lines. They "experienced extreme cold, constant fatigue, contagious diseases, artillery fire, and aerial bombardment. They encountered death and destruction in the closest possible proximity."[99]

Women and girls constituted the majority of volunteer nurses heading to the front, but they also participated in the military in a variety of roles, some of which entailed even greater risk than nursing.[100] Some women answered the call to wield weapons on the battlefield. In August 1939 *Funü shenghuo* reported women from two counties in Sichuan asking to serve in the military, stating that the women of Anyue County "all believe that the men who go to fight are heroes, so they wrote a letter to the Military Affairs Commission asking that women be allowed to fight."[101] Another article in the same issue introduced a whole group of female soldiers who managed to join the front in the north, even though the man in charge rejected their first request to serve, stating that "it is not fitting for women to do this work" because, as he claimed, all the other soldiers were men and life at the front was dangerous and difficult. The women responded, "[O]ur nation is in peril, and you say that women have nothing to contribute. When you say that women cannot eat bitterness or undertake hard work, that we grasp at life and fear death, that is a direct insult to women!"[102] They also called his revolutionary fervor into question, claiming that he had a retrograde attitude that made him unworthy of counting himself a twentieth-century youth. Here they demonstrated their more powerful connection to the legacy of early Republican activism, during which "[m]odern-minded Chinese were coming to expect that women, like men, would be physically more active, assertive, and even vulgar in the role of citizen."[103]

Eventually the women prevailed. They joined the military and over a period of twenty months attracted more than eighty women to their troop. They reported that their commanders "frequently make an example of the female soldiers' work ethic and diligence in their speeches to the [male] soldiers."[104] The (presumably male) commanders' treatment of the female soldiers as exemplars illustrates two types of emotional work at play. On the one hand, in hearing their leaders' praise, the women learned to see themselves as not only capable of being soldiers (which they likely already knew or they would not have joined the military), but capable of being *better* soldiers than men—the presumed standard of soldierly conduct. This entailed an expansion of what it meant to be a woman, what the performance of womanhood could include. On the other hand, it is likely that the commanders highlighted the women's successful adaptation to military life so as to shame the men into improving their own performance lest a woman become a better soldier than they, and the men may indeed have responded to this manipulation.

The women in this troop exhibited what female soldiers who commanded male battalions, served as fighter pilots, and gunned down enemy aircraft for the Soviet Union's Red Army described as legitimate modes of womanhood.[105] Although they met with staunch resistance before receiving support, the fact that they invented identities for themselves as women fighting at the front suggests that they did not subscribe to the traditional gender imaginary of war that posits women as the protected and men as the protectors. The War of Resistance placed women in positions traditionally reserved for men well before the Communist state mobilized women into such roles.[106] This in turn indicates that military "states of exception" create social states of exception that invite the creation of new gender identities. Their story provides one example of how wartime womanhood was performed and observed during the War of Resistance, as women built on the legacy of women's activism in the early Republic.

Not all women who wished to join the battle met with success, however. After proving herself capable of surmounting tremendous hardship in military medical service, Yao Aihua expressed her desire to follow her close family friend to the front. He responded with a pedantic speech about how she, a girl, could not withstand battle and must stay behind the lines to heal wounded soldiers.[107] Since this man had social standing within her own family, Yao did not feel comfortable defying him, and reluctantly accepted his advice. This points to a further reason that war creates opportunities for women to occupy new social roles: the dislocation that it causes places women in contact with men outside their own social circles, whose command they can more readily defy.

Women also had to defy ideas about womanhood that they had internalized over a lifetime of social programing. A photograph taken of female orderlies assisting wounded soldiers at the front in Changsha may display the result of a lost battle against internalized sexism. (See figure 22.) Neither of the two women in this photo has adopted a bodily position that would allow her to accept any of the physical weight of the two wounded soldiers. The woman closest to the viewer even appears to be resting her arm *on* that of the soldier, who in turn rests his weight on a walking stick rather than on the female orderly, while the pained expression on his face suggests that he needs more assistance than the stick can provide. This is understandable given the fact that he appears to bear nearly the entire weight of the other wounded soldier, whose arm is slung around his neck. The two women flanking the soldiers carry the distinctive leather satchels of medical

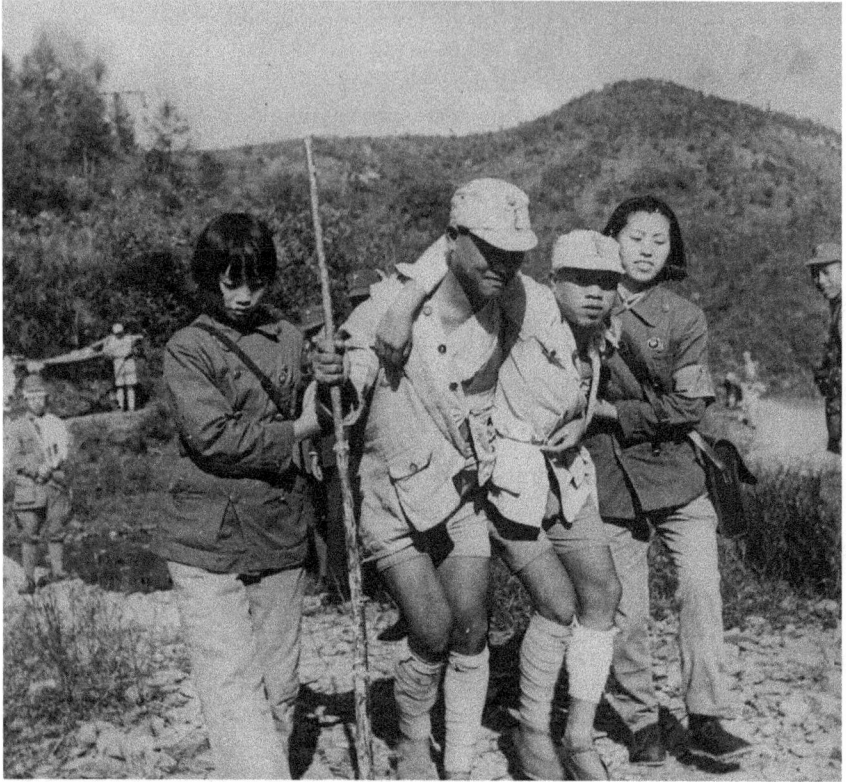

FIGURE 22. Female orderlies assist wounded soldiers in Changsha. Box 77, folder "AMA no. 3." ABMAC Records. Rare Book and Manuscript Library. Columbia University.

orderlies—from which they may have procured the white bandages that now wrap the soldiers' wounds—but in the moment captured here, they do little to help. Several clues that would aid the interpretation of this snapshot are missing. Behind this scene one can see two men carrying a stretcher; did all the soldiers ridicule the women when they said they wanted to carry the stretcher? On the far right, an able-bodied soldier observes in bemusement; is he inwardly laughing at the idea of women helping men, or of men needing the help of women? The woman on the right wears a slight Mona Lisa smile, while her partner looks down and away from the camera; what are the two women feeling in this moment? Humiliation after hearing several taunts from the soldiers? Frustration that they cannot actually perform the work they wish to do? They appear to struggle with something other than the weight of the soldiers, but the photograph does not reveal their secrets.

Many other sources do affirm the persistence of assumptions of female weakness and incompetence. Despite the fact that both men and women contributed to

the war, and all contributions required the acceptance of hardship, personal sacrifice, and the threat of death, many people perceived women as less capable than
men to shoulder the burdens of military life. Therefore, female nurses frequently
advertised their hardiness and courage. One nurse at the 1939 meeting in Chongqing told the following story:

> Our medical team includes both men and women, and at first the men would often
> secretly whisper to each other about the working ability of the women, even to the
> point of looking down on us. In response we women drew closer together, and our
> combined power increased our working capacity such that our work is now equal
> to that of the men, even including heavy tasks, such as stretcher bearing, that we
> frequently do. Whenever a woman loses her grip, we exhort her even more. *In less
> than a month we women were exceeding the men in our work,* and their disregard for
> us disappeared.[108]

This story reveals some details of the process that women had to go through in
order to prove their mettle. First, they "drew close together" so as to gain strength
from each other while they faced the men's whispered remarks. Then they developed a strong sense of teamwork and exhorted one another to work harder. In this
case, the women reportedly gained respect in "less than a month," though one can
easily imagine that other instances required more time and effort. Nonetheless,
even if the nurse quoted here exaggerated her story so as to trumpet her and her
coworkers' abilities, that very hyperbole suggests that women took pride in their
ability to perform womanhood in new ways, and men occasionally responded
with newfound respect. Yet they adopted male behavior as the standard against
which they measured themselves, even as they invented clever ways of working
together and offering moral support to one another.

The assumption of male behavior as the standard in military endeavors sometimes led to confusion about how to read the attributes of actual women at work in
military nursing. In recalling one of her trainees, Zhou Meiyu said:

> To this day I still remember a young woman student named Chang Gexin who was
> hearty and heroic, with *a rather manly spirit* [*poyou nanzi feng*]. One time, her com-
> pany was routing out the Japanese. She rode one horse and trailed two others behind
> her to carry all the medical supplies and surrounded the Japanese; when the Japanese
> came from one side, she ran to that side. She spent two days and two nights doing
> this before she was finally able to safely deliver all of the medical supplies to her
> company. She was very capable.[109]

Clearly, Chang's ability to ride horseback in a war zone did not strip her of her female identity, but her commander, Zhou Meiyu, despite herself being one of the
only women to attain the position of major general within the National Revolutionary Army, described her actions first as "manly," and only then as "capable."[110]

Zhou did not lack proper words for Chang. One early-twentieth-century
feminist activist had invented the term *yingci*—combining the first character in

the masculine term "hero" (*yingxiong*) with the word used for female birds and animals (*ci*)—as a Chinese translation of "heroine."[111] *Yingci* might have quickly fallen out of favor, but the country that had produced the famous story of Hua Mulan possessed a specific expression to describe "women who fulfilled their obligations to their ruler or kin with remarkable deeds in warfare": *jinguo yingxiong* ("hero in a head kerchief").[112] The twentieth-century version interpreted "kin" more broadly, as all members of the "nation-family" (*guojia*). Sun Yat-sen used it in 1912 to honor Qiu Jin as a revolutionary martyr, and a reporter used it in the 1940s to describe the female members of Yao Aihua's volunteer medical corps.[113] Its new usage therefore typifies what chapter 2 theorized as "the romance of the nation"—individual men and women embodying heteronormative gender roles so as to support one another in supporting the nation's ability to kill its enemies. In this context, a woman who suppressed her desire for individual freedom so as to serve the nation could believe that "all her submission and sacrifice acquired new significance."[114]

Nonetheless, by calling attention to a certain type of headdress worn only by women (*jinguo*), the term "*jinguo yingxiong*" distinguishes a woman's actions on a battlefield as distinct from those of men. Neither Qiu Jin nor the military medics could be "heroes" without a gender signifier. Female military nurses had first to outperform their male comrades in order to attain respect. The way in which Zhou understood and narrated the work of the nurses she trained reveals how profoundly her own gendered experience affected her ability to interpret her and her coworkers' reality. Her experience as commander and trainer of military nurses did not suffice to erase her subjectivity as a woman in a patriarchal society, and her choice of words exhibited the limitations that she had learned to place on the female sex. She had learned to believe that the behavior of a "she" must always be gentle and timid, and if otherwise, that the "she" is akin to a "he." Analysis of the language that people used to describe brave and assertive female medical professionals during the war informs a history "that takes the emergence of concepts and identities as historical events in need of explanation." This type of history "insist[s] . . . on the productive quality of discourse"—on the fact that people cannot think outside of the language they have, even if they can (occasionally) act outside of its bounds.[115]

This analysis also points to the fact that women who lived into new ways of performing womanhood spurred such rapid change that it took language a while to catch up with the new social reality. By the time the Communist state created the category of "Iron Women" in the 1960s, the women who defied gender norms to enter traditionally male occupations had long existed, but now they had commonly accepted language with which to describe themselves. Women like Dr. Helena Wong (Huang Ruozhen), pictured in figure 23, had already worked in spaces previously reserved for men alone.

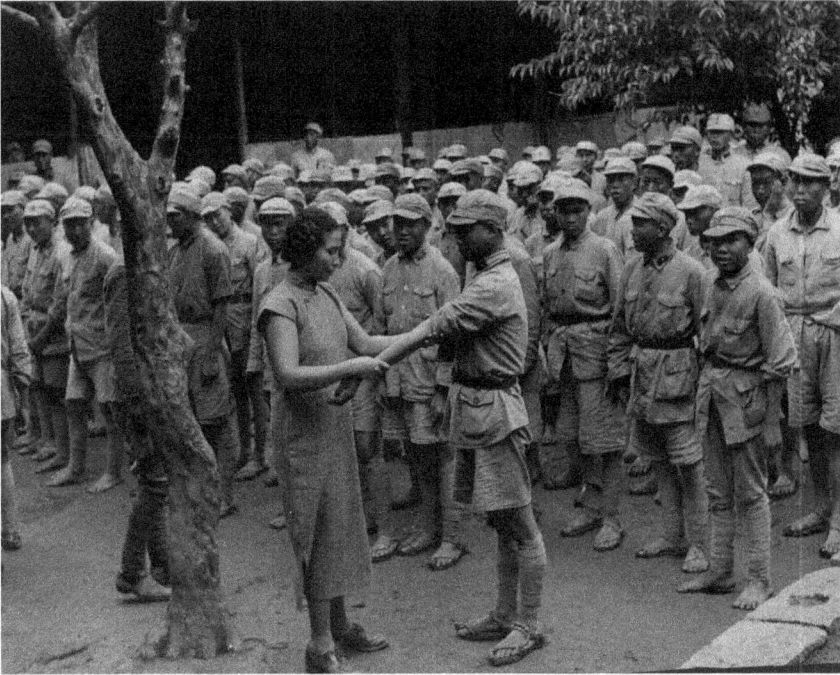

FIGURE 23. Dr. Helena Wong examines soldiers for blood donation, ca. 1944–45. Box 78, folder "Chinese Blood Bank B51–90." ABMAC Records. Rare Book and Manuscript Library. Columbia University.

Dressed in civilian clothes, Dr. Wong stands apart from the soldiers even as she is fully among them. Her permed hair, patent-leather shoes, stockings, and well-fitted *qipao* signal her middle-class status, while the soldiers wear homemade sandals of coarse grass, and some are entirely barefoot. She works on behalf of the ABMAC blood bank established in 1943 to provide fresh blood to wounded soldiers in the field and thereby increase survival rates. Though they first collected blood in New York City's Chinatown (and, unlike the American Red Cross, accepted donations from African-Americans), shipping fresh blood into China proved difficult. Dr. Wong played a key role in relocating the bank to Kunming, Yunnan Province, where it opened in July 1944 with the aim of taking donations from the eventual recipients: Chinese soldiers.[116] The plan looked good on paper, but additional problems arose. Some soldiers and officers believed that blood donation would lead to a loss of physical vitality. Even when commanding officers forced them to participate, so many soldiers could not donate because of poor health (due to malaria, fever, or malnutrition) that some men deemed the whole exercise useless and did not show up even when ordered to do so. Some officers encouraged their men to resist the blood bank personnel. One of the only reliable means of encouraging soldiers to donate blood was to give them nutrition in return: soy milk or an egg. Figure 23 shows Dr. Wong looking for the visible, plump veins of a healthy prospective donor. She has authority not only because their commanding officer lends her some of his by standing close by (just behind the tree), or because of her clear distinction as a middle-class woman, but also because she is the hungry soldiers' ticket to a healthy snack.[117]

Dr. Helena Wong wrote about her experience working in the blood bank in September 1944, providing a rare opportunity to interpret her potential emotional state in this photograph. Her comments affirm that the entire project was marred not only by the poor physical condition of the would-be donors, but also by poor communication between the educated health workers and the uneducated soldiers, many of whom did not understand the reason for storing blood in a bank. One of them asked Dr. Wong directly, "Why keep it in a bottle? Why not just leave it here?"[118] Presumably no one told the soldiers that effective use of the blood bank reduced the death rate to nearly 1 percent in a September 1944 battle in Yunnan, by which time the reputation of fresh plasma "was so great among the Chinese soldiers at the front that the wounded begged for it on arrival at the surgical unit."[119] Dr. Wong's comments, written about her work to collect blood donations in the same month, September 1944, suggest that she herself felt deeply ambivalent about the need to collect blood from young men barely strong enough to perform their military duty. She wrote:

> It takes a certain amount of blind insensitive stubbornness to take blood from these soldiers. It is a sad business; however, I feel we are justified and right because the plasma goes back to them, and the ones that give can afford the amount we take from them. What hurts is that these soldiers are expecting to go to the front soon.[120]

Dr. Wong, distinguished by the privilege of education and material comfort in an impoverished society, believed that she had to exhibit "blind insensitive stubbornness" in order to leverage that privilege for this particular task. Perhaps out of discomfort with this assertion, she immediately justified the work on the grounds of its (quite truthful) ability to save lives, demonstrating her desire to focus on the positive outcome rather than the problematic means of achieving it. She then returned to "what hurts" and evinced sympathy for the soldiers who would soon face a formidable foe. These comments suggest that, at least in that moment, Dr. Wong felt sympathy for the soldiers and recognized that she had to work within a system marred by deep inequality. She certainly would not have used the word "necropolitics," but she did understand that the same society that mobilized her to use her medical training to support organized killing—to keep soldiers alive so that they might kill more enemy soldiers—was the same society that placed young, barefoot, and malnourished men in the line of fire. Though clearly motivated to help her fellow countrymen, at least for a fleeting moment she recognized it as "a sad business," and this recognition caused her emotional pain.

NEW POSITIONS AND OLD EXPECTATIONS: DEAN NIEH AND THE PUMC SCHOOL OF NURSING

The wartime career of Nieh Yuchan (Vera Y. C. Nieh, 1903–98), head of the relocated PUMC School of Nursing and its first Chinese dean, illustrates the limits of the authority of science in helping professional women challenge gender norms. Wartime gender ideology that defined caretaking as a woman's chief role in both her own family and the national family demanded that women contribute to the nation without challenging patriarchy. Despite undeniable gains, women still experienced definitive limits to their professional mobility. Notwithstanding the exception of women like Major General Zhou Meiyu, wartime society placed strict limits on women's professional lives in order to lay claim to female labor while still preserving male claims to positions of authority.

Dean Nieh dealt with a stunning degree of sexism despite her high position and impressive qualifications. In addition to her PUMC School of Nursing degree (class of 1926), she had degrees from Columbia University's Barnard College, the University of Toronto, and the University of Michigan. Prior to her tenure as assistant dean (1938–40) and then dean (1940–46) of the PUMC School of Nursing, Nieh had spent three years as instructor and director of Public Health Nursing at the Beiping First Health Station (1931–33), and had served as secretary of Communication on Nursing Education in the Ministry of Education (1934–35).[121] A woman with such training and experience had much to offer her country. Upon Nieh's first appointment as assistant dean, in 1939, Henry S. Houghton, then president of the China Medical Board, described her as "a highly intelligent woman" with "excellent family and connections" and the "undivided support and good will" of the PUMC School of Nursing alumni.[122] However, the man who assumed leadership of the China Medical Board in January 1943, Claude E. Forkner, felt differently about her.

When the PUMC School of Nursing alumni and administrators met in December 1942, one year after the Japanese Army had occupied their school, they decided that the nation's need for nurses was so great that they would sacrifice their own safety and comfort and move the school to Sichuan. Dean Nieh personally led her faculty and students across enemy lines. Meanwhile, PUMC medical faculty declined to move, and their school remained under Japanese occupation until victory. In September 1943, after much strife in Chongqing, the PUMC School of Nursing finally opened in its third and final wartime location, on the campus of the West China Union University (WCUU) in Chengdu, which had already welcomed Cheeloo (Qilu) Medical College of Shandong Christian University, Yanjing University, Ginling Women's College, and Nanjing University. Simultaneously, twenty-four PUMC medical students matriculated at the WCUU Medical College; ultimately the school trained four classes of undergraduate and one class of postgraduate students during the war. To facilitate clinical training, Dean Nieh became superintendent of nursing services at University Hospital clinics outside of Chengdu, and the school helped WCUU build a new hospital for its clinical training.[123]

Despite her lofty titles, the administration failed to provide Dean Nieh with adequate support from the beginning. The PUMC initially provided no money for the relocated school's operation; the women ran the school for three months without pay or any guarantee thereof. Having initially operated only the OB-GYN ward, the Wartime Advisory Committee did set a date for the opening of the medical ward but changed it at the last minute without notifying Dean Nieh, who had prepared and accompanied all of the staff to the site only to find the door locked.[124]

After this inauspicious beginning, Dean Nieh and Director Forkner immediately entered into conflict. In February 1944, Claude Forkner sent complaints to Dean Nieh and to Y. T. Tsur (Zhou Yichun), a member of the PUMC Board of Trustees and chairman of the Nursing School Advisory Committee, calling the dean "out of order," "insubordinate," and "emotionally unstable."[125] Dean Nieh defended herself; the very next day she cabled a brief message to Chairman Lobenstine of the CMB: "Forkner is great hindrance to nursing school. . . . [S]chool must have budget."[126] She repeatedly asked for the authority and title of principal (xiaozhang) rather than dean, as the (temporary) closure of the PUMC had erased the administrative structure that would have made operation as dean of its nursing school smooth and efficient. She asserted that if she had more autonomy she could more easily complete all of her tasks. She also repeatedly expressed that nurses, not doctors, should be in undisputed charge of the nursing school.[127] Since the PUMC administration consistently ignored her requests for a change in title, she began acting as principal without official permission; she ceased delivering financial and other reports, began speaking directly to those above her within the CMB administration rather than going through their subordinates, and continually resisted Director Forkner's attempts to control her.[128] Forkner concluded that she should be fired and began asking his Chinese colleagues for recommendations of people who might replace her.[129]

Men described Nieh Yuchan as demanding and stubborn, with a bad temper. They also suggested that the war produced a strain she could not handle, rather than admitting that her employment situation might be strain enough. For example, one man suggested that Nieh be replaced and wrote in a letter, "If I may be allowed to say so I am afraid she really needs some psychiatric attention."[130]

Claude Forkner also called her "emotionally unstable" and fit for replacement.[131] The overseas Cantonese doctor Li Ting'an (1899–1948) wrote in a confidential letter:

> There is no doubt that her temperament is bad. This I think is due to her physiological and family conditions which may be improved in a few years. Miss Nieh is capable and honest, and knows her job. It hurts me to state that she is handicapped in the art of dealing with people. I can quite see the reason for the reaction which Dr. Forkner is forced to take at times. I wish Miss Nieh can [sic] be more cooperative and patient.[132]

Dr. Li suggested that Nieh's status as a single woman unpenetrated by a male phallus made her "handicapped in the art of dealing with people." His desire for her to be "more cooperative and patient" indicates that he expected certain behavior from her due to her sex, and therefore could not appreciate her assertiveness as a highly educated woman with an ambition to professionalize nursing and protect it from the meddling of male physicians. Li suggested hiring Zhou Meiyu as Nieh's replacement.

In marked contrast to Dr. Li and his male colleagues, the women who worked with Dean Nieh interpreted their supervisor's assertiveness positively and did not see her status as a single woman—her "family condition"—as a hindrance to her professional aptitude. On March 20, 1944, the faculty of the PUMC School of Nursing wrote a letter in full support of their dean, citing all of the same frustrations that Nieh had been dealing with for months without response.[133] One week later, the all-male Wartime Advisory Committee expressed its full support of Director Forkner.[134] Since the male China Medical Board administrators failed to address Dean Nieh's primary demand for administrative autonomy, several alumnae and nursing school administrators wrote again on May 3, 1944, asserting that the committee members had a marked "lack of confidence in the Dean of the School" and politely requesting a change in attitude. To wit:

> We see no justification for such deviation from established practice by depriving the Dean of the authority and responsibilities that were hers when the School was in Beiping [Beijing]. We wish therefore to suggest that during the present emergency the Dean be given complete charge of the administration of the School. . . . We beg to assure you, Sir, that in our humble opinion we can find no better qualified person than Miss Vera Nieh for the deanship. . . . Miss Nieh has had an excellent record which can well speak for itself. Under the present administrative system we cannot expect her to do her best for the school. For the love of our Alma Mater we take the liberty to request you to do whatever you can to improve the situation and entrust to Miss Nieh the responsibility for the administration of the School.[135]

Two images of Vera Nieh emerge from the documents: one, from male writers, describes her as unduly stubborn, demanding, and emotionally unstable, while the other, from female writers, describes her as professional, assertive, and demonstrably capable. Gender analysis provides one way to interpret these conflicting responses to the same individual. First, women rarely reached high-level positions in professional health care in the war years; in 1941 the NHA had 1,255 male and 762 female employees.[136] In 1945, the Sichuan Provincial Health Administration counted 142 biomedical professionals in the province, of whom 135 were men and only 7 were women.[137] Although women populated the ranks of low-level jobs (as nurses and midwives), any female medical professional in a position of authority operated in a male-dominated world. Second, Director Forkner frequently got into conflicts with the Chinese people with whom he worked and was known for his condescension toward women.[138] This should make one suspicious of Forkner's perception of Nieh, as well as that of other individuals who worked under his direction. Third, male letter writers repeatedly refer to Dean Nieh not by her title but as "Miss Nieh," using language to revoke her professional status and reduce her to her sex and unmarried status, which itself they occasionally cited as a potential source of her "emotionally unstable" behavior. Fourth, male writers interpreted two short cablegrams from Dean Nieh as "attacks" on Claude Forkner in "strong terms," viz.: "Forkner is hindrance to school. Suggest not return," and "Forkner is great hindrance to Nursing School. Not desirable in China."[139] Meanwhile, no such assessment was made of Forkner's comments on Dean Nieh, which included: "Miss Nieh is not suitable to hold the position as dean of the nursing school"; "I think she is emotionally unstable"; "[T]he tone of Miss Nieh's letter is quite insubordinate"; "She cannot talk without losing her temper"; and "Vera Nieh emotionally unstable, fighting everyone, insubordinate."[140] In other words, his male colleagues took Forkner's words at face value, interpreting them as facts, but failed to grant Nieh's words a similar assessment. Nor should it escape one's notice that men have long used the labels "hysterical" and "overly emotional" to demean and silence women, even when the women have justifiable reasons for their ire or frustration.[141] Fifth, Dean Nieh and her faculty felt that professional nurses were fully competent and did not need the input of doctors who wished to control the nursing school. Her case thus illustrates the struggle of nurses in China for professional recognition and autonomy. Sixth, her male colleagues "solved" the situation by silencing her and pressuring her to temporarily abandon her post in Chengdu rather than by admitting any error on their part or making any concessions. Last, even after this resolution Li Ting'an wrote to Claude Forkner, stating, "Some of the ladies [by which he meant other nurses and administrators at the school] are still a little reactive but in general they are cooperating."[142] Still refusing to use titles of respect, the men involved in this drama utterly failed to confer professional dignity upon their female colleagues. Their choice of words—"insubordinate" and "reactive"—indicates a gender politics in which women's refusal to submit to male control constituted inappropriate behavior.

Another way to understand this gender divide between Dean Nieh's proponents and antagonists is in terms of the values that each side held dear. One of the greatest sources of contention between staff of the China Medical Board and the nursing school was the dean's management of rice supports: government-supplied rice given to people who worked in civil service, including public health, in the later years of the war, when astronomical inflation rendered regular salaries practically worthless. Dean Nieh bent the rice support rules in order to keep her staff consistently supplied, further angering Claude Forkner. Letters describing this event illustrate that Forkner believed administrative protocol to be sacred, deserving of reverence even under the extraordinary conditions of the war. On the other hand, as dean of the nursing school, Nieh felt responsible for all of her staff members' well-being, and she did everything in her power—including disrespecting the rules—to fulfill her duty as supervisor and ensure that her staff were well fed and could execute the physically demanding tasks of their jobs.[143] It is not difficult to imagine why her faculty would have appreciated this principle; a total of ten faculty members worked at the relocated school during the war, each of whom started the job with tremendous energy but soon tired under the strain of insufficient nutrition and constant work among the ill. By the summer of 1944, three had contracted tuberculosis.[144] They understood that government rice supports could mean the difference between health and chronic illness, or even between life and death.

Unfortunately for Dean Nieh, soon after the war ended she again faced strident sexism in her already strenuous workplace. In October and November 1945, Ruth Ingram—herself a previous dean of the PUMC School of Nursing—visited the school's Chengdu location to investigate another conflict between Dean Nieh and a male supervisor.[145] This time the conflict involved Dr. Best, general superintendent of the United Hospitals of WCUU, where PUMC nursing students did clinical practice during and after the war. Ingram reported, of her first meeting with Dean Nieh, that she "was eager to talk over her problems. She was candid and quite ready to acknowledge her mistakes."[146] The dean's chief concerns included having had to operate for several years without a clear and delineated protocol regarding her school's partnership with WCUU; having had her problems with this irregular relationship "brushed aside" by the school's Wartime Advisory Committee; personality clashes with Dr. Best; not knowing how to proceed with students' practical training in respect to the upcoming return to Beijing, which could not be firmly scheduled and which did not in fact occur until April 1946;[147] and her uncertainty as to whether or not she had the full support of the Board of Trustees.[148]

As in the previous instance, a man's assessment of the situation stood in direct contrast to the women's assessment, but this time the NHA and NIH cosponsored Ingram's investigative visit to Chengdu, during which she uncovered the falsehood of Dr. Best's claim that "local nurses will not work with Miss Vera Nieh." On the contrary, Dr. Best's "peculiar temperament and strange administrative policies [had] caused trouble continuously with the nurses of his mission for years."[149] Moreover, not a single nurse, under either Dean Nieh's or Dr. Best's supervision, expressed or reported having heard any dissatisfaction with Nieh, but rather voiced discontent with Dr. Best and labeled his rumors about Dean Nieh "propaganda." They also told Ingram about two instances in which Dr. Best had recruited nurses to his staff, instructed them to refuse to work with Dean Nieh, and promised greater pay to sweeten his offer.[150]

In her conversations with Ruth Ingram, Dean Nieh also provided astounding facts about the troubles she had faced in the months when CMB Director Forkner had judged her incapable. Nieh's own narration of her conflict with Forkner presents the perspective that any incapacity she experienced in this period stemmed from the impossible situation in which her own superiors had put her. Ingram concluded that "[o]ne must admire her courage in holding to the standards which she felt were necessary for her students. Her purpose has been to keep up the standard of the school to its prewar level and she has fought everyone whom [sic] she felt was trying to lower the status of the school."[151] Here we see the origin of some of Dean Nieh's reported temper. She had high standards for herself and the organization over which she had elected to take responsibility in very trying times. Though she might have profited from more flexibility, she nonetheless demonstrated admirable tenacity and courage, especially when compared with PUMC faculty and administrators who declined to assume the mantle of leadership under duress of war.

Even after the war ended, Dean Nieh's students and colleagues admired her for that courage, which continued to serve her well in her position as NAC president and simultaneous dean of the PUMC School of Nursing and superintendent of nurses (1947–49).[152] Moreover, at least one man also supported Dean Nieh, writing in 1946 that "[w]hat Miss Nieh and her faculty have achieved during the war has shown the finest quality of Chinese professional women. We all are very proud of them!"[153] A final word of praise for Vera Nieh came in 1972, when John Z. Bowers published his monograph on the PUMC and its nursing school. In the course of his research, Bowers asked why the PUMC had submitted to Japanese occupation while the nursing school had not, and summarized the responses as follows: "that the nurses were a more cohesive group; that Chinese women have an unusually strong character and strong will; and that there was no Vera Nieh to lead the medical faculty."[154] In this reading, Vera Nieh's shrewd professionalism was neither a personality flaw nor a mark of insanity but rather a badge of honor and testament to the undeniable contributions she made to her country in its time of greatest need.

With such evidence at hand, it is indubitable that sexism in the health profession played a major part in the criticisms leveled against Dean Vera Y.C. Nieh. Analyzing these critiques in terms of wartime gender ideology, we see that as a nurse on the caretaking side of the medical profession, Nieh satisfied the demands of both state and society. However, once she pushed for more autonomy as a school administrator she surpassed the bounds of gendered expectations. Dean Nieh's hardships reveal that as long as a woman stayed within the confines of specifically female contributions to the war she received praise and accolades, but once she stepped outside these bounds she might easily receive criticism and blame. The war emergency heightened peacetime gender ideology that charged women with supportive caregiving. Mothering the next generation was a woman's primary duty to the nation, and if she was to work outside the home then she ought to act as a universal mother, dutifully serving the needs of a society regulated by men, not as a professional demanding autonomy in order to materialize her own career goals.

CONCLUSION

The story of wartime nurses underscores the degree to which the war made a particular kind of new womanhood more possible than before. The country's desperate need for help allowed women to cast aside family obligations, ignore social strictures, and proceed to the battlefields without hesitation. Whether they worked on the home front or at the battlefront, women articulated their nursing work as hardship and courageous sacrifice on behalf of their nation in peril, and through it they learned to understand themselves as even more hardy than men and therefore capable of making a unique contribution to their suffering compatriots. Women who entered the medical profession performed womanhood in new ways. This new womanhood comprised not only women entering public spaces, touching the bodies of male strangers, and crossing social boundaries to develop relationships and create the national community, but also women occupying authoritative roles within institutions that themselves claimed the authority of science: hospitals and nursing schools that propagated scientific medicine. The millions of dollars of foreign aid that poured into China aided the indigenization of scientific medicine to an extent that partially explains why the People's Republic of China so readily turned to it in crafting its public health and medical education systems, even in an era of anti-Western xenophobia.[155]

The ways in which China won authorship of its own hygienic modernity put a definitively Chinese stamp on a set of practices that began in Western Europe and Japan. Through the combination of their physical and emotional labor, women did the most to indigenize scientific biomedicine by making it both available and approachable to their compatriots. When the bulk of China's universities and research centers moved to the southwestern provinces, this previously neglected region became home to an active community of international health workers who made important contributions to scientific medicine. The NHA produced vaccines, sera, and sulfa drugs for the local market, and medical researchers worked in Chinese state and university laboratories to develop medicines and public sani-

tation technologies.[156] The concentration of mostly PUMC-trained personnel created international networks along which funds, supplies, and volunteers traveled
from Milan, Miami, and Moscow into China. This wartime network had implications not only for domestic medical practice but also for the postwar development
of an international health community when a handful of Chinese health officials
entered positions of global prominence. In 1948 Minister of Health Jin Baoshan
(P. Z. King) took an appointment with UNICEF in New York City.[157] The World
Health Organization came into existence because of Dr. Sze Szeming's thoughtful
collaboration with Brazilian Dr. Paul de Souza.[158]

From this point the history bifurcates into the distinct stories of mainland China and Taiwan. Zhou Meiyu moved to Taipei, where she served as first director of
the newly formed and relocated National Defense Medical Center (*Guofang yixueyuan*) (NDMC) and continued to lead nurses both locally and internationally.[159]
The China Medical Board (CMB) also treated Taiwan as a center of international
nursing training and applied lessons from working in China to the sponsorship of
public health nursing in the Republic of Korea.[160] Meanwhile, in mainland China,
nursing entered a thirty-year period of decline marked by moments of acute
downturn such as the 1965 disbandment of the Chinese Nurses' Association (CNA)
and closure of all nursing schools. Despite these sea changes, nursing remained a
female profession—for example, of the 213 nurses at the Shanghai Mental Hospital
in 1974, only 30 were male—and women continued to occupy supervisory and
leadership roles.[161]

The feminization of nursing was a direct outcome of the war. In June 1947,
Chongqing's head nurse, Liao Junming, reported a total of 90 female and 6 male
nurses employed in the city's public agencies. Numbers in the recovered capital
Nanjing reflected greater female dominance: 120 women and 2 men. With a total of ten cities reporting, women dominated the nursing profession by a ratio
of seven to one.[162] This owed not solely to the desperate need for women's labor
but also to women's work to professionalize nursing. Perhaps the best expression
of their success is that Lin Sixin (Evelyn Lin) (PUMC School of Nursing, class
of 1926) was chosen as a candidate for superintendent of the Chongqing Central
Hospital.[163] Though the selection committee did not ultimately choose Lin, that
they even considered a nurse capable of leading the entire hospital signaled new
respect for women's capabilities in medicine. As first responders to people's most
immediate health needs, female nurses, through their constant visibility, created
a new public persona for women to embody: a competent, educated professional
who had authority over male (and female) bodies. They achieved this by accepting the primacy of the nation and conceptually hitching their work to national
strength. This remained true in the subsequent civil war, when the nursing educator Wang Xiuying (b. 1908; PUMC School of Nursing, class of 1931) wrote: "Nurses
are the guardians of national health. This is the credo of their work. The nation

cannot do without soldiers for one day, so it equally cannot do without nurses for a single day."[164]

This assertion, far from rhetorical, deeply affected people like Yao Aihua and her fellow volunteer medics. Yao's work as a military nurse did not end when people in the village near her unit beat their drums and announced, "The Japanese devils have surrendered!" She worked throughout the Civil War, during which time the NRA transferred her unit no less than seven times, beginning immediately after "victory." During one of those transfers she carried her third child, for whom her husband had served as midwife a mere five months earlier, while her companion limped along on bound feet for over two hundred miles. In late 1948 her entire medical team voted to join the Communists while stationed in Wenzhou, Zhejiang. Once they switched sides they learned that all of the soldiers they were treating had previously fought for the Nationalists and, along with the soldiers, received training in the famous Three Rules and Eight Points of Attention that formed the bedrock of communist military discipline. In Yao's final transfer, sponsored by the People's Liberation Army (PLA), she was given a choice to go home after a twelve-year absence or continue with her comrades, and she chose the former. Not long thereafter the government called Yao's unit to Korea to serve soldiers of the People's Volunteer Army, but she stayed home because she was pregnant and thereby narrowly missed her death: every single one of her comrades who went to Korea died in the American carpet-bombing campaign. Yao kept her life but suffered the loss of all the friends she had worked with for years, as well as the opportunity to gain veterans' health benefits. The Communist state, lacking complete records on who had served in the NRA, required testimonials from fellow soldiers to enter her in the registers. Nonetheless, she retained her status as "demobilized professional soldier" on her *hukou* household registration form, which saved her from persecution during the Cultural Revolution.[165]

Though Yao's story appears unique, China's story fits a global pattern wherein "changes in [the] scope and authority" of nurses come from "the complicated historical interplay of the needs of the state for more intensive public health systems, the professionalization of [nursing as] a discipline . . . and a willingness on the part of some physicians to see nurses as members of a health care team."[166] In China these forces converged during the war, which forced the Nationalist state finally to fund the military health system, augmented the demand for personnel, encouraged foreign charitable donations that sustained the institutions and individuals who professionalized nursing, and forced (some) male health professionals to make room for women.

Nonetheless, the story of Dean Nieh Yuchan pinpoints the precise location of a glass ceiling. Women predominated in the lower rungs of the medical hierarchy, but those who wished to climb higher faced strident discrimination. This situation was not unique to China; many wartime societies have witnessed simultaneous repudiation and reinforcement of conventional gender ideology, forcing women to continually assert their power even as they assumed new responsibilities and roles on behalf of the fighting men or the state.[167] This occurs not only because of disagreement about women's proper role in society, but also because the new roles for women are often born of a need for their labor rather than of demands for women's self-determination. In China, efforts to mobilize women to contribute to the war fit the state's agenda very well but did not necessarily empower women in their own right.[168]

In this way, too, Republican-era changes in women's professional lives foreshadowed those in the lives of their Communist-era counterparts. While radical feminists purported to "liberate" women from patriarchy, Marxist ideology dictated that women subordinate their demands for self-actualization to the project of working-class liberation, while the party subordinated them to the state.[169] Social changes during the War of Resistance prepared society for women to assume active roles in physically demanding jobs, but true gender equality remained elusive. The same was true in the realm of Maternal and Child Health, another top priority for wartime health officials.

5

Mothers for the Nation

When women are healthy they are more able to give birth, which is indeed that for which society most yearns.

—CHONGQING BUREAU OF PUBLIC HEALTH, ANNOUNCING THE OPENING
OF THE CHONGQING MATERNITY HOSPITAL, MAY 1944

The above sentence from the Chongqing Bureau of Public Health (CBPH) encapsulates wartime public health officials' beliefs about maternity: childbirth was at one and the same time a woman's greatest duty to the nation, and the greatest threat to her health. In other words, from the standpoint of state officials, no woman had a greater need for professional medical care than a laboring mother. Facts affirmed their belief in childbirth as a health threat: China's preeminent specialist in midwifery, Dr. Yang Chongrui (Marion Yang), estimated that 10 to 15 per 1,000 women, and 200 to 250 per 1,000 infants, died in or soon after childbirth, far exceeding the rates in developed countries. Once they survived infancy, Chinese children still faced a high probability of death from disease. Chinese delegates to the Conference of Far Eastern Countries on Rural Hygiene, held in Bandung, Indonesia, in August 1937, reported that 45 percent of rural children died before the age of five.[1] In the public health ecosystem, Maternal and Child Health (MCH) operated like a keystone species indicating the strength or weakness of the overall ecology. Health officials felt a deep attachment to and belief in sterile midwifery because of their genuine concern for the lives of women and children. They worked to assure that more mothers and children could survive childbirth and the tender first months of life even as bombs dropped and epidemics raged.

Although the available services never equaled actual need, they did significantly alter the medical landscape of Sichuan and further the medicalization of childbirth. Before the war, nearly 99 percent of births in Sichuan took place at home. The vast majority of these (over 88 percent) occurred with no midwife in attendance.[2] During the war, the combination of educated health professionals, female medical workers, and foreign funding fueled a rapid construction of hospitals and health centers across Sichuan that shifted childbirth to the clinic. In rural areas most births still took place in homes, but rates of midwifery attendance increased, and these midwives were more likely to be young, unmarried women trained in sterile techniques.

Most of these young women came from eastern cities where hospital birth was already quite common, and where infant mortality rates were lower than the national average.[3] Educated in germ theory at elite schools—principally the Peking Union Medical College (PUMC) or the First National Midwifery School, the latter established in Beijing in 1929—they, like nurses, contributed to the indigenization of scientific medicine.[4] Their flexibility and willingness to adapt to local women's preferences enabled the young midwives to spread lifesaving delivery practices. At the same time their work gradually challenged the social power of elderly midwives, commonly called *chanpo* ("birthing grannies") or *jieshengpo* ("old women who receive the child"), whose prestige derived from their own successful births and record of success at delivering other women's children.[5] While in China the masculinization of midwifery did not attend the medicalization of childbirth, as had occurred in other countries (as well as in China in the Song dynasty), the women who gained professional power in the twentieth century did so at the expense of another group of women.[6]

Midwives also played a central role in expanding the power of the central state in Sichuan. Because their work saved lives, young midwives proved to have particular staying power even in areas where local elites resisted change. Their knowledge of how to aid women through a momentous and potentially lethal event in their lives—parturition—granted midwives special access to women's bodies, homes, and hearts. Midwives, fully convinced of the power of their profession to bring people to health, gladly applied their skills to helping state health officials gain even further access to the people they served. The Nationalist government's move to Chongqing placed even rural areas of Sichuan Province within the reach of MCH workers, who, much like civilian and military nurses, developed relationships with expectant, laboring, and postparturient mothers that further strengthened the Sichuan people's place in the national community. Female midwives employed "scientific midwifery [to] connec[t] family reproduction to state politics."[7]

While the Imperial Japanese Army seized city after city, women could not divorce their domestic and reproductive labor from national concerns any more readily than men could refuse to go to battle. The war's startling death toll intensified the focus on women as "mothers of citizens," who could birth the nation anew with their wombs' issue. Even the country's longest-running women's journal, the progressive *Funü zazhi* (Ladies' journal), had shifted to a stridently pro-natalist stance after male writers took control of the publication in 1921.[8] During the War of Resistance, people's heightened desire for birth amidst all the death charged wives with the responsibility of creating not just healthy children but also healthy homes, managed according to scientific principles of cleanliness and order, in which all family members could flourish as dutiful, obedient citizens. It solidified homemaking as a woman's duty not just to her own family, but also to the "national family"—the literal translation of the term for "nation" (*guojia*) in modern Chinese.[9] In discursive terms, the Chinese woman—herself the "Sick Woman of East Asia"—shouldered the responsibility of healing that same "Sick Woman" through delivering and bearing healthy children for the nation. Happy to play an important role for their nation in need, female midwives and orphanage volunteers worked to transfer women and children from the control of the household patriarch to the control of the state patriarch. In so doing, they became key players in bringing state power into the daily lives and domestic spaces of women and children, just as women had done in Meiji Japan and revolutionary France and were doing in contemporary Germany.[10]

CHILDHOOD UNDER SIEGE

The Japanese invasion endangered all Chinese citizens, but children often suffered the gravest injuries. Children were raped, injured or killed in air raids, orphaned, and captured by both Nationalist and Japanese press gangs looking for soldiers or laborers to carry military supplies. Children also frequently succumbed to infectious diseases to which they had less resistance than adults. In one instance, a reported 60 percent of refugee children got sick while in transit between Wuhan and Sichuan Province, and a high percentage of children under one year of age died in orphanages. Children's suffering had a gendered component as well: girls more frequently suffered rape, while military kidnappers almost exclusively targeted boys.[11]

This section takes children's vulnerability in war as a starting point and argues that childhood was also under siege in another sense. The national emergency compelled many adults to lay claim to children as the physical embodiment of the country's future. The Nationalist Party, with Song Meiling as its representative and spokeswoman, claimed parental authority over the country's "warphans" and built a network of orphanages wherein children learned to hate the Japanese and love the state and party.[12] Forced to shoulder heavy responsibilities on behalf of the entire country and race, and inculcated with obedient patriotism, many of the children who survived the war nonetheless lost their innocence and independence.

The process of evacuating children from their own life-meaning began long before the war. Reformers in the late nineteenth and early twentieth centuries treated women's liberation as a means to a greater end—strengthening the nation; but in fact children were their ultimate targets. Agenda items that appeared on the surface to be for women—girls' education, the abolition of foot binding, and medical care for pregnant women—focused on an end goal of achieving "the nation's survival, . . . its strength . . . , through the education of children."[13] The concept of state ownership of a woman's womb and its issue found its most direct expression in orphan relief, which came under government patronage for the first time during the war. Relief workers focused on fashioning these "parent-free" children into worker-citizens impregnated with nationalism and ready to sacrifice all for their "parent-state." Just as Song Meiling stepped in as the figurative mother of all "warphans," the state she and her husband presided over defined itself as the rightful owner of children who had lost their biological parents in the tragedy of war. The war produced conditions under which the needs of the state took priority, and orphaned children were pressed into service for the national collective.[14]

A cogent if somewhat extreme expression of this idea came from Tang Guozhen, a Nationalist Party member, volunteer in the Wartime Association of Child Welfare (*Zhanshi ertong baoyu hui*) (WACW) and cofounder of the National Association of Chinese Women for the Comforting of War of Resistance Soldiers (*Zhongguo funü weilao ziwei kangzhan jiangshi zonghui*) (NACWCWRS).[15] Tang advocated sending orphans to serve as soldiers on the front lines:

> Special children, such as those who have not had good family education, and have then undergone long periods of vagrancy, as a matter of course do not have the good habits of typical children and controlling them can be particularly difficult. However, since they have long been bathed by the wind and rain, and warmed under the rays of the sun, they are healthier than typical children and their will is tremendously strong, so that not long after they arrive at an orphanage, all of their bad habits undergo quick transformation. Many vagrant children can already bear the responsibilities of a good troop commander [*hao duizhang*]. With a good education and a bit of extra effort to patiently lead them on the right path, one can certainly pick from among this group several children of outstanding talent who can become fresh troops for national salvation [*jiuguo de shenglijun*].[16]

The exigencies of war pressed even young orphans into military service. In what appears to be a subtle move that nonetheless had decades of doctrine behind it, the state that first took the role as these children's protector now put their lives at risk. The Nationalist state's apparently contradictory position as protector-recruiter constituted a cooptation of the parental role, with the nation's rather than the children's interests at heart. Tang Guozhen had borrowed the language of "fresh troops for national salvation" from the contemporary press and used it to express ideas propagated by none other than the child development expert Tao Xingzhi and kindergarten educator Zhang Zonglin, both of whom advocated sending children into the battle zone to serve as covert counterintelligence agents.[17] Indeed, some of the most enthusiastic soldier recruits came from war orphanages, while other child advocates argued that children could serve as military field nurses.[18]

Not all reformers and professional healthcare workers felt the same way. When Major General Zhou Meiyu discovered several eight- and nine-year-old "child soldiers" (*wawa bing*) serving as nurses in a military field hospital, she accused the commander of impropriety. The commander defended himself with the claim that the hospital needed these children's labor because all the adults had gone away to battle. Recognizing her defeat yet still concerned, Zhou recommended that the head physician care for all gravely wounded patients so that the children would not take fright upon witnessing their severe suffering. She also urged hospital staff to allow the children to sleep at night rather than require them to work the graveyard shift, since their growing bodies needed more rest.[19] This story demonstrates that the shortage of laboring hands left even concerned advocates with no choice but to employ children as workers in fields fit for adults.

Another story about a "child soldier" illustrates awe at, rather than concern for, a young boy's dedication to national defense. The young college student Qing, who had volunteered with her classmates to comfort wounded soldiers in rural Guangxi Province, met a fifteen-year-old boy who had been separated from his parents and become a wounded "soldier" through an unfortunate occurrence. The fighting near his village in Zhejiang Province had sent his neighbors scattering, but his family stayed put since his father was too ill to flee. When the Communist guerrilla soldiers came through the village and needed help in navigating the local roads, this young boy bravely volunteered to help them, but in the process of leading the soldiers he was shot in a Japanese ambush. The guerrillas had to retreat quickly, so they carried the boy with them, getting farther from his home with every step. His father had already died, and he surmised that his mother had escaped danger, but the boy still had a bullet lodged in his anus and an unhealed wound with little hope of surgical treatment. Although Qing met this boy in a hospital, he still had not encountered a doctor who could offer him the medical care he needed. Moreover, since Guangxi was over a thousand miles from his home, he faced a slim prospect of reuniting with his mother before the war ended. Qing reported that the war had interrupted this boy's education and he was very eager to get back to school. Though he certainly would have had cause for anger and despair, she did not note any rancor in his heart and recorded his story to mark him as a war hero.[20]

Another boy whose war wound remained untreated almost certainly caused him consternation. Xu Chengzhen's little brother received a severe wound in Chongqing's notorious May 3, 1939, air raid when his elementary school was bombed and a piece of shrapnel flew into his inner thigh and groin area. Xu and her mother rushed him to the nearest medical clinic, where frantic doctors "could only treat people according to the degree of the severity of their wounds." Just as the doctors placed Xu's brother on the operating table, Japanese planes returned for a second round of bombs, and they aborted the procedure. In the end, the clinic ran short of supplies, and the doctor could only place a piece of gauze on the boy's wound. Xu and her mother then took him to a Chinese doctor in the countryside, who however failed to stanch the wound's infection before it left him permanently crippled and sterile. Even though he was not cured, the boy's medical costs and the fact that Xu's father had lost his livelihood in the bombings left the already poor family destitute for the duration of the war.[21]

Many families lived a bare existence on a razor's edge, and the loss of one breadwinner could easily shatter them. After her father died, thirteen-year-old Ye Qingbi had to migrate from Sichuan's Fuling County to Chongqing to find work. Unfortunately, she became a slave at the Yuhua Textile Factory, locked inside the factory with other teenage girls and forced to work twelve-hour shifts. Ye and her coworkers had only poor-quality food to eat, and slept on the cold, damp ground with hundreds of bedbugs. Years of overwork in such conditions gave Ye severe arthritis, but in order to be allowed to leave the factory and return home, where her mother could treat her with herbal medicines, she had to pay the factory owners.[22]

Military families were particularly vulnerable to penury. A 1939 report from the New Life Movement Women's Advisory Council (WAC) in Chongqing claimed that "over 90 percent of military families are rendered destitute by the loss of their primary earner," and attempted to diagnose the problem.[23] Interrupted or long-delayed remittances could leave the homebound family members hungry, and since it generally took six weeks for a letter to get from Chongqing to Beijing, such delays were the norm.[24] Moreover Cui Xiangyu, wife of a military doctor, reported that air raids in Chongqing had destroyed postal facilities and "for months we could not receive either a letter or the promised money. My husband's salary was the family's sole income. Without it, we were starving."[25]

As noted in chapter 3, the greatest military burden already lay on poor families, and although these women volunteering in a government agency did not mention it, corrupt generals in the Nationalist military often deprived fighting men of their pay. More gravely, Japanese (as well as Chinese) troops frequently traveled long distances and, rather than tire their own soldiers with the strain of carrying supplies, stole livestock from villagers or kidnapped boys and men to serve as beasts of burden.[26] The loss of an ox made a family's farm work much more strenuous, and likely had long-term consequences, since replacing a valuable animal was costly. In the case of kidnapping, a family not only lost a valuable laborer, but also received no pay while he was gone.[27] Moreover, Chinese forced to work as coolies for the Japanese Army risked being killed by their own countrymen, since Chinese soldiers might fire indiscriminately on Japanese troops and their stolen coolies in surprise raids.[28] Illness, accidents, opium addiction, sudden death, or flight from conscription gangs could also take a boy or man out of the fields and deprive his family of his labor and income. Coupled with the war era's steep inflation, this could bankrupt a family.[29] Revisiting the question of Chinese nationalism during the War of Resistance in light of such economic hardship suggests that most people simply did not have the luxury of attaching themselves to an abstract concept such as the nation. They had to concern themselves with more-immediate necessities in order to survive. The people who helped them to survive—nurses, doctors, and midwives—stood the best chance of securing their attachment to a national community as a lived and embodied experience, expressed in human caring and intimate interactions.

Most middle-class people failed to comprehend the true needs of their poor compatriots, and instead worked to transform their outward behavior. As members of the working poor, military families became particular targets of reform. WAC women displayed a central feature of most wartime activism. Overwhelmingly from the middle and upper classes, these volunteers "aimed to 'civilize' their rural compatriots" and believed that compelling the poor to adopt a middle-class aesthetic, lifestyle, habits, and attitude would solve the problems of poverty.[30] Women at the 1939 Chongqing meeting cast aspersions on military families for refusing to work, letting their children run free in the streets as unschooled vagrants, and failing to show proper understanding of and dedication to the war effort. Rather than reflect reality, these comments betrayed the women's own class sensibilities and failure to understand the life conditions of the poor and working-class women they wished to reform. They placed their ultimate faith in the power of the state to intervene where the poor had "failed," and suggested that impoverished military families might ameliorate their condition by relinquishing their children to orphanages.[31]

The story of one woman who did just that shows that the state did not necessarily offer superior care. This woman, known as Peng-Wu shi (Mrs. Peng née Wu), both came from and married into a wealthy family, but suffered a series of calamities that left her nearly penniless. She and her husband both became opium addicts, and bandits killed the family's primary earner (the eldest son, a cloth merchant) not long before her husband died. This left Peng bereft of the family land and with six sons to raise on her own. Her eldest surviving son was conscripted into the army, ran away, and received such a severe beating as punishment that the army refused to take him back; her second son had to go in his brother's stead. Peng sent out two more sons to adoptive families and placed her favorite, youngest son in a government orphanage with the hope of retrieving him once she regained solvency. Unfortunately, that son died of dysentery while in the orphanage. In the end only two of her six sons survived.[32]

Wartime conditions were so harsh that even staying at a mother's breast could not guarantee a child's survival. Cui Xiangyu, originally from Hubei, moved with her family to Sichuan in late 1938. Her husband, a military physician, spent the majority of the war far from his family while his wife took care of his parents in Chongqing and gave birth to their two sons, the second on the very day of an air raid. When that son fell ill with a disease he contracted while in the crowded air raid shelter, Cui had no time or money to seek medical assistance for him before he died in her arms, at just three years old. The remaining family of five continued to survive on her husband's single salary, which they supplemented with a family garden.[33] So many pregnant women had to stuff themselves into crowded air raid shelters where contagious diseases flourished that in 1941 the Baoning Maternity Hospital announced the opening of an underground birthing room in Shapingba, just north of Chongqing.[34] Poverty itself also took a toll on human life. Li Shuhua gave birth to six children during the war, but only two survived due to her constant hunger and the anxiety of living in extreme poverty in a frequently bombed city. As she put it, "A woman's body was just a machine for giving birth to babies, even though we had to bury most of them."[35]

The story of a mother who worked in the medical field further illustrates just how vulnerable young children were to infectious disease. Volunteer military nurse Yao Aihua lost her second son in the summer of 1943. Called to assist villagers in delivering children, Yao had had to leave her own child in the care of others. Someone fed him something that gave him an acute intestinal infection resulting in simultaneous vomiting and diarrhea. He died before his second birthday, and Yao recalled, "[W]e couldn't even buy a coffin for him. We were only able to wrap him up in a grass mat and ask people to bury him, but they buried him so shallowly that the wolves came to eat his corpse."[36] This young child never had the chance to live up to his name, (Li) Ji Xing ("Continued Prosperity").

Such stories of poverty and hardship were so common during the war that they came to represent it in Cai Chusheng and Zheng Junli's widely acclaimed 1947 film, *The Spring River Flows East* (*Yijiang chunshui xiang dongliu*). Whereas Ba Jin's novel *Ward Four* reflected dramatic changes in traditional gender roles, this film underscored their perseverance in some popular culture. Despite the fact that more women than men volunteered to serve wounded soldiers on the front, in the film the husband, Zhang Zhongliang ("Loyal and Faithful Zhang"), joins the Chinese Red Cross, while the wife, Sufen, remains at home with her parents-in-law and the couple's infant son, Kang'er ("Son of the Resistance"). Ironically, this puts her in a much more vulnerable position throughout the war, soon rendered more dramatic by the occupying Japanese soldiers' assassination of her father-in-law, leaving the family without a male head of household. Despite her family's own scarcity of food and basic household goods such as soap, Sufen feels compassion for others and volunteers in an orphanage, where she fulfills her role as mother-of-the-nation by day, returning home to care for her mother-in-law by night. Several scenes show Sufen washing and mending clothing, or bathing and feeding the orphans—all with a look of contentment on her face, modeling the emotional labor of happily setting aside all of her own desires in order to work for others. Another scene shows her writing a letter for an illiterate refugee, who dictates the lines "Women have been blown to bits. Bodies have been found in pieces. . . . Our family is so destitute we can't even afford to buy coffins to bury our dead. We have to cover them up with matting." As Sufen writes, she repeatedly stares into the camera, a look of despair on her face. This scene, and many more like it, underscore the theme of women's vulnerability without male protection and erase the strength that Sufen repeatedly demonstrates as she cares for the entire family on her own.

Sufen's son, Kang'er, joins her in the orphanage until he is old enough (at age eight) to start his own job selling newspapers on the street. A scene in the second half of the film dramatizes his defenselessness. He is hawking papers when he encounters his father, now a business mogul recently returned from Chongqing and traveling in a private car, hanging a paper bill out of his car window to request a paper. A flood of desperate hawkers, including his own son, rush toward him, but Zhang Zhongliang does not even recognize the boy, now nine years old, whom the older sellers roughly push aside. At the end of a long day plying his newspapers on the streets of occupied Shanghai, Kang'er collapses in exhaustion. Though she is a diligent and conscientious mother, Sufen cannot save him from these hardships, and his now wealthy but profligate father cannot even recognize him. *The Spring River Flows East* emphasizes civilians' suffering, the functionality of state services (all the children and volunteers in the orphanage are full of smiles), and the traditional housewife's self-sacrificial role as caretaker of two generations—elderly parents-in-law and young children.[37]

DELIVERING THE NEW NATION: MATERNAL AND CHILD HEALTH IN WARTIME

Although the war put grown children at greater risk, notable advancement occurred in combatting the primary vulnerabilities of young children: neonatal and infantile mortality caused primarily by neonatal tetanus. Over the course of the war, Chongqing health officials built eight Maternal and Child Health clinics and one large maternity hospital in the wartime capital, and MCH specialists across Sichuan hosted "well-baby" meetings and family hygiene clinics and visited women in their homes to perform deliveries and both pre- and postnatal checkups. As with nursing, the wave of refugees had unleashed a new supply of personnel, and the threat of national extinction prompted an increase in state funding. Thus, the war placed Chinese children at greater risk, but also created the conditions under which the field of medicine designed to protect them witnessed important achievements.

The problems of maternal and infantile mortality of course predated the war and had been largely attributed to traditional midwifery practices of *jieshengpo*, who without any knowledge of germ theory often spread harmful bacteria quite unawares, inadvertently causing the deaths of the very people whom they wished to protect. They often worked with unwashed hands and soiled nails, which they might use to stretch the vagina or tear the perineum in order to ease the birth.

Many *jieshengpo* worked in rural villages, where farmers saw the soil as a life-giving force capable of bringing tiny seeds to full fruition each year. Accordingly, a *jieshengpo* might plunge a knife into the ground before using it to cut the umbilical cord so as to receive a blessing of earth's life-giving powers. After cutting the umbilical cord, she might use mud, animal dung, or ash from the kitchen stove to dress it. Such practices made perfect sense to people in a farming community with no knowledge of bacteria, but they spread the causative agents of puerperal fever (*Streptococcus* bacteria that enter the body through lesions) and neonatal tetanus (*Clostridium tetani,* which often live in soil or in animals' digestive tracts and hence entered newborns' bodies through their umbilical cord dressings or soiled knives).[38] Furthermore, many people believed that malevolent spirits or angered gods caused a child's death, directing their attention away from the actual cause and from proactively preventing future sorrows.[39]

One woman in particular had long been at work to address this problem. Dr. Yang Chongrui (Marion Yang) (1891–1983) grew up in a wealthy Chinese Christian family in Beijing. She earned her MD from the PUMC when it was still the missionary-run Women's Union Medical College (class of 1917), and later studied obstetrics and gynecology at Johns Hopkins University and the Midwives Institute in Woolrich, England (1925–26) before teaching the subjects at her Chinese alma mater. She also toured midwifery schools and medical facilities in England, Scotland, France, Germany, Denmark, and Canada. All of these experiences made Dr. Yang the most knowledgeable person about her field in early-twentieth-century China.[40] In 1929 Dr. John B. Grant, director of the PUMC Department of Public Health, recommended her to the Nationalist government for an official position as midwifery specialist within the new National Health Administration (NHA). Yang calculated that she could prevent three-quarters of maternal and child deaths if she had solid support. NHA officials, finally convinced, gave her this support; in the single year of 1929 Dr. Yang helped to found and then chaired the National Midwifery Board, became director of the NHA Maternal and Child Health Department, and cofounded (with Dr. Grant), and then directed, the First National Midwifery School (FNMS) in Beijing. Once in these posts, Dr. Yang crafted the education and licensing requirements for new-style midwives and retrained old-style midwives so that they met these requirements, conducting hundreds of trainings.[41]

In this way Yang Chongrui was much like Madame Le Boursier (Angélique Marguerite Le Boursier du Coudray), who 170 years earlier had traveled all over France teaching new-style midwifery to young, unmarried women with the support of Louis XV.[42] This difference of nearly two centuries put Yang on the defensive. Like many modernizers of her era, Yang Chongrui had a powerful sense of being behind the times. In her writings (discussed below) she frequently compared China with "advanced countries" and used the disparity in maternal and infant death rates to incite her compatriots to action. She clearly felt that China would not merit the descriptor "modern" until its people accepted and regularly used the midwifery practices that had become common in many other countries—the same countries whose gunboats had threatened China's shores and whose diplomats had authored humiliating treaties. Under the circumstances it would not have been possible for her to separate conceptually aseptic midwifery from national strength. Hence in her work the two were always conflated, as in virtually all public health texts of the era. Nonetheless, Yang was capable of writing in different registers. For example, when she wrote a report for the American sponsors of her study abroad trip to the United States in 1942, she described China with pride as "the only country on earth where well-educated women bring babies into the world."[43]

Just as the new term *hushi* granted nurses respect by employing the suffix -*shi* that denotes a learned person, Yang Chongrui created the term *zhuchanshi* (birth-helping scholars) to designate the midwives with training in aseptic practices as representatives of a new and respectable profession. In so doing Dr. Yang initiated the transformation of midwifery from a humble occupation of mostly illiterate women to a state-licensed and institutionally recognized profession of educated women.[44] This transformation required associating midwifery with modern science, which Dr. Yang achieved in part by designing a standard midwifery bag that graduates received, containing all the necessary tools for their new trade. Retrained *jieshengpo* received their equipment in a straw basket, while young women trained in aseptic practices received a bag made of black leather, signaling a distinction between the two groups despite their similarity in training and profession. The most important items among their equipment—all of which signaled the medicalization of midwifery—included sterile scissors with which to cut the umbilical cord and a sterile cord tie and dressing; medicines such as alcohol, mercurochrome, Lysol, and silver nitrate eye drops to prevent eye infections in the newborns; a washbasin in which to wash the newborn; soap and a nail brush for the midwife to keep her hands clean; a face mask and apron for the midwife; artery clamps to use in cases of heavy bleeding; and a hypodermic needle and medicine dropper for administering medicine to mother and child. The bag also included a birth report form and a labor record form, signaling the new connection between midwifery and the state.[45]

This connection led the National Institute of Health to include a page for aseptic midwifery in its 1943 public health calendar. (See figure 24.) The image for the month of March shows a young midwife with rosy cheeks carefully cleaning her fingernails with a nail brush and soap prior to attending to the parturient woman, who is also receiving help from her mother. The midwife has placed her iconic black bag on a chair nearby, and its contents—sterile scissors, silver nitrate, and other medicines—lie nearby, as does a pan of hot water, all ready for the delivery. Clean, white linens adorn everything, including the midwife herself, whose attire distinguishes her as a *zhuchanshi* rather than a *jieshengpo*. While the former dressed in white (the color of mourning clothes), the latter usually wore traditional clothing such as a padded jacket and a skirt, making the new-style midwife seem all the more foreign.[46] Like the image, the text below it attempted to introduce a whole new set of childbirth practices with the aim of preventing puerperal fever and neonatal tetanus, "still common in China." The text recommended that all married women go to the doctor if their period stopped, that pregnant women visit the health center for regular prenatal checkups, and that postpartum women take bed rest for ten days followed by a checkup after the first month. It said nothing about "sitting the month" (*zuo yuezi*), the traditional practice of one month's bed rest with a special diet and abstention from washing one's hair or going outside. Taken together, the image and the text for March (the month of International Women's Day) inscribed new practices for the modern mother and signified the indelible connection between womanhood and motherhood in the eyes of the state.[47]

Military nurse Yao Aihua's story of her first birth suggests the power of a midwife trained in aseptic methods. During her pregnancy, Yao's military medical team was stationed in a village outside Laohekou, in northwestern Hubei Province, where a famine had strictly limited the amount of food available and a severe housing shortage meant that she "lived in an old cowshed that stank to high heaven and was full of fleas; [her] body was covered in red bites."

After her fellow medics designated her "a difficult case," Yao went to the city to request the services of a new-style midwife (*zhuchanshi*), who successfully delivered her baby boy. However, she apparently had contracted an illness from the flea bites and had passed it on to her son in utero; most of his skin had rotted away—so much in fact that "his bones were poking through." Once Yao recovered she was able to nurse him, and he soon grew chubby and healthy, even surviving his younger brother, though his arms remained deeply scarred.[48]

Another story illustrates the impact of urban midwifery training in remote Shanxi Province, and in this instance underscores the influence of Rockefeller philanthropy and the PUMC. Hsiao Li Lindsay accompanied her British husband to Yan'an in December 1941 to offer crucial radio services for the Eighth Route Army. In the fall of 1942 she and another woman walked dozens of miles through mountain villages in Shanxi, both eight months pregnant, in search of a safe place to give birth amid shifting battle lines. Although the entire front-line region had only two qualified midwives, the one who eventually came to deliver their babies, Dr. Yang, had graduated from midwifery school and worked at the PUMC with Dr. Lin Qiaozhi, the woman who later became the PRC's foremost midwifery expert. The baby put herself and her mother at great risk by coming out breech, but fortunately Hsiao Li was strong enough to deliver her in so short a time that Dr. Yang had to sterilize her hands with liquor because the water had not yet boiled.[49]

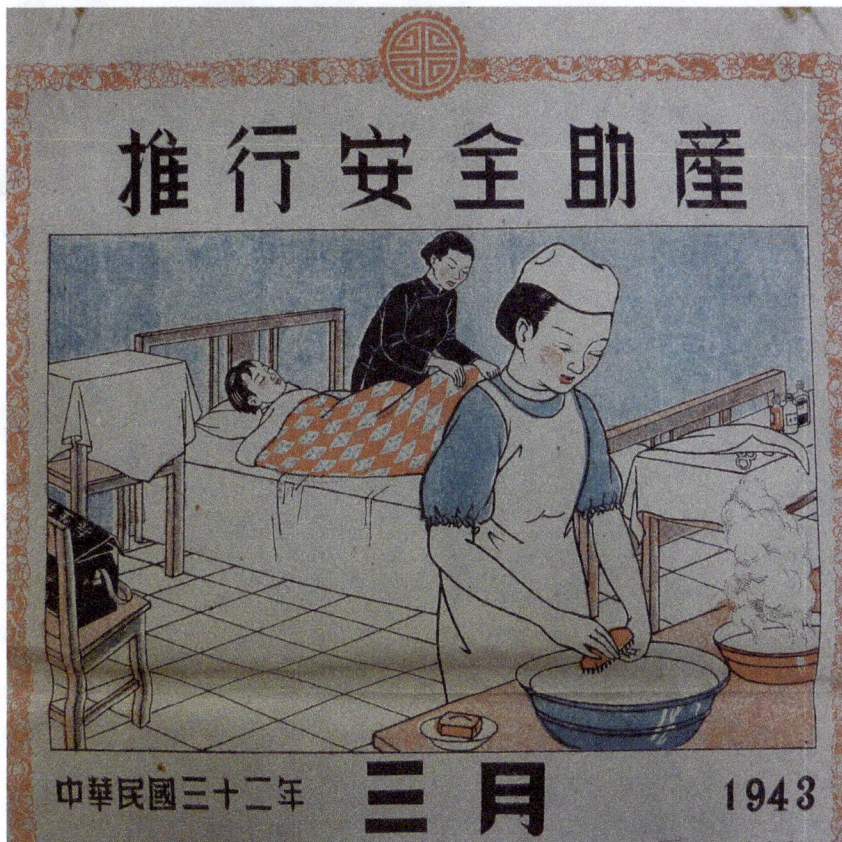

推行安全助產

中華民國三十二年　三月　1943

FIGURE 24. March 1943 page of the National Institute of Health public health calendar, titled "Promote Safe Midwifery." NLM ID 101171294, History of Medicine Division Collection. Courtesy of the United States National Library of Medicine.

Recognizing the lifesaving impact of midwives trained in aseptic methods, Chongqing public health officials built the necessary infrastructure for Mother and Child Health work in the wartime capital. The CBPH set aside resources for MCH from the very beginning of its operation. In early December 1938, bureau staff began planning four MCH clinics, each with one female doctor and one midwife. Over the course of the next year, the bureau made large purchases of medical equipment in preparation for opening all four clinics, but managed to build only two of the four planned facilities. In the first half of 1940 they completed the original four and opened two more MCH clinics, for a total of six; then a seventh by August, and an eighth in October 1940.[50] This gave the wartime capital three more MCH centers than the provincial capital of Chengdu.[51] Over the

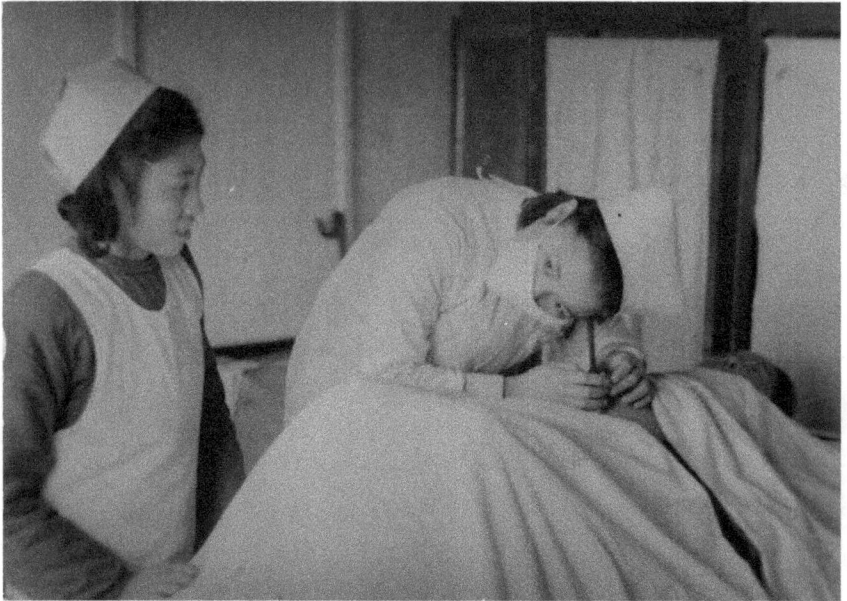

FIGURE 25. Female midwife and nurse conducting a prenatal examination at the National Central Midwifery School in Geleshan, Chongqing. Box 81, folder "Midwifery." ABMAC Records. Rare Book and Manuscript Library. Columbia University.

course of 1940, these eight clinics provided the following services, all free: over 9,000 pre- and postnatal exams, 450 prenatal home visits, over 1,100 births, over 1,100 gynecological exams, and over 1,600 children's health exams.[52] Clinic staff managed to complete this work despite many setbacks: two of the clinics burned down in air raids; several spent most of the year crammed together in a school with inadequate equipment; two others continued operating out of temples; and two were located in frequently bombed areas, so staff had to spend much of their time performing emergency air raid relief at the bombing sites rather than their usual duties.[53]

The central government heartily supported this work. Each of the eight clinics received a start-up fund of nine thousand yuan from the Executive Yuan and operated in cooperation with the National Central Midwifery School (*Guoli zhongyang gaoji zhuchan zhiye xuexiao*) (NCMS), which had relocated to nearby Geleshan. (See figure 25.) Midwifery students received practical training at the clinics, and clinic staff received medical training from the NCMS. The two parties agreed that if the clinics got extremely busy, the NCMS would send additional personnel to lend helping hands, and clinic staff would refer pregnant women with special needs to the better-equipped NCMS hospital.[54] The NCMS maintained high standards of sterility and professionalism.

Local health officials in Chongqing designated the eight MCH clinics as centers of "women's and children's health as well as general healthcare work," so staff also performed air raid relief and gave smallpox inoculations and preventive vaccinations (type unspecified), serving thousands each year.[55] Additionally, in early 1940 the CBPH and the Chongqing Municipal Air Raid Relief Team jointly established a health center (*baojian yuan*) whose services included birthing assistance (*huchan*), an infant nursery, and a nursery school. The bureau also demanded that all municipal clinics perform prenatal exams and postnatal family visits, offer free deliveries, and provide nursing care for pregnant women.[56] The Chongqing Industrial Health Committee also performed seventy prenatal and eighty-three postnatal exams, and assisted twenty-eight births over the course of 1941.[57]

Chongqing still had further need for maternal health services. By 1942 the city's official population had climbed to over 766,000, and the Bureau of Public Health began planning, and in May 1944 finally opened, its own maternity hospital (*chanfuke yiyuan*)—with two physicians, five nurses, two midwives, and three departments (obstetrics, gynecology, and pediatrics)—and reported that sixteen patients had already been admitted.[58] Although the bureau had originally planned for the hospital to have fifty patient beds, it ended up with only thirty, despite the fact that it also spent over two hundred thousand yuan *less* than the budgeted amount on the hospital's equipment.[59] However, it soon got a boost. In May 1945, it was united with the Chongqing Municipal Hospital and became its Obstetrics and Gynecology Department, with forty-five beds.[60] This was the last MCH facility to open during the war era.

The growth of all of these facilities compounded wartime staffing difficulties. To answer this need, the National Institute of Health, officially opened in April 1941 in Geleshan, operated a training institute for doctors, nurses, and midwives that admitted large classes of students, in which nurses and midwives predominated.[61] Meanwhile, the Public Health Personnel Training Institute (PHPTI) in Guiyang, Guizhou, trained doctors, nurses, and midwives for civilian health organizations. A photo of the first and second graduating classes of this institute shows a total of 126 graduates, of which women constitute the majority. (See figure 26.)

As this history shows, any shortcomings in MCH services in wartime Chongqing owed more to wartime circumstances than to lack of earnestness among health authorities and medical professionals. Their perseverance may have been related to the fact that when Dr. Yang Chongrui began midwifery work in Beijing in 1929, that city was designated as a model for the rest of the nation; once the Nationalist government declared Chongqing the wartime capital and Dr. Yang moved there, it became the obvious choice for the new model.[62] Moreover, as the new capital and home to central government institutes, Chongqing had the infrastructure to become a new center of aseptic midwifery. Nonetheless, many obstacles over which they had no control kept officials from fulfilling their goals. These included

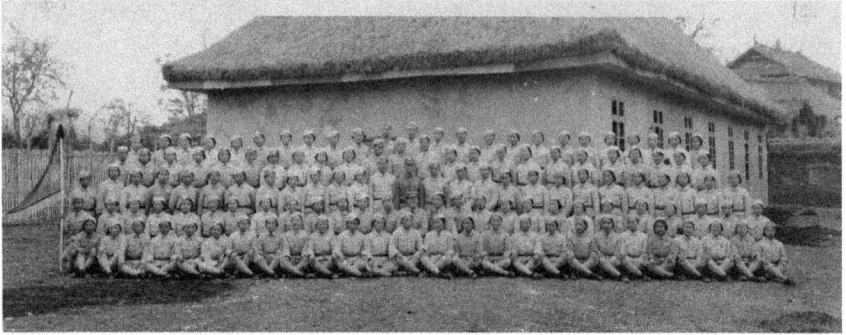

FIGURE 26. First and second graduating classes of doctors, nurses, and midwives at the Public Health Personnel Training Institute in Guiyang, Guizhou. Box 83, folder "NHA and Nursing." ABMAC Records. Rare Book and Manuscript Library. Columbia University.

inflation and financial shortfalls, high staff turnover, bombing and destruction of facilities, and midwives' need during air raid season to divide their time between air raid relief and their usual duties.

Despite these challenges, both local and central health officials committed a remarkable amount of money to institutional midwifery. The resultant quantity of MCH services in Chongqing contrasted sharply with those in the remote and sparsely populated Communist base area. The Shaan-Gan-Ning Border Region government passed progressive regulations about Maternal and Child Health, but still lacked properly trained personnel in this rural region where local sanitary conditions made childbirth extremely dangerous. By the late war years, health workers in the area managed to establish both a successful obstetrics clinic in the Central International Peace Hospital and a training program for midwives that graduated eighty students in July 1945. The immediate postwar period witnessed even more MCH work in the region, demonstrating that lack of resources rather than lack of political will hampered wartime progress.[63] Even in Chongqing, the financial strain of inflation blocked the ambitious plans of the Chongqing Women's Welfare Society (*Chongqing funü fuli she*), established in 1942 with the support of Minister of Finance H. H. Kung and Minister of Education Chen Lifu as well as twenty other social benefactors. When the society attempted to open its own maternity hospital, inflation kept even these political magnates from being able to raise sufficient funds, and the plan failed.[64] Given all of these challenges, it is clear that Chongqing health authorities did everything in their power to improve MCH in their jurisdiction.

Yet convincing all expectant mothers to avail themselves of these services lay outside the power of all but the most patient health workers. Much of the population was unfamiliar with and resisted hospital childbirth, so simply building and staffing the facilities would not ensure their enthusiastic use.[65] As Qi, a woman who earned a respectable monthly salary of forty yuan as a midwife in Chongqing's Red Cross Hospital, explained,

> Women here in the interior do not really like to come to our new-style maternity hospital to seek treatment, so in addition to our regular work we sometimes go to visit pregnant women in their homes and urge them to come to us for checkups since service in our hospital is free, and so far all the women who have used our services are very healthy. Therefore there are some women who come to us, but they're not very enthusiastic about it. As for this, I am hoping that we can increase our education efforts so as to encourage women to better understand our work.[66]

Qi expressed a common mixture of sincerity and didacticism, ending her speech with the declaration that "in the future I hope that we can extend our work into the countryside, because then we can decrease the number of our unlucky sisters who lose their lives. This is our only hope."[67] Like other middle-class female reformers, Qi believed that she could "educate" women into middle-class behavior (i.e., choosing a hospital birth over home birth). Perhaps she did not realize that many women were already doing precisely what she wanted them to do: bringing sterile midwifery practices and hygiene education to "women in the interior." Their experiences suggest that changing cultural practice was anything but easy, and certainly not natural or inevitable.

CITY AND COUNTRY: MATERNAL AND CHILD HEALTH ACROSS SICHUAN

Bishan County, thirty kilometers west of Chongqing proper during the war and now part of Chongqing municipality, had the most successful Maternal and Child Health program in all of Sichuan. Chen Zhiqian (C. C. Chen), as director of the Sichuan Provincial Health Administration (SPHA), established the Bishan County Health Center (BCHC) in October 1939 and granted the center "demonstration" status with a healthy budget underwritten by the Rockefeller Foundation's China Medical Board, the NHA, and the Bishan County government. Director Yu Wei managed a monthly budget of 1,559 yuan and lavish headquarters in the old Jiangxi Guild House. By 1945 its budget exceeded that of any other county health center throughout Sichuan, allowing it to run not only the BCHC in the county seat with a thirty-bed hospital, but also eight hospitals and twelve clinics across the county. In addition to receiving better funding, demonstration centers tended to attract the best staff, and the BCHC boasted more than twice the personnel of the center in the provincial capital of Chengdu, and also trained the greatest number of new colleagues. Its medical staff ran a smallpox vaccination campaign and attained complete vaccination across the county by 1940.[68] Bishan's superior medical services trouble the narrative of Nationalist state neglect of rural areas and suggest that further study of Republican-era health work can illuminate the rapid growth of post-1949 health services.[69]

Although the Bishan MCH center (*fuying baojiansuo*) was not established until December 1943, the BCHC trained new midwives prior to this date and by 1942 performed an average of twenty-five deliveries per month.[70] In choosing its midwifery students, the BCHC accepted only literate local women around twenty-five years of age, healthy in body and pure in mind (*sixiang chunzheng*), with gentle spirits (*taidu wenrou*) and without any previous experience in midwifery. These qualities presumably made the women impressionable and ready to accept the training without questioning the differences between its foundational principles and those of traditional village midwifery. The two-and-a-half-month training's explicit goals included fostering a "spirit of obedience" (*fucong jingshen*) and training the students to "understand the importance of new-style midwifery [*xinfa jiesheng*] and decide to earnestly promote it," as well as learn how to "eat bitterness, endure hardship, and obey orders" (*chiku nailao fucong zhihui*). Graduates had to remain in their village after graduation and continue to work there, reporting on their work monthly, lest they be required to forfeit their diplomas and reimburse the center for all instructional fees.[71]

Stated in this manner, the midwifery training appeared closely tied to the New Life Movement in its aim to produce dutiful citizens who remained devoted to the Nationalist Party. Moreover, it strongly suggests that new-style midwives were charged not only with physical but also emotional labor, since "[o]ne indication of the rising importance of affective labor . . . is the tendency for employers to highlight education, attitude, character, and 'prosocial' behavior as the primary skills employees need. A worker with a good attitude and social skills is another way of saying a worker adept at affective labor."[72] Since the state saw women as the gateway to the family, and midwives had the power to earn their trust by aiding them in the potentially dangerous moment of childbirth, midwifery clearly signaled its importance to building the affective community of the nation.

Bishan's MCH programs garnered success from the staff members' willingness to honor people's preference for a familiar environment when submitting to a new medical practice. In 1940, personnel made 120 home visits that included fifty-five home hygiene lessons. While far more women received their prenatal exams in hospital (150) than at home (22), midwives attended forty-seven home births and only eighteen hospital births, and conducted home-based postnatal exams for forty-eight women and hospital-based exams for only four women. These numbers show that MCH workers often succeeded in getting women to their hospital once, but frequently had to follow up with women in their own homes. (See figure 27.) The staff most likely recorded the women's home addresses at the first visit and might have shown up uninvited if the time came for a follow-up appointment and the women failed to appear at the hospital.[73]

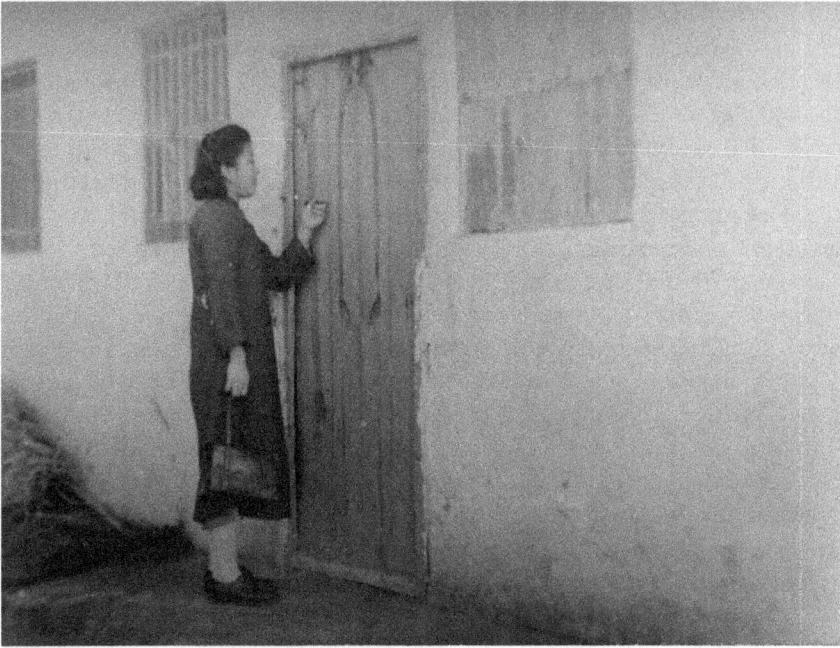

FIGURE 27. A traveling midwife knocks on the door of a private residence, midwifery bag in hand. Box 81, folder "Midwifery." ABMAC Records. Rare Book and Manuscript Library. Columbia University.

When patients did come into the clinic, staff took full advantage of their presence in the waiting room, delivering 115 public health talks to their captive audiences over a six-month period. Mothers [initially] showed reluctance to attend mothers' meetings where staff gave parental advice, with only four people appearing at the sole meeting in 1940, but avidly participated in well-baby competitions (two competitions with 338 people in attendance), and also took greater advantage of the clinic's outpatient services than did men.[74] By 1945 Bishan MCH workers had made such an impression that over four hundred women attended mother's meetings, and well-baby meetings continued to draw large crowds.[75] Furthermore, staff in Bishan performed the greatest number of pre- and postnatal exams and delivered the most babies of any county health center, including that of Lu Zuofu's progressive city, Beibei.[76]

Nonetheless, even at a successful county health center such as this, staff conducted far more general public health activities—such as hygiene lectures and scabies treatments at the county seat's bus terminal—than sophisticated medical services.[77] Nurse Zhu Baotian (PUMC, class of 1938) worked in Bishan for several years on treating and preventing trachoma, one of the most common ailments among children in both urban and rural China in the war years. This approach therefore accorded with both the dominant model of rural health development at the time and the needs of rural communities.[78]

The BCHC also served as a base from which to conduct work in the county's villages; its forty-eight village health workers accomplished much more by going to the people than by waiting for the people to come to their clinics. This work followed the commitment of Yang Chongrui to bring aseptic midwifery to the people rather than restrict it to elite and exclusive locales.[79] It also demonstrates the growing influence of the program of roving public health nurses that Zhou Meiyu created in Dingxian (described in chapter 2). County health staff traveled to villages to set up mobile clinics in canvas tents, just as missionaries had done decades before (often traveling illegally to parts of China they were not supposed to visit). They also conducted community health talks, home visits, mothers' meetings, and children's health contests.[80] In the 1960s, the barefoot doctor program followed this model, with well-equipped clinics in county seats serving as the institutional headquarters for village-based barefoot doctors.[81]

Health work in one village of Bishan County, Xinglong ("Prosperity"), began in late 1939 when the National Christian Council (NCC) launched a Rural Reconstruction project that attracted bright young volunteers. The NCC, with wartime headquarters in Chongqing, aimed to fight rural poverty while discouraging communism and expanding the influence of the Christian church. (The first opened in Xinglong in 1928.) Zhu Xiuzhen's midwifery clinic became the most successful part of NCC work in Xinglong, outlasting the collapse of every other project (the salt cooperative, the church community project, education, and house-to-house economic surveying).[82] Yet it did not start out this way. It took a lot of work and a bit of luck for Zhu to gain the local women's trust.

Originally trained at the PUMC School of Nursing and the Canadian-run South Henan Union Hospital, Zhu Xiuzhen received her pay from the organization that sponsored most missionary health work in rural Sichuan, the American Methodist Episcopal Mission (AMEM). As a Christian trained in scientific medicine in foreign schools, Zhu embodied a mixture of Chinese and Western values, yet as a Chinese woman she had a better chance of gaining the trust of the suspicious. Zhu's clinic, which opened in early 1940, was Xinglong's first scientific medicine establishment. Being entirely new, it received little attention from most villagers, who barely gave it a sideways glance when passing by, and the first people who sat on its benches asked for no treatment but merely used it as a convenient place to chat with their friends.[83]

Zhu's first success resulted from her patience and understanding that she should allow the village women to use the clinic as they best saw fit: as a gathering place. Once the clinic did become operational, women's positive associations with it made it simultaneously a site of social cohesion and a site for medical care. Regarding the latter, Zhu Xiuzhen eventually got her lucky break. A local doctor failed to cure his own infant son of an ailment that Zhu managed to treat, and thereafter referred some of his patients to her and gave her public recognition. Yet it remained even more challenging to make any headway in midwifery, since local women strongly preferred home births attended by *jieshengpo*. Ignored for six months, Zhu had the chance to redeem herself from negligence when a family called her in as a last resort for a difficult case and she safely delivered the mother a healthy baby. In another difficult case around the same time, the family did not call on Zhu, and the woman died. After this nearly all parturient women wanted Zhu by their side, and by November 1940 she had a midwifery case almost every single day.[84] No records document how the local *jieshengpo* reacted to this loss of business, or what they did thereafter to supplement their incomes.

Meanwhile, back in Chongqing, local health officials' emphasis on MCH produced results. Women in wartime Chongqing went to the hospital infrequently, and stayed as inpatients even less often, unless they were giving birth. In 1940, the Chongqing Municipal Hospital reported 527 female and 904 male patients.[85] Men constituted 63 percent of the hospital's patients, whereas women constituted 37 percent. In the second half of 1944, 144 women and 434 men received treatment at the Contagious Disease Hospital; its patients were 75 percent male and 25 percent female.[86] Records from January 1944 through June 1945 at the Chongqing Municipal Hospital show that male patients outnumbered female patients throughout this eighteen-month period, during which men constituted 62 percent of the outpatients and women accounted for 38 percent. The gender imbalance is steeper for inpatients, most of whom paid for their medical services; among this group the male–female ratio was 2.54 to 1.0.[87]

On the other hand, available evidence suggests that adult women in Chongqing considered parturition worthy of a hospital visit. In the last two months of this period, May and June 1945, female inpatient and outpatient numbers leapt ahead of previous averages, precisely because women flocked to the hospital's new Obstetrics and Gynecology Department, which had opened on May 1. In the first month of its operation, department staff tended to 318 outpatients and 56 inpatients. The following month, June 1945, the department serviced 708 outpatients and 56 inpatients.[88] All available statistics and numbers reported from the MCH clinics, into the postwar period, show a similar trend, marking a shift in women's preference for a sterile, professional environment rather than their own homes.[89] In other words, these numbers show a gradual medicalization and institutionalization of childbirth in wartime Chongqing. They likely also reflect social valorization of motherhood as a woman's most important life role, suggesting that family members believed that a woman's own ailments did not justify medical costs, but the arrival or care of a new child did.

Disaggregating female hospital attendance from widespread resistance to new medical practices is challenging. Women who knew about infectious diseases, or whose wealth and social status made them inclined to patronize a maternity hospital as a form of conspicuous consumption, might have accounted for this spike in visits to the Chongqing Municipal Hospital. Wealthy mothers around the country preferred to give birth in hospitals and clinics "instead of at home attended by what they considered unlearned and unclean traditional midwives," with annual attendance at one women's hospital reaching nearly twelve thousand on the eve of the war in 1937.[90] Wartime Chongqing certainly did have enough wealthy women to account for the sudden interest in the city's first large MCH facility.

These included women such as Zhang Rongzhen, who came from a large middle-class family (with five sons and three daughters) in Shanghai. In 1938 she and her newly betrothed husband moved to Chongqing along with a family servant. A "new woman," Zhang had attended a mission school and joined the girls' volleyball team before entering Shanghai's music conservatory, where she studied choral singing. Once she arrived in Chongqing, she performed as a soloist at a big fund-raising event for the NACWCWRS, affirming her place among middle-class wives whose contribution to the war effort took the shape of financial donations rather than sending family members to battle.[91] Her husband worked a short while in a factory in the city that produced medical equipment for the military. However, the intensity of the Chongqing air raids in this early period scared the family into hiding in Geleshan, living off savings and pawned jewelry until they had nothing left and chose to return to occupied Shanghai. Roughly one year before they left, Zhang Rongzhen gave birth to their first child, and she chose a small hospital with a famous physician recommended by a friend.[92]

Chongqing had many private midwifery clinics that an expectant mother of means could choose from. Dozens of specialists in obstetrics, gynecology, and children's medicine advertised their services in the *Dagongbao*, Chongqing's largest, twice-daily newspaper. These included private midwifery clinics, such as those of Drs. Zhang Lianghui, Zhang Yaoxian, Liang Guifang, and Li Shiwei.[93] Other doctors advertised women's and children's medicines (*fuke, xiao'erke*) as specialties without mentioning parturition, including Chinese medicine doctors Zhao Fengqiao and Wang Liujie, and scientific medicine doctors Yang Tingmei, Wang Lanfang, Zheng Tuixian, Li Shifang, Huan Shi'an, and Liang Zheng.[94] Some of these doctors may have made house calls, since their advertisements did not always list a clinic address. Other doctors mentioned particular hospitals, such as Drs. Chen Yuanchao and Chen Hui at the Red Cross Hospital, and female doctor Lu Jin, who had been head physician at the National Central Midwifery Hospital in Nanjing.[95] Some advertisements added to a doctor's prestige by listing his or her overseas education, but public letters of gratitude constituted the most special category of medical advertisement. A letter published twice in January 1943 honored children's doctor Tang Shaoqian.[96] Another praised Chinese medicine doctor Wu Huaibai for curing a little boy who at age four contracted a serious illness that many other doctors of both Chinese and scientific medicines had not been able to treat. Dr. Wu, on the other hand, possessed "the power to bring [the boy] back to life" (*you huitian zhili*) and cured him in a short time.[97] The director of the Central Institute of National (Chinese) Medicine, Jiao Yitang, wrote a letter thanking Dr. Zhou Muying for treating his wife's ovarian tumor. He likened Dr. Zhou, head physician of obstetrics and gynecology at National Central Hospital, to legendary physician Hua Tuo of the late Han dynasty, writing, "[W]ithout a doubt she is Hua Tuo come back to life, such is her mastery in women's medicine."[98]

These stories of midwifery in Chongqing, Bishan County, and Xinglong reveal two key things: that the war brought new medical services to Sichuan, and that women played a central role in spreading those services. Like Hua Tuo reincarnate, female midwives possessed the right skills to inspire awe and confidence, which proved essential to gaining the trust of people who believed cosmological rather than bacterial forces to be at the root of illness. As midwives they needed to gain the trust of women first and foremost, and the fact that women had always played a central role in community health (usually home based rather than clinic based) aided them in this regard.[99] Young midwives with training at elite educational institutions could introduce new, sterile practices without upsetting local gender dynamics, though they did challenge the power of elderly *jieshengpo*. While in Chongqing they performed most deliveries in hospital, in the Bishan County Health Center most births occurred at home, and in Xinglong village every woman gave birth at home.

Comparative analysis also reveals a gradation of medicalization wherein rural areas required medical professionals to make the greatest amount of adaptation to local preferences. This owed not to a failure of villagers to be adequately accepting of new medical practices, but rather to a success of villagers and their medical providers alike, who accommodated one another's preferences and found common ground on which to stand together. Yang Chongrui documented some of the adaptations made by the roughly two thousand women who graduated each year from fifty-five schools in twenty-six provinces across China. Yang reported that "ancient customs helped us most, and we observed all of them," citing the opening of something in the room (a door, clothing trunk, or box) to smooth the passage of the child into the world, and preparation of a special meat dumpling "with the dough ends pinched together" on the twelfth day after childbirth to ensure the mother's complete recovery.[100] Through the vernacularization of praxis—the application of aseptic midwifery in the traditional setting of the parturient woman's home and the adoption of local customs to ease the mother's mind—midwives and mothers saved lives and gradually changed their relationships to each other and to childbirth itself.[101]

CREATING MOTHERS OF THE NATION: DR. YANG CHONGRUI'S WARTIME WRITINGS

Yang Chongrui did not serve continuously as head of the Maternal and Child Health Department at the National Institute of Health (NIH). She spent some time furthering her studies in the United States, fulfilled Song Meiling's demand that she work with war orphans, and briefly resigned from her post in protest of the appointment of a man she interpreted as a political lackey (Zhu Zhanggeng, or C. K. Chu) as director of the NIH.[102] However, throughout these interruptions she maintained a continuous presence in the field as an author. Dr. Yang wrote no less than six texts during the war: *Diyi zhuchan xuexiao shi zhounian jinian kan* (The First National Midwifery School tenth-anniversary memorial publication; 1939); *Zhongguo fuying weisheng guoqu yu xianzai* (The past and present of maternal and children's health in China; 1940); *Fuying weisheng gaiyao* (An outline of maternal and children's health; 1943); *Zhufu xuzhi: Jiating weisheng ji jiazheng gaiyao* (What a housewife must know: An outline of family hygiene and home economics; 1934, 1940, and 1943); *Fuying weisheng xue* (The study of maternal and children's health; coauthored with Wang Shijin; 1944); and *Fuying weisheng jiangzuo* (Lectures on maternal and children's health; 1945). Her work also reached a broad audience: individual lectures from this last book appeared, from January to December 1944, in serial format in *Funü Xinyun* (Women's New Life Movement), a monthly journal published in Chongqing.[103] While working at the NIH, she simultaneously served as technical expert on aseptic midwifery to the NHA and to the League of Nations Health Organization.[104]

A close examination of Yang Chongrui's wartime writings reveals several key aspects of new-style midwifery, including the reaffirmation of conventional gender roles. In her preface to the second edition of *Zhufu xuzhi*, a general home-economics text originally published by the NHA in 1934 and republished in 1940 and 1943, Dr. Yang premised the book on the idea that women contributed to the nation primarily as homemakers. She wrote, "[P]ersonal health begins with the body, but environmental sanitation, health education, maternal and children's health, school health, and so forth all rely upon the housewife for promotion and implementation. Therefore, in pursuing public health, the training of mothers is a crucial duty." Yang defined personal health as an individual's responsibility, and public health—the health of the national community—as the responsibility of housewives. Put in concrete terms, mothers bore the primary responsibility of "fostering national-racial consciousness" (*guojia minzu guannian*) in their children.[105]

Dr. Yang also reinforced traditional gender roles by asserting the usefulness of man and the uselessness of woman. She began the section on families and economic prosperity with the declaration that "[i]n China, men are more highly valued because they contribute to the family's economy, while women spend the

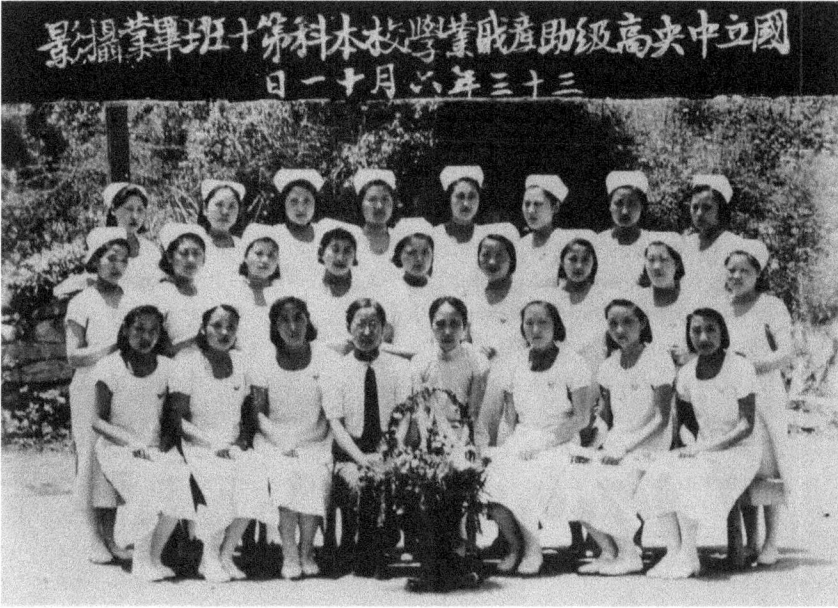

FIGURE 28. Dr. Yang Chongrui (Marion Yang) with the 1944 graduating class of midwives in Chongqing. Box 83, folder "NHA and Nursing." ABMAC Records. Rare Book and Manuscript Library. Columbia University.

majority of their time taking care of the children and thus cannot become productive workers and consumers."[106] This equation stood even though it contradicted the ideological premise of the entire book: that a mother's work in the home is the very foundation of a healthy nation. Moreover, she wrote that a mother must raise her children to be financially independent and thus able to contribute to the national economy, making child-rearing itself economically productive, but she did not directly acknowledge this fact in her text.[107] Yang also blamed wives for overstraining their husbands by having too many children, as if wives faced no pressure from the greater family to procreate but made unilateral decisions to get pregnant repeatedly on their own (though she neglected to explain how such an immaculate conception could occur). Despite describing housewives as a useless strain on the family, Yang charged them with responsibility over all matters pertaining to the health of all family members, including everything from food safety and regular bowel movements to avoiding public napkins and teacups so as to guard against contagion of tuberculosis, trachoma, and "venereal disease." This led to the conclusion that a family's weakness all originated with an ignorant housewife, and that only an educated and (re)trained housewife could strengthen the family.[108] Yang's attitude accorded with that of home economists, who "viewed management of Chinese homes (domesticity) as central to national concerns."[109] In other words, Yang outlined the duties of "mothers of the nation" and reinforced the idea that a mother's sphere of influence extended far beyond her own home to encompass the entire "national family" (*guojia*), even as she described housewives as profligate idlers.

Yang Chongrui's other texts offer some clues for resolving this apparent contradiction between a housewife presumed ineffectual in her own home while simultaneously carrying the weight of the entire nation. Simply stated, her writings betray her class prejudice. Like other highly educated middle-class women, particularly those who had traveled or studied abroad, Yang believed that she knew the proper way of doing things, that this way differed almost entirely from the manners of her poor compatriots, and that she therefore bore the responsibility of schooling them in "proper" behavior. This attitude had characterized the scholar-officials of imperial times as well as their descendants, the intellectuals of the May Fourth generation, and in the 1930s it found its best expression in the New Life Movement (NLM). As previously explained, middle-class ideals dominated the NLM and gave activists a source of self-righteous pride in transforming the poor into "self-respecting and worthwhile citizens."[110] In other words, Yang Chongrui and her fellow activists believed that lower-class housewives had the potential to deliver the nation to prosperity, but only once educated women had transformed their thinking and behavior patterns to conform to middle-class ideals.

This attitude appeared in a midwifery textbook that Yang coauthored with Wang Shijin, a public health lecturer in the National Central Midwifery School (NCMS). First published in Chongqing in 1944, and again in Nanjing in 1947, *Fuying weisheng xue* (The study of maternal and children's health) originated with a request from the Ministry of Education's Medical Education Committee for a suitable textbook for the NCMS. This project addressed the great need for textbooks that schools in Free China experienced during the war, and replaced a 1943 text that Dr. Yang had written for that purpose but believed inferior, *Fuying weisheng gaiyao* (An outline of maternal and children's health).[111] Given that it was designed to serve as the primary textbook for the central government's own midwifery school, *Fuying weisheng xue* provides a good snapshot of contemporary political ideology and how it inflected the original goal of diminishing maternal and infant mortality toward strengthening the nation and race. The very first lines in the book illustrate this dynamic:

> Maternal and children's health is an important part of public health. It utilizes science and technology to implement health and sanitation for neonates, infants, and young children. . . . It prevents diseases, promotes health, lowers mortality, ensures the complete physical and emotional health of the next generation, and promotes a healthy physique in the entire nation-race [*minzu*].[112]

This formulation completely effaced the women themselves, transforming them into ovaries and uteruses designed to carry the next generation into a healthy and prosperous future. While a mother may appear to be at the center of motherhood, "she is often evacuated from this position by a discursive focus on the child."[113] Moreover, the discursive focus on the child-as-nation and child-as-race constitutes a double evacuation, since the child in utero is already displaced from his or her own existence and representative of—and physically responsible for the health of—the entire nation and race, even before its birth.

The story from Sichuan's Bishan County illustrates how the double evacuation of women and children from their life-meaning could occur alongside life-affirming practices. Recall that in the small town of Xinglong, foreign and Chinese volunteers from the National Christian Council launched a variety of social welfare projects. They performed local surveys, taught adult literacy classes in the church, opened an aseptic midwifery clinic, and planned a salt cooperative to provide affordable salt to the local community. None of their work proceeded without the explicit approval of local members of the well-established secret society, the Paoge ("Robed Brothers"), and because the salt cooperative threatened the society's profits in black market salt, one influential man shut everything down. Everything, that is, except for the midwifery clinic. Because the work of the midwife did not challenge but affirmed local patriarchy, and because she had demonstrated to the fathers that she could keep their wives and infants alive through complicated deliveries, the midwife alone continued her work after this disastrous social conflict.[114] Aseptic midwifery simultaneously protected women's and children's lives and affirmed patriarchy, and it therefore survived the demise of all other social work in Xinglong. Likewise, Yang Chongqrui and Wang Shijin wrote in this manner because they were describing their own social reality in a culture that placed so much emphasis on children that women appeared absent from their own physical experiences, and so much emphasis on the nation's future that children were absented from their own childhoods.

Yang and Wang also lay bare their devotion to science, writing that between the childbearing ages of fifteen and forty-five, women "require the work that personnel trained in professional, scientific medicine and technology can perform in order to protect their health."[115] This formulation empowered not women, but scientifically trained personnel, who treated the parturient woman as a *patient,* with the Chinese term meaning literally "sick person" (*bingren*).[116] The use of this term clearly signaled the medicalization of childbirth, and constituted a not-so-veiled critique of all elderly midwives who had not undergone retraining to learn aseptic techniques. In this manner, while maintaining the overall focus on saving women's and children's lives and improving their health, MCH professionals, compelled by a love of science, utilized a means of achieving this goal that could easily have been more disempowering than empowering to an expectant mother, particularly for those who preferred to labor at home with the aid of a *jieshengpo* respected in the community.

The authors described both women and children as in a compromised state, in constant danger of contracting life-threatening diseases, and therefore in need of "professional science and technology" to step in for their own "relatively weak immune systems" and save them from puerperal fever or lifelong gynecological disorders, and their offspring from neonatal tetanus or conjunctivitis.[117] In this sense wartime discourse on MCH mirrored the Song-dynasty argument of women ruled by blood and inherently weaker than men—a medical discourse that male physicians had challenged in the Ming and Qing dynasties.[118] In a discussion on menstrual health in *Zhufu xuzhi,* Yang advised menstruating women, "[T]o care for your nerves, do not read overly stimulating texts or picture books so as to avoid arousal. One must also endure and control the excitement of romantic feelings (since during this period it is easiest to be overstimulated, making one's happiness, anger, sorrow, and joy abnormal)."[119] By depicting women as particularly volatile and prone to emotional abnormalities during menses, Yang recycled centuries-old notions of female weakness and refuted more recent challenges thereto.[120]

In other ways Yang Chongrui was fully embedded in her era. Like other intellectuals coming of age in the early twentieth century, she believed so fully in the power of science and its indispensable tool—data—that she exhibited a "passion for facts" and a certainty that all successful work began with gathering statistics.[121] In their textbook, Yang and Wang backed their depiction of the dangers of childbirth with statistics on maternal and infant mortality. Citing first the NHA estimates for China with which this chapter opened, they then compared their own country with 1926–36 data from "other countries with advanced health," including Australia, Austria, Chile, England, Wales, France, Italy, Japan, New Zealand, Scotland, Spain, Sweden, Germany, and the United States. They then referenced the argument of an Englishman in order to affirm their claim that high mortality eroded the foundation not only of individual families, but of the entire nation and race.[122] In addition to painting China as "Europe *manqué,*" Yang Chongrui and Wang Shijin used this international comparison to leverage their position as MCH specialists who spent their days worrying about how to save mothers and newborns from premature deaths.[123] This framing also demonstrated that Yang and Wang paid close attention to the worldwide discussion of MCH and saw themselves as contributors thereto. As such it further legitimized their own role as specialists and impressed upon student readers the idea that China needed to "catch up" to the "advanced" countries in order to be considered part of the civilized world. In the authors' view, this process began with women and children—or, stated more honestly, with professionals such as themselves teaching women and children how to behave. Thus they argued that, just as a house needs a solid foundation, the nation needs a base of strong women and healthy children in order to build its future prosperity. This required "improving racial health" by conducting premarital examinations to determine the genetic fitness of a couple; if either partner was determined to be a carrier of a contagious disease, then, the authors declared, "we can encourage them not to marry or sterilize them." Yang and Wang resorted to eugenics in order to establish the importance of MCH to "strengthening nation-building and establishing a healthy racial family" (*zengqiang guojia jianshe, shuli jianquan jiazu*).[124]

Pithy texts such as this can easily obfuscate the authors' true intentions. In an era of heightened ideology and propaganda, people often learn to couch their arguments in fashionable clichés, regardless of their own feelings about the subject.[125] Intelligent use of politically permitted metaphors and culturally approved analogies can win adherents to a health policy or medical practice far more readily than can resisting the demands of the day. Therefore, Yang Chongrui and Wang Shijin's copious discussion of the nation and race in a textbook written at the behest of a central government agency does not necessarily preclude the possibility of a female-empowering project—by and for women—masquerading as a nation-empowering one. Nonetheless, Yang and Wang likely did believe in eugenics, or *youshengxue,* the "study of optimal birth." A popular ideology in Republican China, eugenics merged with the earlier concept of fetal education (*taijiao*) to stress the pregnant or parturient woman's vulnerability and imperfection, as well as the idea that her responsibility as mother began with conception rather than birth.[126] But while fetal education drew on Confucian morality to reinforce a mother's central importance in the creation of life, here the authors used science as a lever with which to unseat women from their own birthing process.

In addition to their belief in eugenics, Yang and Wang clearly wished to empower the state in its role as health provider. The promise of state medicine had charmed nearly all health professionals by the early twentieth century, and since the Japanese assault made the achievement of a powerful Chinese state not only a cultural and political goal but also a military and economic imperative, few dared to speak out against state medicine in the war years.[127] Thus, our two authors argued that MCH workers wove a veritable red carpet upon which the state could march into people's homes:

> Improving mothers' and children's health can be the way inside the homes of the people whom we wish to touch with other health measures. For example, the work that is involved in educational propaganda, moral cultivation, and other health work, such as epidemic prevention and environmental hygiene, can be brought before the people smoothly and effectively by mothers' and children's health workers who have earned the housewives' trust.[128]

This framing both legitimized MCH as a potent tool for extending state power and affirmed the link between health work and central governance. The authors assumed the voice of the state when they referenced "people whom we wish to touch with other health measures." This points to an unavoidable dynamic of twentieth-century health activism. No one, not even Rural Reconstruction activists, could do effective work without the support of the state, yet inviting state support required rendering themselves and their work legible to male politicians who prioritized the state's needs. Thus, motherhood and childbirth had to bear upon state building, national salvation, and social reform in order to gain political legitimacy and state funding.[129]

In other words, in order to gain a place for themselves in the professional world, public health nurses and MCH workers had to channel state power into the home, but in so doing they extended the power of state patriarchy into spaces that had previously belonged to the family patriarch (the home and the womb). In effect they transferred power over women's wombs and their issue from individual men of the family to the male collective of the state, all while preserving gender hierarchy. The assertion that caring for the family constituted service to the greater collective squared with home economists' esteem for women's domestic work as a cornerstone of a strong nation. Moreover, treating families as "legitimate targets for public reform" allowed professional women—home economists, nurses, and midwives alike—to "[clear] the way for a smoother operation of state power."[130] In this way, both home economics and MCH paralleled general public health work in linking individual units—such as the nuclear family and the individual body—to the collective nation and race. Yet the manner in which they arrived at this goal affirmed the goals of state patriarchy and robbed them of any opportunity for true gender equality.

The last line in this passage indicates the most crucial issue in aseptic midwifery: the authors placed their own faith in, and asked state officials to believe in, health workers who had "earned the housewives' trust." Trust was the fulcrum on which all the work of strengthening the race and building the nation rotated. As with nurses whose tender healing touch transformed irate soldiers into willing fighters, young midwives equipped to perform the emotional labor of "earn[ing] the housewives' trust" served as a proxy of the masculinist, necropolitical state in the most intimate moment in the life of a woman and child: birth. By entering a woman's home and body, a young midwife trained in aseptic techniques accomplished a triplicate task: securing the lives of the mother and child even as she opened them to the discursively life-negating effects of state control and severed their relationship to well-known elderly midwives in their community. As long as the pregnant woman trusted her and focused on the first of the three goals, a midwife's labor could multiply to produce an outcome that far exceeded the event and space of childbirth. Like military nurses, midwives simultaneously affirmed and denied life (though in the latter case the denial hinged on discursive evacuation from life meaning, rather than augmenting a direct threat to physical safety).

The centrality of trust in women's health care echoes its centrality in the making of scientific meaning. Trust did more than empirical evidence to solidify faith in science, at least for seventeenth-century natural philosophers in England, and the same principle operated in wartime midwifery: a trusted midwife like Zhu Xiuzhen, who respected rather than upset local custom, experienced a sudden explosion in demand for her previously ignored services. In other words, just as seventeenth-century Englishmen gained access to the status of truth maker in the early days of science by adhering to codes of gentlemanly conduct so as to be perceived as trustworthy, the empirical evidence that young midwives could save lives was not interpreted as such until they had gained the trust of the community.[131]

Once young midwives and public health nurses gained a trusted status within a given microcommunity in China (a network of villages or an urban network like that of Zhang Rongzhen, whose members recommended trusted physicians to each other), their work proceeded smoothly. This was the foundational principle of the barefoot doctor program, in which young people who already had the respected status of the peasant class in Maoist China worked in their own communities.[132] Likewise, the health work in Dingxian and other model sites rested on community members' trust of the people offering the otherwise foreign services, and the most successful activists fully understood this principle. Zhou Meiyu's public health nurses ate and slept with the people they served and deputized schoolchildren to recruit their family members to vaccination drives. Chen Zhiqian carefully selected the people who taught village health workers out of recognition of the importance of trust. He wrote in his memoir, "I was well aware that the success of the training program depended not only on what was taught but also on the personality of the teacher . . . [because] mutual respect and confidence must be developed on an individual basis."[133]

The role of trust in establishing scientific "truth" also offers a clue for unraveling the failure of spreading aseptic midwifery in Dingxian, the same place where general public health work resulted in resounding success. In Chen Zhiqian's reporting, midwifery reform "was impeded by prevailing social attitudes and economic conditions," of which he cites mothers-in-law's insistence that their daughters-in-law give birth at home (even if the latter were willing to go to the clinic), and local midwives' resistance to retraining classes. Yet Chen directed his incisive analysis of the cultural effects of "social attitudes" only at the villagers, and not at himself or his coworkers. In contradistinction to his frequent declarations of admiration for the villagers, he described the elderly *jieshengpo*—who, it must be emphasized, had gained that title by earning the trust of their community members—as "ignorant old women," betraying his utter lack of respect for them and their place in local society. They responded in kind; they "resented the young, unmarried woman we selected as the trainer . . . [and] regarded her as an inexperienced upstart." As "an outsider of only twenty-five years of age," the trainer could not gain the status of "a trustworthy person." The reformers eventually learned to gain elder midwives' trust by training one of their own young family members, who "would receive the older woman's support in her new role"; but they could not ensure that these young women had enough time to devote to midwifery, so even that innovation failed.[134] In the end, the very reformers who understood the necessity of trust "themselves had a hard time trusting midwives," and the work of promoting aseptic midwifery constituted a notable failure in Dingxian.[135] They also faltered in reforming marriage practices, and in the analysis of Kate Merkel-Hess, both failures resulted from the fact that villagers experienced the attempts to change childbirth and marriage practices as an effort "to trample [their] power and expertise," so they resisted mightily.[136]

CONCLUSION

In 1929, in his capacity as the first vice minister of health, Liu Ruiheng (Dr. J. Heng Liu) expressed a hope for "the gradual extinction of old-style midwives and the substitution for them by the modern-trained."[137] From the perspective of modernizing health officials, wholly wedded to germ theory and committed to using this knowledge to fulfill what they deemed their responsibility to the public, the war constituted a dangerous interruption of lifesaving work. Yet the threat of conquest brought the discursive meaning of motherhood to the fore. Charged with mothering the nation, women came under special scrutiny as the targets of social and political reform. Both MCH workers and state officials believed that childbirth and motherhood should be performed in a specific fashion that adhered to the tenets of germ theory and middle-class values. This aligned MCH with the broader aims of public health and enlisted midwives and orphan relief workers in the project of creating not just healthy but also dutiful citizens. The war pushed people to prioritize the needs of the national collective and treat individual men, women, and children as possessions of state and society. This manifested itself in efforts to put orphans in the battlefield, Yang Chongrui's writings on scientific midwifery, and statements such as that of British-educated physician Sze Szeming (Shi Siming), who expressed regret that Song Meiling had gone to the United States in late 1944 with the claim that "[s]he belongs to China and should be with her husband."[138] As the foremost shaper of Chinese midwifery, Dr. Yang had a powerful influence on her readers. Dr. Sze's opinions also mattered. As personal secretary to Foreign Minister Song Ziwen (T. V. Soong) during the war, Washington, DC–based staff member of the United Nations Relief and Rehabilitation Administration (UNRRA) after the war, and one of the three men who engineered the creation of the World Health Organization in 1948, Dr. Sze had a profound influence on Chinese statecraft and postwar global health.[139] In one sweeping statement he implied that marriage is a man's ownership of his wife and equated this conjugal possession to a country's proprietary relationship with its (female) head of state.

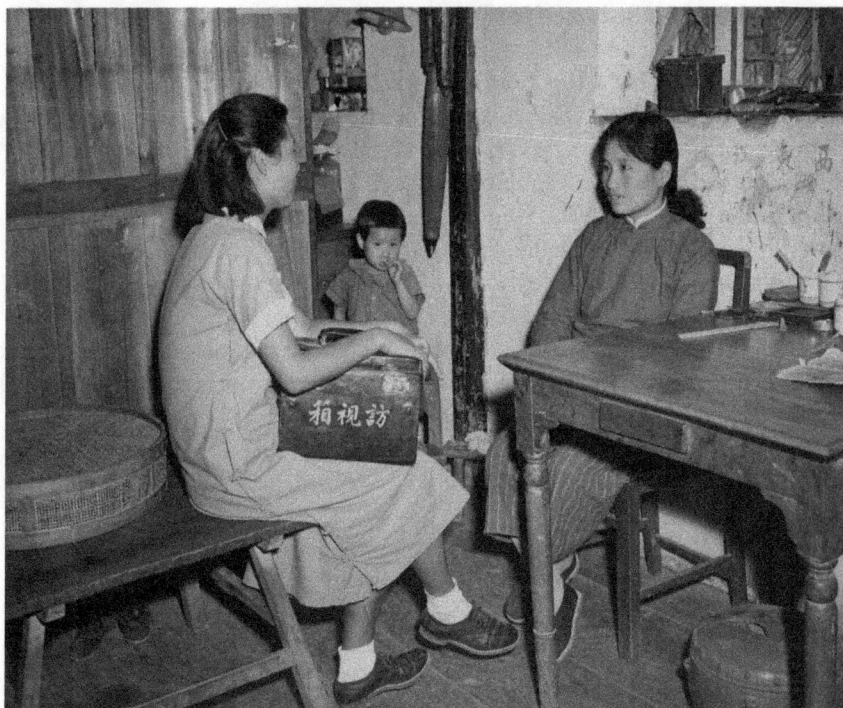

FIGURE 29. A visiting nurse instructs a mother in her home near Nanjing, late 1940s. Box 80, folder "Health Station Clinics." ABMAC Records. Rare Book and Manuscript Library. Columbia University.

Aside from the power of discourse, women's contributions to the national family through motherhood and midwifery exceeded the rhetorical. Women working in the field of Maternal and Child Health made notable achievements that saved the lives of birthing women and children across Sichuan Province, even in remote villages. Rural women actively chose aseptic midwifery once they recognized it as a lifesaving practice, and midwives' willingness to accommodate to rural culture made this resource available to them. In the village of Xinglong, midwife Zhu Xiu-zhen patiently cultivated her relationships with local women, whose absolute trust she needed in order to do her job. At the same time, midwives' status as women working in a traditionally female field allowed them access to private homes. They therefore became indispensable servants in the mutually reinforcing projects of enveloping the southwest into the national body and introducing state power into the home.

A photograph of a traveling public health nurse visiting a young mother in her home near Nanjing in the late 1940s documents a continued need for trust in medical encounters, as well as a postwar continuation of women's role in state-sponsored, home-based care. (See figure 29.) While the facial expressions and body language of mother and child suggest a measure of shyness and trepidation, the nurse sits comfortably across from the mother in a posture that implies humility, with a "house-call box" (*fangshi xiang*) perched on her lap. The photo tells us nothing of the words that they exchanged, but does show mother and nurse in similar attire, apparently deep in conversation. This photograph was taken a few years before Yang Chongrui, who had long worked with and in the Nationalist government, acquired the status of political pariah while her most talented student, Lin Qiaozhi, became the beloved, iconic heroine of modern midwifery in the People's Republic.[140] With this apparently smooth transition from one representative leader to the next and one state regime to another, the work of promoting aseptic midwifery continued in intimate encounters inside women's homes across China.

Conclusion

During wartime, the best way that a woman can properly and satisfactorily serve her country is through nursing. I believe that this is the most noble profession that a woman can undertake at any point in her life.

—TRANSLATED ARTICLE IN *FUNÜ GONGMING* (WOMEN'S ECHO), CHONGQING, DECEMBER 1944

Far from being a fringe issue of little importance during a pitched battle, a gendered history of civilian and military medicines during the War of Resistance elegantly narrates the making of modern China. It reflects the enduring obsession with hygiene as a central component of political sovereignty, cultural pride, and national modernity—an obsession that endured well after the war's end. Most importantly, by highlighting the duality of "Sick (Wo)Man" speak—and the centrality of the distinctly female "Sick Woman" in the story of modern China—it clarifies how a new national community formed when women took charge of instituting hygienic modernity on their own terms. As millions of refugees left their homes and soldiers marched to battle, traveling farther than ever before, they discovered their fellow Chinese in settings and contexts that they never would have experienced in peacetime. They tasted each other's cuisines, learned to understand other dialects, and began to follow similar sartorial fashions. Refugees who gathered in Sichuan and the greater southwest coupled their energy and expertise with foreign donations to create civilian and military medical systems out of collaborative efforts. Military and public health nurses played the most important role in rendering operable the donated dollars and newly built structures. Their labor of preserving life and limb cemented new relationships that formed the fabric of a national community born in the midst of fire, a community that enabled China to withstand the pressure of yet another war. Rather than tear asunder an already splintered country, the War of Resistance put enough pressure on Chinese society to form it into a durable structure, as surely as extreme heat transforms sand into glass.

When Chinese women undertook "the most noble profession" to serve as the caring arm of a state bent on organized killing, they joined a global choreography of military medicine.[1] Their story helps to unravel several puzzles of twentieth-century China's development. It explains, at least partially, the unexpected endurance of the Nationalist state during prolonged warfare. It furthermore helps to clarify the rapidity with which the Communists built functional state structures and established control of local society. The bonds of trust that people developed through wartime medical encounters, and the role that women played in the construction of the national community, help to explain the near-perfect adherence of contemporary China's political boundaries to those of the Qing empire. This endurance over the *longue durée* easily escapes notice because the short-term devastation was so wrenching. It has also escaped notice because it took place among the seldom examined: women and the unlettered in the inland provinces.

Theirs is not a heroic story of triumph, nor did all the hard work of the people whose stories appear in these pages come to any satisfactory conclusion in 1945. Quite the opposite; a national community needs continual remaking.[2] The abundant evidence that scholars have amassed of factional strife, regional prejudices, and self-serving and treacherous behavior before, during, and after the War of Resistance does not so much call into question the parallel process of making the national community as illustrate the salient need for that community in an era of constant conflict.[3] The war therefore placed both the Nationalist and Communist parties on a similar trajectory of development, one in which each had to "create a new social contract based on greater obligations between the state and the citizen."[4] For the Nationalists this process was most crucial in Sichuan, its wartime base and the country's rice bowl for the duration of the war.

Controlling Sichuan had never been easy, at least for nonlocals. Its place at the foot of the Tibetan Plateau made it a strategic location for attempting to control Tibetans throughout the Qing dynasty, though the province played a key role in ending that dynasty in 1911.[5] After this point, "no outside military or political force was able to govern all of Sichuan," and Chiang Kai-shek's "unification" of China in 1927 ironically left local leaders "stronger and freer from outside interference than they had ever been before."[6] Decades of internecine warfare between local militarists turned the province into a bloodbath.[7] Only the Nationalist government's westward move in 1938 enabled Chiang to lay claim to Sichuan's land and labor, especially after the most prominent warlord at the time, forty-seven-year-old Liu Xiang, had the courtesy to die a somewhat mysterious death from illness in January 1938.[8] Even then, as the story of rural reconstruction work in Bishan indicates, local power holders—members of the famous Paoge ("Robed Brothers") secret society—proved most formidable, particularly outside of Chengdu and Chongqing. Paoge rituals, liturgy, and origin story all celebrated a Han nativism that, in Sichuan, often manifested itself as strident localism.[9] Sichuan Paoge members frequently perceived fellow Chinese as outsiders, and in 1949–50 they led staunch resistance to the People's Liberation Army.[10]

Clearly, wartime health services did not do much to fuse a social contract between the people and the central state, at least in Sichuan. People in both Chengdu and the nearby village of Gaodianzi responded to news of the Communist takeover with great trepidation and gave the soldiers of both the turncoat Nationalist-cum-Communist General Deng Xihou and the actual PLA troops a very tepid welcome.[11] Local strongmen who had held power and commanded armies in the prewar years returned to postwar prominence, as if the war had done nothing to change the local power structure.[12] However, turning attention away from the power holders to the common people reveals that an increasing number of people—particularly in Chongqing and Chengdu, but also in other parts of the country—began during the war to understand central state officials less as an occupying force bent on maximum extraction of resources and more as a source of useful services. More importantly, they learned a new way of relating to one another in moments of bodily intimacy, personally experienced the exchange of care, and in some cases even learned to speak one another's dialects.[13]

This powerful affective attachment, embedded in the relationships people had developed with each other, unfolded in intimate medical encounters. In countless instances female health workers were the first to offer a message of respect for the human dignity of poor refugees, rural women, and wounded urbanites and soldiers. Their ability to deliver lifesaving services at the most vulnerable moments in people's lives—as they began labor with the fresh memory of a previous stillbirth, faced the possibility of losing life or limb to infection, suffered through third-degree burns from incendiary bombs, or pawned a family heirloom to buy medicine for their child—affirmed the affective ties that bound a nation primarily comprised of illiterate farmers. These encounters occurred in the interstices of life as well as in moments of miracle and misfortune—childbirth and death—and cemented the interpersonal bonds of the national community.

Discussions of hygienic modernity triggered an unrequited desire for the very type of modernity that defined Chinese bodies, in the language of Japanese imperialism, as always already inferior and deficient, and Chineseness as a "problem" to be solved or a limitation to be overcome. Once the term *eisei/weisheng* existed as "hygienic modernity" (which Ruth Rogaski pinpoints as the year 1900), even as other interpretations of the phrase circulated in discourse, no Chinese could escape the fate of being *not* "hygienically modern."[14] For the first three and a half decades of the twentieth century, the stinging pain of this realization led people of all political stripes and medical training to fiercely debate the best path toward attaining the unattainable prize. Yet almost all of them belonged to one social class—that of the intellectual elite—and from this limited perspective they almost universally derided lower-class and poor Chinese as the true source of the "problem." Even when they attempted to reach the poor with a politics of empowerment, most elite Chinese did so from a distance, both physical and cultural.

It is therefore sweetly ironic that these predominantly male and universally elite reformers inadvertently backed their way into a solution: by creating a highly gendered discourse of hygienic modernity and reifying Woman as the keeper of tradition, bearer of healthy babies, and maker of a hygienic household, they invited actual women to play a powerful role in constructing a hygienically modern nation. When China faced its greatest threat of all—total war and the possibility of complete loss of sovereignty—women seeking simultaneously to uplift themselves and their country entered medical service and performed the low-paid, back-breaking, and often life-threatening labor of building the nation, one relationship at a time. True national strength was born when these women dared to touch and physically heal the "unhygienic" bodies of soldiers, refugees, and the rural poor.

Just as creating a new standard of Asian civilization had been Japan's strategy for repelling Western imperialism and winning national autonomy, the pursuit of this new Asian standard—hygienic modernity—became China's winning strategy for repelling the Japanese invaders and achieving national strength. Yet it did not work well until women altered the terms of its practice. Trained to perform the emotional labor of suppressing certain emotions (such as disgust and anger) so as to produce others (such as patience and kindness), and thereby produce a positive response in their charges, female medical workers did not recoil from the signs of poverty or disdainfully deride the poor and diseased as the indelibly dirty embodiment of antimodernity. Instead they willingly touched their bodies, which touched their hearts.

That the Communists but not the Nationalists understood this adds an important emotional dimension to the story of modern Chinese politics. Unlike Nationalist rightists, who demonized and feared people who committed themselves to serving the poor, Communist officials promoted such behavior because it affirmed what is arguably the single most important tenet of international communism: the inherent humanity of poor people. Adding emotion to this analysis also informs a fresh understanding of the Chinese state and women's role therein. Many gender scholars have challenged the narrative of "feudal oppression" during all periods predating the Communist Party's victory and interrogated the claim that the party "liberated" Chinese women, establishing that the process was incomplete, deferred, and founded on a false narration of Chinese history.[15] This book furthers such scholarship by turning this formula on its head to ask not what the state did (or did not do) for women, but what women did for the state: specifically, how they created "new visions of gender" through wartime health work that shaped the modern Chinese state itself.[16]

Chinese women did not need the Communist state to liberate them. Rather, the Communists desperately needed women to enact their state-building projects, particularly as they "liberated" cities and desired immediate access to the intimate details of their residents: names, ages, occupations, and number of people in each household; stories of people's political pasts and likely alliances; reports of family finances and whether children were attending school. The new state promoted Li Dequan to Minister of Health (the first woman to hold this position), and at the grassroots level relied on women to deliver state services like relief for military personnel; "street sanitation, public hygiene, and immunization"; sewer dredging and street lamp repair; literacy classes; and scrap metal collection.[17]

The two cities where civilian women's work in the 1950s anchored regulatory control of the populace—Beijing and Shanghai—had enormous political and symbolic significance for the new Communist state. For five hundred years Beijing had been the capital of two imperial dynasties, with the massive imperial palace at its architectural and ritual center; in 1949 the state, purporting to deliver people from the shackles of "feudal society," wished to transform it into the capital of New China. As the infamous heartland of bourgeois decadence and chief center of Nationalist Party power, Shanghai had to be stripped of its moniker "Paris of the Orient" and motley crew of foreign residents. It is therefore telling that the Communist state mobilized women to establish control of these two cities' populations, and that public health work was an instrumental means by which women "proved an effective vehicle for the government to 'penetrate the masses'"[18] and "build the socialist grassroots governance"[19] in both metropolises.

These women performed a laundry list of tasks that closely mirrored that of the predominantly male baojia heads in the war period. In Beijing, "[w]omen were put in charge of the process of dismantling the old control system and instituting the new one," and by January 1953, women held 69 percent of the representative seats in the new residents' committees (juweihui) with which the Communist state replaced the baojia system.[20] They performed many key functions of the new state, including promulgating and explaining the 1950 Marriage Law, "mediating domestic disputes," organizing and hosting the celebration of International Women's Day, "organizing lectures on women's health and childcare practices," and conducting a variety of propaganda work, particularly during the Korean War (known in China as the War to Resist America and Aid Korea).[21] In Shanghai, women, organized into nearly four thousand residents' committees by 1952, served as direct liaisons between state officials and 85 percent of the city's population, or 4.21 million people.[22] These women—urban housewives—formed the personnel and structure of a "democratic government" that distinguished the Communist state from what it slyly labeled the Nationalists' "reactionary dictatorship." Their intimate work in quotidian encounters with their neighbors affirmed the legitimacy of the Communist state, helped to "establish effective state control over local society," and made the "socialist state appear humane in the eyes of the residents."[23]

Women in Beijing and Shanghai residents' committees accomplished the same work of intimacy that medical professionals had done during the war, soothing with their attentive care the rough disciplinary edges of the masculinist, necropolitical state. Not surprisingly, this type of work, of which public health work was a central feature, gave women "a space where they formed lasting personal relationships with residents." The women performed (or asked neighbors to perform) such tasks as "sterilizing sewer lids to prevent disease, setting up medicinal bonfires to kill mosquitoes, leading inspection teams to check residential cleanliness," recruiting people to public health campaigns, managing vaccination drives, and supervising street cleaning.[24] The responsibility for instituting urban hygienic modernity now lay firmly on the shoulders of women, and at least in postwar Beijing and Shanghai it worked much better than the masculinist system in wartime Chongqing. The distinction lay in the fact that, more than a simple domestication of public space, the postwar work enlisted women to continually reproduce national sentiment by bringing the emotional community of the family into the public space of the state, which "turned urban anonymity into semikinship."[25] This rested on the same principle of family making that had characterized the battlefield experience of so many women during the war, and the same construction of intimacy that had typified medical encounters in civilian hospitals and clinics.

Although the 1950s mobilization schemes followed what readers by now recognize as a well-worn script, Communist officials designated themselves the original revolutionaries by "charg[ing] that the Nationalist regime suppressed women by denying them a voice in politics and crushing their class-consciousness."[26] They were half right. The Nationalist state had faced the same pressure to supply state services under straitened circumstances and, like its successors would later do, had mobilized women to provide cheap labor. During the war, just as in the 1950s, some women cleverly maneuvered through a world tightly circumscribed by power structures that privileged men's values and found the means of seeking personal liberation therein.[27] These women had a (tightly controlled, heavily scripted) "voice in politics" during the war. The crucial difference lay in the fact that the Communists focused on mobilizing working-class women and thereby uplifting them as important members of the national community, whereas the Nationalists had marshaled women of all social strata but asked them to support a class structure that privileged middle-class values and lifestyles.[28]

The various failures in Chongqing, Bishan, Dingxian, and Zouping recounted in chapters 1, 2, and 5 underscore the importance of this distinction, since the difference between success and failure turns out to have been not so much about locale—rural versus urban—as about power and attitude. Rural Reconstruction activists adopted certain "habits of thought" that "reflected the broader ethos of blaming villagers' supposed backwardness on tradition rather than examining the ways reform agendas sat at cross-purposes . . . with local power structures," and therefore failed to effect change in marriage and childbirth practices in their model rural counties of Dingxian and Zouping.[29] The failure of all reform efforts in rural Bishan save the midwifery work that affirmed local patriarchs' desire for healthy children shows not only the necessity of obtaining local power holders' approval, but also that nurse Zhu Xiuzhen's patience with local women's reticence and her decision to let them take the lead paid off.[30] As argued in chapter 1, Nationalist state officials' insistence on employing public health regulation as a means of securing political sovereignty by disciplining the people to satisfy the foreign gaze as well as their own dreams of universalizing a middle-class lifestyle, rather than as a means of meeting the real needs of the people, led to multiple failures in Chongqing.

These microhistories of defeat in specific locales across China demonstrate the instrumentality of women's emotional labor in the history of healthcare. They indicate that if the recipient perceived a public health measure as a power play—an attempt either to outright deny her control over her own body or to define her behaviors as incorrect—she routinely resisted. If, on the other hand, a reform came without "preformed ideas about what was good, modern, and healthful"[31] and did not upset local power structures, a recipient could more readily perceive its promise of personal benefit and become an active participant therein. As long as women in the medical field inserted themselves into existing power structures— to support family patriarchy with safe childbirth, or state patriarchy with healthy soldiers, for example—they attained support from both the patrons and recipients of their work. On the other hand, if like Dean Vera Nieh they wished to use their authority for other means, men systematically blocked and belittled them.

There are two important lessons here. First, performing medical work during the war placed women at the center of the national story, but also decentered them from their own story. Most women labored under the assumption that their work earned its primary significance from its ability to serve the needs of the nation-state; in this respect it marked the triumph of a conservative gender ideology that forced women continually to place other people's needs before their own. It schooled women in governmentality, training them to bend their intimate care to the requirements of the state, and habituated them to consistent deferral of their own desires for the sake of the "real" revolution. Although many women escaped arranged marriages and gained education and employment, they also made personal sacrifices for their wartime careers. They accepted lower pay, status, and authority than the majority of their male colleagues. They lived far away from their families and exposed themselves to deadly risks on a daily basis, and quite a few of them died.[32] The fact that thousands of women routinely worked under such duress proves that they had the stamina to endure what many people at the time believed only men could endure; indeed, many women took pride in demonstrating their hardiness and believed it a means of proving their equality to men. Their work transformed the "Sick Woman" from the nation's problem into its strength and salvation, but in hitching themselves to the nation and anchoring their contribution in intimacy, they inadvertently contributed to and helped to solidify an iconic version of womanhood that inhibited women's liberation. Men writing in the 1980s backlash against socialist feminism expressed nostalgia for the archetypal woman that female medical professionals had partaken in crafting during the war: women, they argued, have "their own special charm, for example exquisiteness and depth of emotions."[33] They advised their female compatriots to "sacrifice themselves for the nation." They placed "men's masculinity" and "women's tenderness" neatly at two opposite poles of a gender binary and insisted that any movement on one end would automatically trouble the other.[34]

The second important lesson pertains to the intersectionality of gender and class. This book has argued that China's national community began to emerge when female medical professionals reached across social boundaries such as gender and class to develop intimate relationships, transforming strangers into friends. It has furthermore posited that Communists' celebration of this emotional labor, and Nationalist Party rightists' fear thereof, gave strength to the former in the Civil War. If the modern subject as national subject did not begin to take shape until women moved away from the masculinist state model to alter the terms of medical practice during the War of Resistance, perhaps mass mobilization of women in the 1950s to take the place of *baojia* heads was the requisite move to solidify the national community as an inclusive emotional community in the People's Republic. If this is the case, then any departure from inclusivity has the potential to weaken the Communist state. Examining the 1980s backlash against feminism with this in mind highlights the fact that it was just as much about middle-class men's dislike of working-class culture as about their dislike of "strong women who could outperform men," because the two go together. Among the agricultural working class, where a woman's brawn secures economic benefit, "there is no evidence that rural women and men have ever worried that women would be masculinized by performing physical labor," and many women continue to express pride in physical capabilities that their middle-class compatriots frequently deem undesirable in a woman.[35] From its founding in 1949 through the Cultural Revolution (1966–76), the Communist Party–state celebrated working-class culture and saturated public spaces with beautiful and emotionally evocative artistic representations thereof, creating a sensory experience that "was (and is) in practice and experience liked and enjoyed by many."[36] Beginning in the late 1970s, economic reforms made space for people to advocate a return to the normalization and privileging of middle-class aesthetics, as the Nationalists' New Life Movement had done decades prior. One way to think of the working- and middle-class aesthetics is as fuel for two distinct emotional communities, each anchored in a specific version of how a woman shows love for her family. In the former, a woman does so with her physical strength (which therefore makes her attractive), while in the latter a woman does so by retreating from public space to secure the domestic.[37] It is perhaps no accident that at the same time that neoliberal economic policies began harming China's working-class laborers, respectful representations of working-class definitions of beauty were subject to attack. These dual processes may have begun to erode the Communist Party's winning support of the victorious emotional community of inclusion. Multiple emotional communities operate in the same space-time, and no one can guarantee that the party *shuole suan* ("has the last word").[38]

This book cannot serve as the definitive study of women's role in medicine, in wartime or otherwise, so I end with a series of questions with the goal of inspiring further scholarship. How many women had to defy their families in order to get to the front lines, and what did this do to family structure? Did witnessing the failures and foibles of either political party up close influence women's own politics, and if such a shift took place, what role did it play in local and national politics? What happened to healthcare during the Civil War, when the briefly feminized profession once again accepted men into the fold for want of labor, and China witnessed an even greater increase in the numbers of registered midwives and nurses? How did treatment of soldiers' sexually transmitted diseases affirm or trouble the politics of intimacy? How or *did* nurses speak, to their loved ones or to the public, about their traumatic experiences of working on the front lines and in frequently bombarded cities? What language could they use to describe this experience in the Maoist period when political campaigns so sharply defined the available vocabulary, and no one could openly discuss having worked for the Nationalists? Did women speak privately—in diaries, letters, memoirs, or whispered conversations—about this experience, or simply hold it all inside, as did Yao Aihua (who upon finally encountering a journalist interested in her story after sixty-five years of silence admitted, "before, I never dared speak about the War of Resistance, not even with my own children. It wasn't honorable.")?[39] What happens to a woman's sense of self when she builds the very country that subsequently refutes her contributions?

NOTES

PROLOGUE

1. Agnes Smedley, *China Fights Back: An American Woman with the Eighth Route Army* (London: Victor Gollancz Limited, 1938), 23.

2. Ad placed in *Dagongbao*, nos. 13755 and 13759 (March 13 and 17, 1942). Many thanks to David Knight for his invaluable assistance with the translation.

INTRODUCTION

Yao Aihua, "Memoir of Yao Aihua," in Fang Jun, *Zuihou yi ci jijie* (The last concentration of troops) (Shenyang: Liaoning renmin chubanshe, 2012), 208.

1. Yao Aihua, "Memoir of Yao Aihua," 201–14, esp. 205.

2. Diana Lary, *Warlord Soldiers: Chinese Common Soldiers, 1911–1937* (New York: Cambridge University Press, 1985). From 1912 to 1928, more than thirteen hundred individuals qualified as warlords who commanded their own territory and fighting forces. See S.C.M. Paine, *The Wars for Asia, 1911–1949* (New York: Cambridge University Press, 2012), 18.

3. Odd Arne Westad calculates only two million military deaths and twelve million civilian deaths. Odd Arne Westad, *Restless Empire: China and the World since 1750* (New York: Basic Books, 2012), 248–49. Diana Lary uses pre- and postwar population estimates to calculate a population deficit of eighteen million. Diana Lary, *The Chinese People at War: Human Suffering and Social Transformation, 1937–1945* (New York: Cambridge University Press, 2010), 173.

4. This process was neither smooth nor simple. See, e.g., Neil J. Diamant, *Revolutionizing the Family: Politics, Love, and Divorce in Urban and Rural China, 1949–1968* (Berkeley: University of California Press, 2000).

5. The foundational work on emotional labor of women in the workforce focuses on American flight attendants. See Arlie Russell Hochschild, *The Managed Heart: Commercialization of Human Feeling* (Berkeley: University of California Press, 2003).

6. Stephen MacKinnon has called this "the greatest forced migration in Chinese history," perhaps echoing assessments of the Atlantic slave trade. Stephen R. MacKinnon, *Wuhan, 1938: War, Refugees, and the Making of Modern China* (Berkeley: University of California Press, 2008), 46–47.

7. Revenue had come from customs duties, the salt tax, and other commodity taxes in the highly populated and well-developed coastal regions that the Japanese army occupied. Lloyd E. Eastman, "Nationalist China during the Sino-Japanese War 1937–1945," in *The Cambridge History of China*, vol. 13, *Republican China 1912–1949, Part 2*, ed. John K. Fairbank and Albert Feuerwerker (Cambridge: Cambridge University Press, 1986), 584–85.

8. Chou Chun-yen, "Funü yu kangzhan shiqi de zhandi jiuhu" / "Women and battlefield first aid during the Second Sino-Japanese War," *Jindai Zhongguo funüshi yanjiu / Research on Women in Modern Chinese History* 24 (December 2014): 208–9; Sean Hsiang-lin Lei, *Neither Donkey nor Horse: Medicine in the Struggle over China's Modernity* (Chicago: University of Chicago Press, 2014), 130.

9. On women's public appearance as transgressive in the Republican era, see David Strand, *An Unfinished Republic: Leading by Word and Deed in Modern China* (Berkeley: University of California Press, 2011), 45, 121, 144–45; and Zhao Ma, *Runaway Wives, Urban Crimes, and Survival Tactics in Wartime Beijing, 1937–1949* (Cambridge, MA: Harvard University Asia Center, 2015), 280.

10. Interestingly, while in China in the 1930s public health nurses rose to prominence in the medical system, by the early 1930s in the United States, public health nurses had been sidelined in the field of healthcare that they had created. See Karen Buhler-Wilkerson, *False Dawn: The Rise and Decline of Public Health Nursing, 1900–1930* (New York: Garland Publishing, 1989); and Karen Buhler-Wilkerson, *No Place Like Home: A History of Nursing and Home Care in the United States* (Baltimore: Johns Hopkins University Press, 2001).

11. In his classic work on nationalism, Benedict Anderson cites print capitalism as the origin of national consciousness in Europe, and the intelligentsia as the instigators of Asian nationalisms. Benedict Anderson, *Imagined Communities: Reflections on the Origin and Spread of Nationalism*, 2nd ed. (London: Verso Press, 1991), esp. 37–46, 116. The specific quote is on p. 141.

12. This situation remains despite many outstanding works on rural China. Notable works include Gail Hershatter, *The Gender of Memory: Rural Women and China's Collective Past* (Berkeley: University of California Press, 2011); Isabel Brown Crook and Christina Kelley Gilmartin with Yu Xiji, *Prosperity's Predicament: Identity, Reform, and Resistance in Rural Wartime China*, comp. and ed. Gail Hershatter and Emily Honig (Lanham, MD: Rowman and Littlefield, 2013); Kate Merkel-Hess, *The Rural Modern: Reconstructing the Self and State in Republican China* (Chicago: University of Chicago Press, 2016); William T. Rowe, *Crimson Rain: Seven Centuries of Violence in a Chinese County* (Stanford, CA: Stanford University Press, 2007); G. William Skinner, *Marketing and Social Structure in Rural China* (Ann Arbor, MI: Association for Asian Studies, 1965); and Ralph A. Thaxton Jr., *Catastrophe and Contention in Rural China: Mao's Great Leap Forward Famine and the*

Origins of Righteous Resistance in Da Fo Village (Cambridge and New York: Cambridge University Press, 2008).

13. R. Keith Schoppa, *In a Sea of Bitterness: Refugees during the Sino-Japanese War, 1937–1945* (Cambridge, MA: Harvard University Press, 2011), 15, 135, 308–11.

14. Parks M. Coble, *China's War Reporters: The Legacy of Resistance against Japan* (Cambridge, MA: Harvard University Press, 2015), 36–37.

15. Lary, *Warlord Soldiers.* Warlords did not only devastate the people in their regions, however; they also sponsored many progressive modernization schemes. For examples in Sichuan, see Kristen Stapleton, *Civilizing Chengdu: Chinese Urban Reform, 1895–1937* (Cambridge, MA: Harvard University Asia Center , 2000).

16. Crook and Gilmartin, Prosperity's Predicament, 67, 77–78, 86.

17. Merkel-Hess, *The Rural Modern*, 4.

18. Prasenjit Duara, *Culture, Power, and the State: Rural North China, 1900–1942* (Stanford, CA: Stanford University Press, 1988), esp. 73–74. Duara restricted his study to North China, but other areas likely suffered from a similar process, particularly as warlords exacted heavy taxes to pay for their militaries.

19. Ara Wilson, "Intimacy: A Useful Category of Transnational Analysis," in *The Global and The Intimate: Feminism in Our Time,* ed. Geraldine Pratt and Victoria Rosner (New York: Columbia University Press, 2012), 46.

20. Barbara H. Rosenwein, "Worrying about Emotions in History," *American Historical Review* 107, no. 3 (June 2002): 842. See also Barbara H. Rosenwein, *Emotional Communities in the Early Middle Ages* (Ithaca, NY: Cornell University Press, 2006).

21. Eugenia Lean, *Public Passions: The Trial of Shi Jianqiao and the Rise of Popular Sympathy in Republican China* (Berkeley: University of California Press, 2007), 3–4.

22. Ibid., 89.

23. Ibid., 181–93, 210.

24. Haiyan Lee, *Revolution of the Heart: A Genealogy of Love in China, 1900–1950* (Stanford, CA: Stanford University Press, 2007), 16.

25. Norman Kutcher, "The Skein of Chinese Emotions History," in *Doing Emotions History,* ed. Susan J. Matt and Peter N. Stearns (Urbana and Chicago: University of Illinois Press, 2013), 67–68.

26. Lary, *Chinese People at War,* 4, 7, 16, 22, 38, 44, 56, 101.

27. The present work does not engage with the rich literature on the history of emotions in premodern China. See esp. the works of Paolo Santangelo, but also Dorothy Ko, "Thinking about Copulating: An Early-Qing Confucian Thinker's Problem with Emotions and Words," in *Remapping China: Fissures in Historical Terrain,* ed. Gail Hershatter, Emily Honig, Jonathan N. Lipman, and Randall Stross (Stanford, CA: Stanford University Press, 1996), 59–75. Nor, as a historian, do I engage as deeply with the work on emotions in Chinese literature. See esp. Halvor Eifring, ed., *Minds and Mentalities in Traditional Chinese Literature* (Beijing: Culture and Art Publishing House, 1999). Other key concepts of emotions history—Bill Reddy's "emotional regime" and "emotional refuge"—do not adequately fit the present work. See William M. Reddy, *The Navigation of Feeling: A Framework for the History of Emotions* (Cambridge: Cambridge University Press, 2001).

28. Stephen R. MacKinnon, Diana Lary, and Ezra F. Vogel, eds., *China at War: Regions of China, 1937–45* (Stanford, CA: Stanford University Press, 2007), esp. 12.

29. The highest estimate of six million Holocaust deaths is half that of China's most conservative estimate of twelve million civilian deaths. Donald L. Niewyk, *The Columbia Guide to the Holocaust* (New York: Columbia University Press, 2000), 421.

30. These calculations combine estimated military and civilian deaths, for the following totals: Japan, 1.74 million troops and approximately one million civilians (John Dower, *Embracing Defeat: Japan in the Wake of World War II* [New York: W. W. Norton, 1999], 45); British Empire, 580,500 (Commonwealth War Graves Commission, *Commonwealth War Graves Commission Annual Report, 2014–15*); United States, 405,399 (Bernard D. Rostker, *Providing for the Casualties of War: The American Experience through World War II* [Santa Monica, CA: RAND Corporation, 2013], 268); Soviet Union, twenty-six million, or according to some perhaps as many as forty-three to forty-seven million (Richard Overy, *Russia's War: A History of the Soviet Effort, 1941–1945* [London: Allen Lane, 1998], 5). Almost all tallies are gross estimates, but the general comparison between China's losses and those of other belligerent nations still stands.

31. Ruth Rogaski, *Hygienic Modernity: Meanings of Health and Disease in Treaty-Port China* (Berkeley: University of California Press, 2004), esp. 13–14, 137–38, 160, 164. Rogaski points out that late-Qing officials moved very quickly to indigenize hygienic modernity, copying colonial institutions and placing Chinese in positions of power (ibid., 186). This process occurred in colonial Korea as well; see Todd A. Henry, *Assimilating Seoul: Japanese Rule and the Politics of Public Space in Colonial Korea, 1910–1945* (Berkeley: University of California Press, 2014).

32. Hu Cheng, "The Modernization of Japanese and Chinese Medicine (1914–1931)," *Chinese Studies in History* 47, no. 4 (Summer 2014): 78–94, esp. 80–81; Paula Harrell, *Sowing the Seeds of Change: Chinese Students, Japanese Teachers, 1895–1905* (Stanford, CA: Stanford University Press, 1992).

33. Ann Janetta, *The Vaccinators: Smallpox, Medical Knowledge, and the "Opening" of Japan* (Stanford, CA: Stanford University Press, 2007), 177–78; Rogaski, *Hygienic Modernity,* 160, 163.

34. Iijima Wataru, "The Establishment of Japanese Colonial Medicine: Infectious and Parasitic Disease Studies in Taiwan, Manchuria, and Korea under Japanese Rule before WWII," *Aoyama rekishigaku* (Aoyama University historical studies), no. 28 (March 2010): 78.

35. Strand, *Unfinished Republic,* 172.

36. Rana Mitter, "Classifying Citizens in Nationalist China during World War II, 1937–1941," in "China in World War II, 1937–1945: Experience, Memory, and Legacy," special issue, *Modern Asian Studies* 45, no. 2 (2011): 243–75.

37. Helen M. Schneider, *Keeping the Nation's House: Domestic Management and the Making of Modern China* (Vancouver: University of British Columbia Press, 2011).

38. On how this occurred in Tianjin, see Rogaski, *Hygienic Modernity,* 187–92.

39. Ibid., 105, 165–92, esp. 175–76.

40. Tong Lam, "Policing the Imperial Nation: Sovereignty, International Law, and the Civilizing Mission in Late Qing China," *Comparative Studies in Society and History* 52, no. 4 (2015): 881–908.

41. Arif Dirlik, "The Ideological Foundations of the New Life Movement: A Study in Counterrevolution," *Journal of Asian Studies* 34, no. 4 (August 1975): 945.

42. Federica Ferlanti, "The New Life Movement at War: Wartime Mobilisation and State Control in Chongqing and Chengdu, 1938–1942," *European Journal of East Asian Studies* 11 (December 2012): 189.

43. Elizabeth J. Remick, "Introduction to the *JAS* at AAS Roundtable on 'Sexuality and the State in Asia,'" *Journal of Asian Studies* 71, no. 4 (November 2012): 919–27, esp. 921.

44. In this aspect women's wartime experience was similar to that of contemporary German women under the Nazi regime, though I contend that women in China had more room for their own agency. Claudia Koonz, *Mothers in the Fatherland: Women, the Family and Nazi Politics* (New York: St. Martin's Press, 1987).

45. Two maps, from 1937 and 1942, vividly illustrate this geographic shift. See "Distribution of Health Organizations in China, 1937" and "Distribution of Health Organizations in China, 1942," ABMAC archives, box 83, folder "NHA and Nursing," RBML.

46. Some scholars have asserted that the dynamism of the war period was largely limited to Chongqing. See Bridie Andrews, *The Making of Modern Chinese Medicine, 1850–1960* (Vancouver: University of British Columbia Press, 2014), 206; and Ka-che Yip, "Disease and the Fighting Men: Nationalist Anti-Epidemic Efforts in Wartime China, 1937–1945," in *China in the Anti-Japanese War, 1937–1945,* ed. David P. Barrett and Larry N. Shyu (New York: Peter Lang, 2001), 172. However, small health organizations built during the war had a seemingly outsized influence. See Nicole Elizabeth Barnes and John R. Watt, "The Influence of War on China's Modern Health Systems," in *Medical Transitions in Twentieth-Century China,* ed. Bridie Andrews and Mary Brown Bullock (Bloomington: Indiana University Press, 2014), 227–42.

47. On Lanzhou, Kunming, and Guiyang, see Mary Augusta Brazelton, "Vaccinating the Nation: Public Health and Mass Immunization in Modern China, 1900–1960" (PhD diss., Yale University, 2015); and John R. Watt, *Saving Lives in Wartime China: How Medical Reformers Built Modern Healthcare Systems amid War and Epidemics, 1928–1945* (Leiden: E. J. Brill, 2014).

48. Chou Chun-yen, "Funü yu kangzhan," 133; Schneider, *Keeping the Nation's House,* 172; Yang Shanyao, *Kangzhan shiqi de Zhongguo junyi* (China's military medicine during the War of Resistance) (Taipei: Academia Historica, 2015), 6.

49. Timothy Mitchell, "Society, Economy, and the State Effect," in *State/Culture: State-Formation after the Cultural Turn,* ed. George Steinmetz (Ithaca, NY: Cornell University Press, 1999), 81.

50. On homemaking, see Schneider, *Keeping the Nation's House.* On orphan relief, see M. Colette Plum, "Unlikely Heirs: War Orphans during the Second Sino-Japanese War, 1937–1945" (PhD diss., Stanford University, 2006).

51. Nicole Elizabeth Barnes, "Disease in the Capital: Nationalist Health Services and the 'Sick (Wo)man of East Asia' in Wartime Chongqing," *European Journal of East Asian Studies* 11 (December 2012): 286–87.

52. Song Meiling, telegram of August 2, 1937, quoted in Chou Chun-yen, "Funü yu kangzhan," 173.

53. Frank Dikötter, *The Discourse of Race in Modern China* (London: Hurst and Company, 1992), 98–101; Joan Judge, *The Precious Raft of History: The Past, the West, and the Woman Question in China* (Stanford, CA: Stanford University Press, 2008).

54. Gail Hershatter, "Making the Visible Invisible: The Fate of 'The Private' in Revolutionary China," in *Wusheng zhi sheng (I): Jindai Zhongguo de funü yu guojia (1600–1950)* (Voices amid silence (I): Women and the nation in modern China, 1600–1950), ed. Fangshang Lu (Taipei: Academia Sinica Institute of Modern History, 2003), 259.

55. On this process in India, see Partha Chatterjee, *The Nation and Its Fragments: Colonial and Postcolonial Histories* (Princeton, NJ: Princeton University Press, 1993), esp. 6–11 and chap. 6. On Japan, see Sharon H. Nolte and Sally Ann Hastings, "The Meiji State's Policy toward Women, 1890–1910," in *Recreating Japanese Women, 1600–1945*, ed. Gail Lee Bernstein (Berkeley: University of California Press, 1991), 151–74. On China, see Prasenjit Duara, *Sovereignty and Authenticity: Manchukuo and the East Asian Modern* (Lanham, MD: Rowman and Littlefield, 2003), esp. 131–69.

56. Duara, *Sovereignty and Authenticity,* 133; Judge, *Precious Raft of History,* 8.

57. Judge, *Precious Raft of History,* 115, 118.

58. Sarah Elizabeth Stevens, "Hygienic Bodies and Public Mothers: The Rhetoric of Reproduction, Fetal Education, and Childhood in Republican China," in *Mapping Meanings: The Field of New Learning in Late Qing China,* ed. Michael Lackner and Natascha Vittinghoff (Leiden: E. J. Brill, 2004), 659–84.

59. Helen Schneider articulates the effects of this most clearly in her examination of home economists in twentieth-century China. See Schneider, *Keeping the Nation's House.*

60. Qing, "Weilao fushang zhuangshi" (Comforting wounded heroes), *Funü shenghuo* (Women's lives) 8. no. 5 (December 1939): 15–16.

61. Watt, *Saving Lives,* 65–67, esp. 67.

62. Ranajit Guha argued that a historian must read colonial records "backwards" in order to interpret the actions of the colonized. For example, if colonial record keepers created precise calorie charts for recipients of famine relief, we can interpret not only that British scientific values dominated colonial works of charity, but also that Indian recipients had different ideas about diet and nutrition, which the colonizers attempted to alter with the imposition of precise measures. In such a manner we might interpret the image of low-caste Indians left to us in the "distorting mirror" of archival documents. Ranajit Guha, *Elementary Aspects of Peasant Insurgency in Colonial India* (Delhi: Oxford University Press, 1983), 333.

63. Essays in James L. Watson and Evelyn S. Rawski, eds., *Death Ritual in Late Imperial and Modern China* (Berkeley: University of California Press, 1988), identify "the existence of an agreed-upon normative sequence of funeral rituals . . . as central to Chinese identity" (x).

1. POLICING THE PUBLIC IN THE NEW CAPITAL

Khwaja Ahmad Abbas, *And One Did Not Come Back! The Story of the Congress Medical Mission to China* (Bombay: Sound Magazine, 1944), 63.

1. Quoted in Lloyd E. Eastman, "Nationalist China during the Sino-Japanese War 1937–1945," in *The Cambridge History of China*, vol. 13, *Republican China 1912–1949, Part 2,* ed. John K. Fairbank and Albert Feuerwerker (Cambridge: Cambridge University Press, 1986), 561.

2. Jeffrey N. Wasserstrom, *Student Protests in Twentieth-Century China: The View from Shanghai* (Stanford, CA: Stanford University Press, 1991), 16.

3. Quoted in Frederic E. Wakeman Jr., "Licensing Leisure: The Chinese Nationalists' Attempt to Regulate Shanghai, 1927–1949," in *Telling Chinese History: A Selection of Essays*, ed. Lea H. Wakeman (Berkeley: University of California Press, 2009), 222. Emphasis added. Ironically, the War of Resistance both curtailed and aided Chiang's negotiations of foreign treaties, since Japanese occupation of cities with foreign concessions made Chinese sovereignty a moot point, but China's new status as an ally during the Pacific War ultimately led the US Congress to end American extraterritoriality in China in December 1943.

4. Janet Y. Chen, *Guilty of Indigence: The Urban Poor in China, 1900–1953* (Princeton, NJ: Princeton University Press, 2012), 82–83, 116, 120; Zwia Lipkin, *Useless to the State: "Social Problems" and Social Engineering in Nationalist Nanjing, 1927–1937* (Cambridge, MA: Harvard University Asia Center, 2006), 12–15, 54, 86–87; Rebecca Nedostup, *Superstitious Regimes: Religion and the Politics of Chinese Modernity* (Cambridge, MA: Harvard University Asia Center, 2009), 36–37.

5. The treaty designating Chongqing a treaty-port city was signed in November 1890, but negotiations took years, and the local government secured a short, thirty-year concession period. When the treaty expired on September 4, 1931, local workers, students, and business-people organized a strike and blockaded the concession area, forcing the Japanese residents to flee the following month. Zhang Jin, *Quanli, chongtu, yu biange: 1926–1937 nian Chongqing chengshi xiandaihua yanjiu* (Power, conflict, and reform: The modernization of Chongqing, 1926–1937) (Chongqing: Chongqing Publishing House, 2003), 48–52.

6. CBPH Work Report, January–June 1940, CMA, 66-1-3, 176.

7. John R. Watt, *Saving Lives in Wartime China: How Medical Reformers Built Modern Healthcare Systems amid War and Epidemics, 1928–1945* (Leiden: E. J. Brill, 2014), 240.

8. CBPH Work Report, October 1946, AH, 90–183, 1; CBPH Work Report, December 1938, CMA, 66-1-2, 181, 188; Danke Li, *Echoes of Chongqing: Women in Wartime China* (Urbana and Chicago: University of Illinois Press, 2010), 89, 105. Some water pipes had been laid in the mid-1930s, but they never covered the whole city, and soon after the air raids began many of these pipes were destroyed. Mary Lee McIsaac, "The Limits of Chinese Nationalism: Workers of Wartime Chongqing, 1937–1945" (PhD diss., Yale University, 1994), 44. When the Nationalist government collaborated with the League of Nations Health Organization (LNHO) in 1929–30 to establish its own sovereign National Quarantine Service (NQS) with operations at major port cities, Chongqing was excluded because it had no extant service; however, the Shanghai headquarters of the NQS moved first to Wuhan and then to Chongqing during the war. See Ka-che Yip, *Health and National Reconstruction in Nationalist China: The Development of Modern Health Services, 1928–1937* (Ann Arbor, MI: Association for Asian Studies, 1995), 116–18. Between May 1939 and August 1940, Japanese planes bombed the following hospitals in Sichuan: Chongqing Red Cross Hospital (May 3, 1939); Canadian Mission Hospital dispensary in downtown Chongqing (severely damaged in 1939, then completely destroyed in 1940); Canadian Mission Hospital dispensary in Leshan (Fall 1939); Canadian Mission Hospital and two Chinese hospitals in Luzhou (September 11, 1939); Canadian Mission Hospital in Ziliujing (in October 1939, bombs fell directly on the men's wing of the hospital, killing three patients; on August 12, 1940, bombs destroyed the women's wing and severely damaged the men's wing); Women's Missionary

Society Hospital in Chengdu (May 8, 1940); Canadian Mission Hospital in Fuzhou (July 31, 1940). See the following records, all held at UCC: Mrs. Winifred Harris to Mrs. H. D. Taylor in Toronto, May 7, 1939, 83.058C, 61–11, ser. 5; A. Stewart Allen to Dr. Jesse H. Arnup, Secretary, Board of Foreign Missions, September 23, 1939, 1983.047C, 7–160; A. C. Hoffman, Gordon R. Jones, and James G. Endicott, "The Bombing of Luchow, Sichuan, China," September 1939, 1983.047C, 7–160; Loraine Edmonds to Dr. Arnup and Friends of the Mission Rooms' Staff, October 30, 1939, 1983.047C, 7–160; Gerald Bell to Jesse Arnup, May 8, 1940, 1983.047C, 8–165; Gerald Bell to Jesse Arnup, August 9, 1940, 1983.047C, 8–165; Gerald Bell to Jesse Arnup, August 16, 1940, 1983.047C, 8–165.

9. Kristin Stapleton, *Civilizing Chengdu: Chinese Urban Reform, 1895–1937* (Cambridge, MA: Harvard University Press, 2000), 4.

10. National Institute of Health, Public Health Calendar, 1943, NLM.

11. Sean Hsiang-lin Lei, "Habituating Individuality: Framing Tuberculosis and Its Material Solutions in Republican China," *Bulletin for the History of Medicine* 84 (2010): 248–79.

12. Omar L. Kilborn, *Our West China Mission: Being a Somewhat Extensive Summary by the Missionaries on the Field of Work during the First Twenty-Five Years of the Canadian Methodist Mission in the Province of Szechwan, Western China* (Toronto: Missionary Society of the Methodist Church, 1920), 224.

13. Mary Lee McIsaac, "The City as Nation: Creating a Wartime Capital in Chongqing," in *Remaking the Chinese City: Modernity and National Identity, 1900–1950,* ed. Joseph W. Esherick (Honolulu: University of Hawai'i Press, 1999), 175.

14. Robert A. Kapp, "Chungking as a Center of Warlord Power, 1926–1937," in *The Chinese City between Two Worlds,* ed. Mark Elvin and G. William Skinner (Stanford, CA: Stanford University Press, 1974), 152. See also McIsaac, "City as Nation," 177.

15. Han Suyin, *Destination Chungking: An Autobiography* (Boston: Little, Brown, and Company, 1942), 208–9.

16. Quoted in Frances Wood, *The Lure of China: Writers from Marco Polo to J. G. Ballard* (New Haven, CT: Yale University Press, 2009), 236.

17. Theodore H. White and Annalee Jacoby, *Thunder Out of China* (New York: Da Capo Press, 1946), 16.

18. Joseph Warren Stilwell, *The Stilwell Papers,* ed. Theodore H. White (New York: William Sloane Associates, 1948), 199–200.

19. Li, *Echoes of Chongqing,* 35, 52–53, 158–70.

20. Graham Peck, *Through China's Wall* (Boston: Houghton Mifflin, 1940), 157; R. de Muerville, *La Chine du Yang-tse* (Paris: Payot, 1946), 143.

21. Freddie Guest, *Escape from the Bloodied Sun* (London: Jarrolds, 1956), 161,

22. Kapp, "Center of Warlord Power," 151; Li, *Echoes of Chongqing,* 13, 117–19; Adet Lin, Anor Lin, and Meimei Lin, *Dawn over Chungking* (New York: John Day, 1941).

23. Peck, *Through China's Wall,* 164, 167.

24. McIsaac, "Limits of Chinese Nationalism," 40.

25. Luo Zhuanxu, ed., *Chongqing Kangzhan dashiji* (Grand record of Chongqing's War of Resistance) (Chongqing: Chongqing Publishing House, 1995), 21.

26. Diana Lary and Stephen MacKinnon, eds., *Scars of War: The Impact of Warfare on Modern China* (Vancouver: University of British Columbia Press, 2001), plate 8.

27. Edna Tow, "The Great Bombing of Chongqing and the Anti-Japanese War, 1937–1945," in *The Battle for China: Essays on the Military History of the Sino-Japanese War of 1937–1945*, ed. Mark Peattie, Edward Drea, and Hans van de Ven (Stanford, CA: Stanford University Press, 2011), 256.

28. Although the term "strategic bombing" was first used during World War I, during World War II British and American airmen used it "to distinguish the strategy of attacking and wearing down the enemy home front and economy from the strategy of directly assaulting the enemy's armed forces." See Richard Overy, *The Bombing War: Europe 1939–1945* (New York: Penguin Books, 2013), 9.

29. Marshall C. Balfour, officer's diary, May 21, 1939, record group 12.1, RF, RAC, 17; Associated Office for Chongqing Emergency Air Raid Relief Outline of the Physicians and Nurses Council and Air Raid Medical Relief Plans for the Bureau of Public Health, SHA, May 1939, 11.8727.

30. Ding Rongcan, *Peidu fangkong shilüe* (A brief history of air raid defense in the wartime capital) (Taipei: Academia Historica, August 8, 1985), 9; Joshua H. Howard, "Workers at War: Labor in the Nationalist Arsenals of Chongqing, 1937–1949" (PhD diss., University of California at Berkeley, 1998), 246.

31. Richard Overy writes, "The local records make it clear that if the Blitz had begun on 3 September 1939, the consequences would have been much worse than they proved to be a year later" (128). He does get the chronology wrong, however, and incorrectly asserts that "[t]he British people were the first to experience a heavy and prolonged campaign of independent bombing" (126). Overy, *Bombing War*, 126, 128.

32. Chongqing Women's Federation, Chongqingshi funü hui liangnianlai zhi gongzuo baogao (Chongqing Women's Federation work report for the past two years) (Chongqing: Chongqing Women's Federation, 1942), 5; *Chongqingshi tuixing xialing weisheng yundong qingxing de youguan wenshu* (Records on promoting the Summertime Health Movement in Chongqing), May 1941–July 1943, SHA, 11.7595. Each year after 1939 the government attempted to relocate three hundred thousand people and offered financial incentives to voluntary movers. Tow, "Great Bombing of Chongqing," 271.

33. CBPH Work Report, 1940, CMA, 66-1-3, 167; CBPH Work Report, 1944, CMA, Chongqing, 66-1-2, 61–62; CBPH Work Report, September 20–26, 1944, CMA, 66-1-2, 90; Chongqing Municipal Government, *Chongqingshi tongji tiyao* (A summary of Chongqing statistics) (Chongqing: Chongqing Municipal Government, 1942), table 41. Air raids in Chengdu also triggered a months-long setback after the bombing of the Women's Missionary Hospital. See Gerald Bell to Jesse Arnup, October 3, 1940, 1983.047C, 8–166, UCC.

34. Luo Zhuanxu, *Chongqing Kangzhan dashiji*, 76.

35. Sometimes the Japanese employed Chinese civilians to guide their pilots. Hired civilians were to dress in white beneath a dark cloak, then run out into the open and doff the cloak when they saw a bomber approaching, using their bright white clothing to attract the pilot to a bombing site. For this reason, missionary nurses in Chongqing changed into blue nurses' uniforms during an air raid, lest they unwittingly attract bombers to their hospital grounds. Sonya Grypma, *Healing Henan: Canadian Nurses at the North China Mission, 1888–1947* (Vancouver: University of British Columbia Press, 2008), 170–71.

36. Chen Lansun and Kong Xiangyun, eds., *Xiajiangren gushi* (Stories of downriver people) (Hong Kong: Tianma Book Publishing Company, 2005), 453.

37. Overy, *Bombing War,* esp. 398–409.

38. Sichuan Chongqing Cultural History Research Committee, eds., *Chongqing kangzhan jishi, 1937-1945* (A record of Chongqing events in the War of Resistance, 1937–1945) (Chongqing: Chongqing Publishing House, 1985), 170; Luo Zhuanxu, *Chongqing Kangzhan dashiji,* 17, 147. The numbers were derived from statistics of the Chongqing Air Raid Defense Ministry, wartime newspapers, and reports from the Japanese Defense Ministry Wartime History Office. These numbers are widely cited, but other sources cite different statistics; the differences stem largely from various interpretations of the wartime capital's boundaries. Note that from September 21, 1941, until the last air raid on August 23, 1943, the city enjoyed a respite that lasted nearly two years (ibid., 108).

39. Thomas Hippler, *Governing from the Skies: A Global History of Aerial Bombing* (New York: Verso, 2017). On changes to the Nationalist state's governance of refugees as a result of air raids, see Rana Mitter, *Forgotten Ally: China's World War II, 1937–1945* (New York: Houghton Mifflin Harcourt, 2013), 178–80.

40. The first newspaper report of the August 13 incident, printed in the *Dagongbao* on the following day, cited rumors that at least four hundred people had perished. *Dagongbao* no. 13179 (August 14, 1940). On August 15 the Chongqing Municipal Air Raid Relief Team released its official report, citing only eight dead, thirty-six seriously wounded, and five "severely disoriented" people. "Letter from the Chongqing Air Raid Relief Corps," August 15, 1940, Chongqing Asphyxiation Cases file, AH. The newspaper responded, citing the Air Raid Relief Corps's numbers along with those from another report, which stated that nine had died and over one hundred had been wounded, while also citing eyewitness accounts claiming that "the number of dead and wounded certainly exceeded 100." *Dagongbao* no. 13181 (August 16, 1940). On the death toll of the June 5, 1941, asphyxiation case, see Ding Rongcan, *Peidu fangkong shilüe,* 11; and Chen Lifu, *Suidao zhixi an shen weiyuan baogao fabiao* (Tunnel Asphyxiation Case Investigative Committee report), 1941, AH, 8b-10a.

41. *Dagongbao* no. 13181 (August 16, 1940).

42. Chen Lifu, *Suidao zhixi an shen weiyuan baogao fabiao,* 3b, 8b.

43. Kate Merkel-Hess, *The Rural Modern: Reconstructing the Self and the State in Republican China* (Chicago: University of Chicago Press, 2016).

44. Mitter, *Forgotten Ally,* 173.

45. Lu Ping, "De Xiansheng he Sai Xiansheng zhiwai de guanhuai: Cong Mu Guniang de tichu kan Xinwenhua yundong shiqi daode geming de zouxiang" (Beyond Mr. Democracy and Mr. Science: The introduction of Miss Moral and the trend of moral revolution in the New Culture Movement), *Lishi yanjiu* (Historical research) 2006, no. 1:79–95.

46. Arif Dirlik, *Anarchism in the Chinese Revolution* (Berkeley: University of California Press, 1991), 120; 73–74. Noted anarchists included Wang Zhihui, Li Shizeng, Zhang Ji, Cai Yuanpei, and Wang Jingwei.

47. Arif Dirlik, "The Ideological Foundations of the New Life Movement: A Study in Counterrevolution," *Journal of Asian Studies* 34, no. 4 (August 1975): 945.

48. Prasenjit Duara, *Sovereignty and Authenticity: Manchukuo and the East Asian Modern* (Lanham, MD: Rowman and Littlefield, 2003),137.

49. Chen Ruoshui, "Guanyu Huaren shehui wenhua xiandaihua de jidian xingsi: Yi gongde wenti weizhu" (Some reflections on Chinese society, culture, and modernization: Focusing on the question of public virtue), in *Gonggong yishi yu Zhongguo wenhua* (Public consciousness and Chinese culture) (Taipei: Linjing chubanshe, 2005), 57–78. New research has shown that traditionalism among intellectuals also grew after 1932, increasing their support for the NLM. Yiyun Ding, "Traditionalism and Wartime Education: The New Life Movement, 1934–1935," paper presented at the annual meeting of the American Historical Association, January 2018.

50. Watt, *Saving Lives,* 170, 240.

51. Samuel C. Chu, "The New Life Movement, 1934–1937," in *Researches in the Social Sciences on China,* ed. John E. Lane (New York: Columbia University Press, 1957), 3.

52. Lipkin, *Useless to the State,* 11–12, 164, 210–11.

53. Chen, *Guilty of Indigence.*

54. Michel Foucault, *Discipline and Punish: The Birth of the Prison,* trans. Alan Sheridan, 2nd ed. (New York: Vintage Books, 1995).

55. See, e.g., "Improve Your Living Environment," August 1943 page of the NIH public health calendar, NLM.

56. Zhou Yong, ed., *Chongqing tongshi* (A comprehensive history of Chongqing), vol. 3 (Chongqing: Chongqing Press, 2002), 1160.

57. Li, *Echoes of Chongqing,* 86, 90, 93.

58. CBPH Work Report, November 1943, CMA, 66-1-2, 198.

59. These two photos can be seen in the US Library of Congress Prints and Photographs Division online catalog, http://www.loc.gov/pictures/. See LC-USZ62–131090 and LC-USZ62–131091.

60. Li, *Echoes of Chongqing,* 88.

61. CBPH Work Report, November 1943, CMA, 66-1-2, 198–202.

62. Foucault, *Discipline and Punish.* Positive power, biopower, and governmentality together constituted Foucault's central intellectual contribution to the analysis of modern French society. As such they appear and take further shape in virtually all of Foucault's writings, but the central argument about (self-) punishment appears in the work cited here.

63. Foucault's theories have spawned a massive literature on Western societies, as well as a much smaller number of important works on Asia. Salient Foucauldian works on Western societies include Willem de Blécort and Cornelie Usborne, eds., *Cultural Approaches to the History of Medicine: Mediating Medicine in Early Modern and Modern Europe* (New York: Palgrave Macmillan, 2004); and Colin Jones and Roy Porter, eds., *Reassessing Foucault: Power, Medicine and the Body* (London and New York: Routledge, 1994). Foucauldian works on China include Huang Jinlin, *Lishi, Shenti, Guojia: Jindai Zhongguo de shenti xingcheng (1895–1937)* (History, body, nation: The formation of the modern Chinese body, 1895–1937) (Beijing: New Star Press, 2006); David Luesink, "Anatomy and the Reconfiguration of Life and Death in Republican China," *Journal of Asian Studies* 76, no. 4 (November 2017): 1009–34; and Malcolm Thompson, "Foucault, Fields of Governability, and the Population-Family-Economy Nexus in China," *History and Theory* 51, no. 1 (2012): 42–62.

64. "F. C. Yen to Mayor Jiang [Zhicheng]," November 18, 1938, CMA, 53-1-386, 182–83.

65. "Wartime Capital Chinese Medicine Hospital" files, 1944–1945, CMA, 163-2-19; 163-2-24; CBPH Work Report, 1938, CMA, Chongqing, 66-1-2, 182; CBPH Work Report, January–June 1940, CMA, 66-1-3, 171; CBPH Work Report, 1940, CMA, Chongqing, 66-1-3: "Table of Private and Public Hospitals in Chongqing Proper and in the Suburbs," August 1940, CMA, 66-1-3, 182–83; CBPH Work Report, September 1940–February 1941, CMA, 66-1-3, 198.

66. "Yen to Mayor Jiang," November 18, 1938, CMA, 53-1-386.

67. Hsiung Ping-chen, interviewer, and Cheng Li-jung, recorder, *Yang Wenda xiansheng fangwen jilu* (Reminiscences of Dr. Yang Wen-ta), Oral History Series no. 26 (Taipei: Academia Sinica Institute of Modern History, 1991), 32; Mei Zuwu and Lu Yuan, "Meishi jiazu yu qishouwei shihao yuan" (The Mei family at the Standard Bearer no. 10 Court), *Zhongguo dang'an bao* (China Archives news), October 22, October 29, and November 5, 2004; Yang Shanyao, *Kangzhan shiqi de Zhongguo junyi* (China's military medicine during the War of Resistance) (Taipei: Academia Historica, 2015), 50, 54. Mei Yilin was directly transferred from his Central Field Health Station post to his directorship of the CBPH ("F. C. Yen to Mayor Jiang," November 18, 1938, CMA, 53-1-386).

68. Ruth Rogaski, *Hygienic Modernity: Meanings of Health and Disease in Treaty-Port China* (Berkeley: University of California Press, 2004).

69. Sean Hsiang-lin Lei, *Neither Donkey nor Horse: Medicine in the Struggle over China's Modernity* (Chicago: University of Chicago Press, 2014), 21–44; the quote is on p. 44.

70. Bridie Andrews, "Tuberculosis and the Assimilation of Germ Theory in China, 1895–1937," *Journal of the History of Medicine* 52 (January 1997): 134.

71. Lei, *Neither Donkey nor Horse*, 42–44; Yip, *Health and National Reconstruction*, 9.

72. On the national survey, see John R. Watt, *A Friend in Deed: ABMAC and the Republic of China, 1937–1987* (New York: American Bureau for Medical Advancement in China, 1992), 3.

73. CBPH Work Report, December 5–10, 1938, CMA, 66-1-2, 184, 187–88.

74. Lei, *Neither Donkey nor Horse*, 101–17.

75. Survey of Physicians, Pharmacists, and Midwives in Chongqing City, February 1939, SPA, 113-1-637, 1–35. Given that most Chinese drugstores employed one or two druggists, pharmacists, or physicians to write and fill prescriptions, there must have been more druggists and pharmacists in the city, but they may have been entered in the survey under the category of "physicians of Chinese medicine." See app. B for the full survey in translation.

76. Tong Lam, *A Passion for Facts: Social Surveys and the Construction of the Chinese Nation-State, 1900–1949* (Berkeley: University of California Press, 2011).

77. CBPH Work Report, December 5–10, 1938, CMA, 66-1-2, 181–89.

78. See, e.g., CBPH Work Report, 1940, CMA, 66-1-3, 167, 223.

79. National Health Administration, *Jiuzhong fading chuanranbing qianshuo* (A brief introduction to the nine notifiable infectious diseases) (Nanjing: National Health Administration, July 1937), 1–2.

80. CBPH Work Report, December 5–10, 1938, CMA, 66-1-2, 189.

81. CBPH 1939 Summertime Cholera Prevention Plan, 1939, CMA, 162-1-20, 45–46.

82. Ibid.; also SPA, 113-1-639. In addition to the police, other entities that assisted the CBPH included the Bureau of Social Affairs, the Central Party Bureau and Municipal Party

Bureau, the Three People's Principles Youth Corps, and the New Life Movement Promotion Committee.

83. CBPH Work Report, March–August 1940. CMA, 66-1-3, 167–68; CBPH Work Report, August 1940, CMA, 66-1-3, 101; P. Z. King, "China's Civilian Health," in *Looking after China's Civilians*, United China Relief Series, no. 6 (Chungking: China Publishing Company, 1941), 2. King reported that the NHA had inoculated two and a half million people against cholera between the beginning of the war in July 1937 and May 1941.

84. Nicole Elizabeth Barnes, "Disease in the Capital: Nationalist Health Services and the 'Sick (Wo)man of East Asia' in Wartime Chongqing," *European Journal of East Asian Studies* 11, no. 2 (December 2012): 283–303.

85. Chongqing Municipal Government, *Chongqingshi tongji tiyao*, tables 43, 46. The gender differential in these vaccinations is huge: 113,513 men and 37,356 women were vaccinated.

86. CBPH Work Report, November 1943, CMA, 66-1-2, 204.

87. CBPH Work Plans for 1944, CMA, 66-1-4, 12; CBPH Work Report, January–March 1944, CMA, 66-1-2, 16; CBPH Work Report, 1944, CMA, 66-1-2, 15, 25, 50. Curiously, no numbers were reported for April–June, the high vaccination season.

88. CBPH Work Reports, July–October 11, 1944, CMA, 66-1-2, 81, 84, 86, 87.

89. CBPH Work Reports, November 1–7 and November 8–14, 1944, CMA, 66-1-2, 96, 99.

90. CBPH Work Report, October 1946, AH, 90–183, 12b; Record of Meeting to Expand Disease Prevention in Chongqing, June 29, 1945, CMA, 66-1-67; CBPH Work Report, n.d., CMA, 66-1-2, 4.

91. Chen, *Guilty of Indigence*; Lipkin, *Useless to the State*; Nedostup, *Superstitious Regimes*; Wakeman, "Licensing Leisure," 218.

92. This echoes David Strand's assertion that in Republican-era Beijing, "the government of the street and the courtyard was the police force." David Strand, *Rickshaw Beijing: City People and Politics in the 1920s* (Berkeley: University of California Press, 1989), 65.

93. Bruno Latour, *The Pasteurization of France*, trans. Alan Sheridan and John Law (Cambridge, MA: Harvard University Press, 1988), 123.

94. Jordan Goodman, Anthony McElligott, and Lara Marks, eds., *Useful Bodies: Humans in the Service of Medical Science in the Twentieth Century* (Baltimore: Johns Hopkins University Press, 2003), 11.

95. Dipesh Chakrabarty, "Postcoloniality and the Artifice of History: Who Speaks for 'Indian' Pasts?," in *A Subaltern Studies Reader, 1986–1995*, ed. Ranajit Guha (Delhi: Oxford University Press, 1998), 288.

96. Dorothy Porter, introduction to *The History of Public Health and the Modern State*, ed. Dorothy Porter (Amsterdam: Rodopi, 1994), 6; Matthew Ramsey, "Public Health in France," in *The History of Public Health and the Modern State*, ed. Dorothy Porter (Amsterdam: Rodopi, 1994), 46; Paul Weindling, "Public Health in Germany," in *The History of Public Health and the Modern State*, ed. Dorothy Porter (Amsterdam: Rodopi, 1994), 122.

97. Ramsey, "Public Health in France," 55. The Paris Conseil de Salubrité took charge of "noxious industries . . . , [such as] quacks, garbage, sewage, and adulterated food" (ibid.);

George Rosen, "The Fate of the Concept of Medical Police, 1780–1890," *Centaurus* 5, no. 2 (June 1957): 97 (article republished in 2008).

98. Mahito H. Fukuda, "Public Health in Modern Japan: From Regimen to Hygiene," in *The History of Public Health and the Modern State*, ed. Dorothy Porter (Amsterdam: Rodopi, 1994), 391.

99. Stapleton, *Civilizing Chengdu*, 56, 136; Di Wang, *Street Culture in Chengdu: Public Space, Urban Commoners, and Local Politics in Chengdu, 1870–1930* (Stanford, CA: Stanford University Press, 2003), 59, 98, 131–60.

100. Ran Minhui and Li Huiyu, *Minguo shiqi baojia zhidu yanjiu* (Research on the *baojia* system in the Republican era) (Chengdu: Sichuan University Press, 2005), 60, 65, 122–23.

101. Lloyd E. Eastman, *Seeds of Destruction: Nationalist China in War and Revolution, 1937–1945* (Stanford, CA: Stanford University Press, 1984), 148; Zhao Ma, *Runaway Wives, Urban Crimes, and Survival Tactics in Wartime Beijing, 1937–1949* (Cambridge, MA: Harvard University Asia Center, 2015), 163; Rana Mitter, "Classifying Citizens in Nationalist China during World War II, 1937–1941," in "China in World War II, 1937–1945: Experience, Memory, and Legacy," special issue, *Modern Asian Studies* 45, no. 2 (March 2011): 266.

102. Michael Shiyung Liu, *Prescribing Colonization: The Role of Medical Practices and Policies in Japan-Ruled Taiwan, 1895–1945* (Ann Arbor, MI: Association for Asian Studies, 2009), 81; Zhao Ma, *Runaway Wives*, 162–64; Yip, *Health and National Reconstruction*, 84, 177, 182, 195.

103. Chongqing Municipal Government, *Chongqingshi tongji tiyao*, table 21.

104. Records from Chongqing Bureau of Police Investigating and Punishing Yang Xuegao's Crime against Public Health, July 21, n.d., CMA, 61–15–408.

105. Letter to Chongqing no. 10 Police Bureau Regarding Fines for Crimes against Public Health, October 7, 1942, CMA, 61–15–5012.

106. List of Crimes against Hygiene from the Chongqing no. 2 Police Bureau, March 10, 1944, CMA, 61–15–630.

107. Letter to the Chongqing no. 10 Police Bureau Promising Never Again to Harm Public Health, June 27, 1944, CMA, 61–15–1075.

108. List of Crimes against Hygiene from the Chongqing no. 10 Police Bureau stationed at Xiangguo Temple, September 25, 1944, CMA, 61–15–774. The records do not explain the nature of the public savings account in which Chen and his chef were required to invest.

109. List of Crimes against Hygiene from the Chongqing no. 2 Police Bureau at Dayanggou, March 10, 1944, CMA, 61–15–630. Emphasis added.

110. The man in Chengdu had not only rebuked but also punched the police officer who attempted to arrest him for urination. He was later apprehended and arrested. Wang, *Street Culture in Chengdu*, 135–36. Wang takes the perspective of the archival sources and faults "residents' ignorance of sanitation" for continued conflict (ibid., 135).

111. Yip, *Health and National Reconstruction*, 35–39.

112. See, e.g., CMA 61–15–443, 53–4–56, 61–15–408, 61–15–852, and 61–15–2800.

113. CBPH Work Report, January–June 1940, CMA, 66–1–3.

114. Petition from the Chongqing Municipal Night Soil Porters' Professional Labor Union to the Sichuan Provincial Governor, March 1940, SPA, 59–60.

115. McIsaac, "Limits of Chinese Nationalism," 94.

116. For an example, see reports on sending workers to clear away garbage and excrement from the toilets, 1943, CMA, 66–1–63.

117. Letters Regarding Sending Personnel to Clear away Trash and Toilet Waste, April 22, 1943, and June 5, 1943, CMA, 66–1-63; Order to Clean Garbage off the Sidewalk Facing National Government Offices, May 1944, CMA, 61–15-5051, 395(2).

118. Order #16816, November 1943, CMA, 66–1-2, 202.

119. This drawing appears in Urgent Order to no. 10 Chongqing Police District Regarding Public Trashcan Designs, June 4, 1946, CMA, 61–15-1409.

120. Cleanliness Regulations Outlawing Trash in Chongqing, August 1939, CMA, 61–15-5091; revised in March 1941 (see CMA, 61–15-5145); CBPH Work Report, January–June 1940, CMA, 66–1-3, 175.

121. CBPH Work Report, January–June 1940, CMA, 66–1-3, 175.

122. The 1940 total was slightly less than 882,000 tons (CBPH Work Report, September 1940–February 1941, CMA, 66–1-3, 212), and the 1941 total was 993,926 tons (Chongqing Municipal Government, *Chongqingshi tongji tiyao*, table 44.).

123. Letter Regarding Trashcan Placement in the Domain of the No. 10 Police District, May 1940, CMA, 61–15-5091. The Number Ten District Police Office complied with the regulation and placed eighteen receptacles in strategic locations throughout its domain.

124. Trash Prohibition Cases, April 14, 1944, CMA, 61–15-5051, 392(1).

125. Li, *Echoes of Chongqing*, 84.

126. This chain of command appears in the notes of a December 1945 meeting of government staff on the issue of trash collection. Urgent Order to No. 10 Chongqing Police District Regarding Public Trashcan Designs, June 4, 1946, CMA, 61–15-1409.

127. Rogaski, *Hygienic Modernity*, 174–75.

128. CBPH Work Plans for 1944, CMA, 66–1-4, 19.

129. CBPH Work Report, January–March 1944, CMA, 66–1-2, 15.

130. CBPH Work Report, March–August 1940, CMA, 66–1-3, 181.

131. Li, *Echoes of Chongqing*, 89.

132. CBPH Work Report, March–August 1940, CMA, 66–1-3, 181.

133. Chongqing Municipal Hospital: Patient Treatment Statistics and Work Report, 1944, CMA, 165–2-5, 13.

134. Karl Eskelund, *My Chinese Wife* (London: George G. Harrap, 1946), 214.

135. On NHA cessation of Mei's salary, see Telegram from Chongqing Municipal Government to CBPH, February 13, 1942, 53–19-2660, CMA, 38–39. On Mei Yilin's December 1942 resignation, see Huang Yanfu and Wang Xiaoning, eds., *Mei Yiqi riji: 1941–1946* (Diary of Mei Yiqi: 1941–1946) (Beijing: Qinghua University Press, 2001), 119. On Wang assuming CBPH directorship in September 1943, see Executive Yuan order to Chongqing Municipal Government, September 17, 1943, CMA, 53–32-42. Wang had earned his credentials as a member of the board of directors of the Chongqing branch of the Chinese Red Cross, and head of the chief epidemic prevention team. In late 1946 Wang left Chongqing for Guangzhou, where he served as director of the relocated NHA; in 1949 he went to Taiwan to direct the newly relocated NIH. See Chinese Red Cross Chongqing Branch Name List and Work Report, 1940–49, CMA, 97–1-7, 84; and Watt, *Saving Lives*, 249.

136. James L. Watson and Evelyn S. Rawski, eds. Preface to *Death Ritual in Late Imperial and Modern China* (Berkeley: University of California Press, 1988), x–xi.

137. Ibid., xi.

138. Chinese Red Cross Chongqing Branch Name List and Work Report, 1940–49, CMA, 97-1-7, 83.

139. Although Shanghai employed female police officers as early as 1929, and Beijing in 1933 (Zhao Ma, *Runaway Wives*, 292), I have found no evidence of women working for the Chongqing police force.

140. Rogaski, *Hygienic Modernity*, 205.

2. APPEARING IN PUBLIC: THE RELATIONSHIPS AT THE HEART OF THE NATION

Chang Peng-yuan, interviewer, and Lo Jiu-jung, recorder, *Zhou Meiyu xiansheng fangwen jilu* (The reminiscences of Professor Chow Mei-yu), Oral History Series no. 47 (Taipei: Academia Sinica Institute of Modern History, 1993), 112.

1. Xie Bingying claimed that nine out of ten of the women she recruited for her auxiliary corps for the Northern Expedition joined in order to escape arranged marriages and the control of their families, just as she did. See Xie Bingying, *A Woman Soldier's Own Story*, trans. Lily Chia Brissman and Barry Brissman (New York: Berkeley Books, 2001), 52.

2. Arlie Russell Hochschild, *The Managed Heart: Commercialization of Human Feeling* (Berkeley: University of California Press, 2003), 5. Emphasis in original.

3. This is a relationship that persists in many societies, wherein nursing is a typically female profession, along with other jobs that include care for others such as teaching and social work. See Arlie Russell Hochschild, "Introduction: An Emotions Lens on the World," in *Theorizing Emotions: Sociological Exploration and Applications*, ed. Debra Hopkins, Jochen Kleres, Helena Flam, and Helmut Kizmics (Frankfurt am Main: Campus, 2009), 32.

4. Ba Jin, *Ward Four: A Novel of Wartime China*, trans. Haili Kong and Howard Goldblatt (San Francisco: China Books, 2012).

5. Margaret Strobel, *European Women and the Second British Empire* (Bloomington: Indiana University Press, 1991), 29–30.

6. Rosemary Wall and Anne Marie Rafferty, "Nursing and the 'Hearts and Minds' Campaign (1948–1958): The Malayan Emergency," in *Routledge Handbook on the Global History of Nursing*, ed. Patricia D'Antonio, Julie A. Fairman, and Jean C. Whelan (New York: Routledge, 2013), 223–24, 231.

7. Alison Bashford, "Medicine, Gender and Empire," in *Gender and Empire: The Oxford History of the British Empire*, ed. Philippa Levine (Oxford: Oxford University Press, 2004), 113.

8. Benedict Anderson, *Imagined Communities*, 2nd ed. (London: Verso, 1991), esp. chap. 8.

9. On traveling drama troupes, see Chang-tai Hung, *War and Popular Culture: Resistance in Modern China, 1937–1945* (Berkeley: University of California Press, 1994). On professional letter writers, see Diana Lary, *The Chinese People at War: Human Suffering and Social Transformation, 1937–1945* (New York: Cambridge University Press, 2010), 105. On public speeches as an essential repertoire of political culture in the Republic, which women in particular understood as a way to reach illiterate women, see David Strand, *An Unfinished Republic: Leading by Word and Deed in Modern China* (Berkeley: University of California Press, 2011), 94–96. On rumors in market towns, see G. William Skinner, *Marketing and Social Structure in Rural China* (Ann Arbor, MI: Association for Asian Studies, 1965). On teahouses in Sichuan, see Di Wang, *The Teahouse: Small Business,*

Everyday Culture, and Public Politics in Chengdu, 1900–1950 (Stanford, CA: Stanford University Press, 2008), 121, 144.

10. Haiyan Lee, *Revolution of the Heart: A Genealogy of Love in China, 1900–1950* (Stanford, CA: Stanford University Press, 2007), 7.

11. Norman Kutcher, "The Skein of Chinese Emotions History," in *Doing Emotions History,* ed. Susan J. Matt and Peter N. Stearns (Urbana and Chicago: University of Illinois Press, 2013), 58.

12. Partly for this reason, Sichuan teahouses hired female waitresses for the first time during the war. See Wang, *Teahouse,* 90–92. Wang makes an important point about the shift during the war years but misses the presence of female medical workers in his assertion that "[e]ntertainers and prostitutes . . . were the only women who earned a living in public places" in Chengdu at this time (90). Oddly, in an earlier book Wang asserts that "through the late Qing, women were restricted from most public places" in Chengdu, but by the 1920s and '30s "it was no longer novel for women to appear in public." Di Wang, *Street Culture in Chengdu: Public Space, Urban Commoners, and Local Politics in Chengdu, 1870–1930* (Stanford, CA: Stanford University Press, 2003), 180, 184. Teahouses and restaurants in Beijing had begun to hire female servers only in 1928, and hired many more in the 1930s for the simple economic reason that female employees were cheaper. See Zhao Ma, *Runaway Wives, Urban Crimes, and Survival Tactics in Wartime Beijing, 1937–1949* (Cambridge, MA: Harvard University Asia Center, 2015), 67–68.

13. On women's participation in the 1911 Revolution, see Louise Edwards, "Narratives of Race and Nation in China: Women's Suffrage in the Early Twentieth Century," *Women's Studies International Forum* 25, no. 6 (November–December 2002): 619–30. On women's participation in the 1927 Northern Expedition, see Xie Bingying, Woman Soldier's Own Story.

14. "Different Types of Medical Personnel Registered with the National Health Administration of China, 1929–1941," ABMAC records, box 83, folder "NHA and Nursing," RBML.

15. Chou Chun-yen, "Funü yu kangzhan shiqi de zhandi jiuhu" / "Women and Battlefield First Aid during the Second Sino-Japanese War," *Jindai Zhongguo funüshi yanjiu / Research on Women in Modern Chinese History* 24 (December 2014): 138–39.

16. Margaret Humphreys, *Marrow of Tragedy: The Health Crisis of the American Civil War* (Baltimore: Johns Hopkins University Press, 2013), 48–75, esp. 74.

17. Bridie Andrews, "From Bedpan to Revolution: Qiu Jin and Western Nursing in China," in *Women and Modern Medicine,* ed. Anne Hardy and Lawrence Conrad (Amsterdam: Rodopi, 2001): 54; Bridie Andrews, *The Making of Modern Chinese Medicine, 1850–1960* (Vancouver: University of British Columbia Press, 2014), 68; Chen Kaiyi, "Missionaries and the Early Development of Nursing in China," *Nursing History Review* 4 (1996): 143–44; Chou Chun-yen, "Funü yu kangzhan," 138–41; Sonya Grypma, "Neither Angels of Mercy nor Foreign Devils: Revisioning Canadian Missionary Nurses in China, 1935–1947," *Nursing History Review* 12 (2004); John Watt, "Breaking into Public Service: The Development of Nursing in Modern China, 1870–1949," *Nursing History Review* 12 (2004).

18. Chou Chun-yen, "Funü yu kangzhan," 144.

19. Ibid., 140; Chang Peng-yuan and Lo Jiu-rung, *Zhou Meiyu xiansheng fangwen jilu,* 21–29.

20. The Executive Committee and the Committee on Science and Publication of the Ninth Congress of the Far Eastern Association of Tropical Medicine, *A Glimpse of China* (Shanghai: Mercury Press, 1934), 74.

21. Connie A. Shemo, *The Chinese Medical Ministries of Kang Cheng and Shi Meiyu, 1872–1937: On a Cross-Cultural Frontier of Gender, Race, and Nation* (Bethlehem, MD: Lehigh University Press, 2011).

22. Andrews, *Modern Chinese Medicine,* 114–15, 141.

23. Hu Ying, *Burying Autumn: Poetry, Friendship, and Loss* (Cambridge, MA: Harvard University Asia Center Press, 2016), 97. Qiu Jin is known to posterity not because of her sensational life or even her dramatic death, but thanks to the dedication and courage of her two closest friends, Wu Zhiying and Xu Zihua, who gave her a proper burial—seven times in all—and memorialized her in their own poetry and essays.

24. Chang Peng-yuan and Lo Jiu-rung, *Zhou Meiyu xiansheng fangwen jilu,* 21–29.

25. Olga Lang, *Chinese Family and Society* (New Haven, CT: Yale University Press, 1946), 201; Danke Li, *Echoes of Chongqing: Women in Wartime China* (Urbana and Chicago: University of Illinois Press, 2010), 170; Kristin Stapleton, "Warfare and Modern Urban Administration in Chinese Cities," in *Cities in Motion: Interior, Coast, and Diaspora in Transnational China,* ed. Sherman Cochran et al. (Berkeley: University of California Press, 2007), 70.

26. Zhao Ma, *Runaway Wives,* 40, 58. Ma finds that in Beijing and the surrounding areas, even lower-class and peasant women did not like to engage in factory work at least until 1950 because it was considered dishonorable and "a sign of economic destitution and desperation" (40).

27. From the early Republic, hair became "a political statement," allowing one to "make your point in public without even opening your mouth." Short, bobbed hair on a woman frequently marked her as a "new woman" with more radical politics. Strand, *Unfinished Republic,* 93.

28. National Institute of Health, Public Health Calendar, 1943, NLM.

29. On poor sanitation in teahouses as a problem that the Chengdu government attempted to regulate, see Wang, *Teahouse,* 50–52.

30. Zhao Ma, *Runaway Wives,* 280–81.

31. Ibid., 280, 315. Ma narrates this cultural shift among lower-class women in wartime Beijing and argues that "mobility became a survival tactic that helped women eke out a precarious livelihood" (315).

32. Watches became a marker of modernity in urban China in the mid–nineteenth century. The bob was both the most popular hairstyle for women in the 1930s and a common signal of radical politics. Antonia Finnane, *Changing Clothes in China: Fashion, History, Nation* (New York: Columbia University Press, 2008), 65, 157–60.

33. Strand, *Unfinished Republic,* 131.

34. Li, *Echoes of Chongqing,* 72. Song's roles included chairing the Wartime Association for Child Welfare (*Zhanshi ertong baoyuhui*) (WACW) and its parent organization, the National Association of Chinese Women for Comforting War of Resistance Soldiers (*Zhongguo funü weilao ziwei kangzhan jiangshi zonghui*) (NACWCWRS).

35. On the *qipao* as a marker of modernity, see Finnane, *Changing Clothes in China,* 5–6. On women and philanthropy, see Xia Shi, *At Home in the World: Women and Charity in Late Qing and Early Republican China* (New York: Columbia University Press, 2018).

36. Former missionary to China Geraldine Fitch in 1943, cited in Karen J. Leong, *The China Mystique: Pearl S. Buck, Anna May Wong, Mayling Soong, and the Transformation of American Orientalism* (Berkeley: University of California Press, 2005), 106.

37. Leong, *China Mystique*.

38. Song Meiling had an even stronger southern accent in Chinese—that of Zhejiang and Jiangsu Provinces. Most Nationalist Party officials came from southern China, so her accent marked her as a Nationalist leader.

39. May-ling Soong Chiang, *War Messages and Other Selections by Madame Chiang Kai-shek* (Hankow [Hankou]: China Information Committee, 1938), 1–2.

40. Helen M. Schneider, "Mobilising Women: The Women's Advisory Council, Resistance and Reconstruction during China's War with Japan," *European Journal of East Asian Studies* 11, no. 2 (December 2012): 213–36.

41. Chou Chun-yen, "Funü yu kangzhan," 173.

42. Song Meiling, *Madame Chiang Kai-shek on the New Life Movement* (Shanghai: China Weekly Review Press, 1937), 69. Emphasis added.

43. Federica Ferlanti, "The New Life Movement at War: Wartime Mobilisation and State Control in Chongqing and Chengdu, 1938–1942," *European Journal of East Asian Studies* 11, no. 2 (December 2012): esp. 192.

44. Stephen R. MacKinnon, *Wuhan, 1938: War, Refugees, and the Making of Modern China* (Berkeley: University of California Press, 2008), 55–58; Li, *Echoes of Chongqing*, 20–21.

45. Gail Hershatter, "Making the Visible Invisible: The Fate of 'The Private' in Revolutionary China," in *Wusheng zhi sheng (I): Jindai Zhongguo de funü yu guojia (1600–1950)* (Voices amid Silence (I): Women and the Nation in Modern China, 1600–1950), ed. Fangshang Lu (Taipei: Academia Sinica Institute of Modern History, 2003), 259.

46. Sean Hsiang-lin Lei, "Habituating Individuality: Framing Tuberculosis and Its Material Solutions in Republican China," *Bulletin for the History of Medicine* 84 (2010): 248–79.

47. Mary Colette Plum, "Unlikely Heirs: War Orphans during the Second Sino-Japanese War, 1937–1945" (PhD diss., Stanford University, 2006), 203–9. Plum interviewed adults who had grown up in orphanages during the war, and notes that her interviewees frequently recited the text of four particular lessons from memory.

48. Ibid., 182.

49. Helen M. Schneider, *Keeping the Nation's House: Domestic Management and the Making of Modern China* (Vancouver: University of British Columbia Press, 2011), 152–55. Specific quotes are on pp. 153 and 154.

50. Ibid., 156.

51. Martha C. Nussbaum, *Political Emotions: Why Love Matters for Justice* (Cambridge, MA: Belknap Press of Harvard University Press, 2013), 210–11.

52. Ibid., 211.

53. Kate Merkel-Hess, *The Rural Modern: Reconstructing the Self and State in Republican China* (Chicago: University of Chicago Press, 2016), esp. 2. Work in Dingxian began in 1929 and ended in 1937 when the war forced rural reconstructionists to abandon their model county.

54. Zhou Meiyu, *Zhongguo junhu jiaoyu fazhan shi* (History of the development of military nursing education) (Taipei: Jianhe yinshua chang, 1985), 3.

55. Sean Hsiang-lin Lei, *Neither Donkey nor Horse: Medicine in the Struggle over China's Modernity* (Chicago: University of Chicago Press, 2014), 231–37.

56. C.C. Chen, "A Statement of the Szechuan Provincial Health Administration," December 1, 1939, p. 1, folder 161, box 18, series 601, record group 1.1, RF, RAC. On the public health nurse as kingpin worker, see John R. Watt, *Saving Lives in Wartime China: How Medical Reformers Built Modern Healthcare Systems amid War and Epidemics, 1928–1945* (Leiden: E.J. Brill, 2014), 65–67.

57. C.C. Chen in collaboration with Frederica M. Bunge, *Medicine in Rural China: A Personal Account,* (Berkeley: University of California Press, 1989), 77–78. It should be noted that Chen modestly credited not the system he had a hand in creating, but the ingenuity of Chinese villagers who "since time immemorial . . . had been seeking medical counsel and obtaining their medication from other villagers whose knowledge of medicine was only slightly greater than their own" (78).

58. Chang Peng-yuan and Lo Jiu-rung, *Zhou Meiyu xiansheng fangwen jilu,* 11, 106–11.

59. Cited in Lei, *Neither Donkey nor Horse,* 237.

60. Ibid., 254.

61. Elizabeth Fee and Mary Garofalo, "Florence Nightingale and the Crimean War," *American Journal of Public Health* 100, no. 9 (September 2010): 1591.

62. It seems not accidental that one document called Zhou Meiyu Asia's Florence Nightingale. ABMAC, *The Story of a Unique Institution and Its Heroic Students: Asia's Florence Nightingale* (New York: ABMAC, n.d.), ABMAC Archives, RBML, box 32, folder "Chow Mei-yu."

63. Jonathan Hagood, "*Agentes de Enlace:* Nursing professionalization and public health in 1940s and 1950s Argentina," in *Routledge Handbook on the Global History of Nursing,* ed. Patricia D'Antonio, Julie A. Fairman, and Jean C. Whelan (New York: Routledge, 2013), 183–97.

64. Steven Palmer, "Windsor's Metropolitan Demonstration School and the Reform of Nursing Education in Canada, 1944–1970," in *Routledge Handbook on the Global History of Nursing,* ed. Patricia D'Antonio, Julie A. Fairman, and Jean C. Whelan (New York: Routledge, 2013), 131–50.

65. Patricia D'Antonio, Julie A. Fairman, and Jean C. Whelan, introduction to *Routledge Handbook on the Global History of Nursing,* ed. Patricia D'Antonio, Julie A. Fairman, and Jean C. Whelan (New York: Routledge, 2013), 6.

66. Chang Peng-yuan and Lo Jiu-rung, *Zhou Meiyu xiansheng fangwen jilu,* 5.

67. M.B. Hadley, L.S. Blum, S. Mujaddid, S. Parveen, S. Nuremowla, M.E. Haque, and M. Ullah, "Why Bangladeshi Nurses Avoid 'Nursing': Social and Structural Factors on Hospital Wards in Bangladesh," *Social Science and Medicine* 64, no. 6 (March 2007): 1166–77, esp. 1166 and 1168.

68. Chang Peng-yuan and Lo Jiu-rung, *Zhou Meiyu xiansheng fangwen jilu,* 111–12.

69. Ibid., 13.

70. Chen, *Medicine in Rural China,* 94.

71. Julie Livingston, *Improvising Medicine: An African Oncology Ward in an Emerging Cancer Epidemic* (Durham, NC: Duke University Press, 2012), 6, 96.

72. Ibid., 1, 100, 104, 105, 108–12, 115, 118.

73. Ibid., 100.

74. Ibid., 97.

75. Chang Peng-yuan and Lo Jiu-rung, *Zhou Meiyu xiansheng fangwen jilu,* 112.

76. This is a central argument in Livingston's book (as reflected in its title, *Improvising Medicine*), wherein she describes another setting characterized by chronic resource scarcity yet facing continual demand.

77. Hochschild, *Managed Heart,* 7.

78. Rachel Jewkes, Naeemah Abrahams, and Zodumo Mvo, "Why Do Nurses Abuse Patients? Reflections from South African Obstetric Services," *Social Science and Medicine* 47, no. 11 (1998): 1781–95. The authors describe a situation that was widely discussed for decades but never corrected. South African nurses thereby earned a reputation for being "cruel."

79. Livingston, *Improvising Medicine,* 115.

80. Ibid., 110.

81. Hochschild, *Managed Heart,* 8.

82. It is important to note that one male nurse worked in the Botswana cancer ward, and Livingston did not note any failure on his part to perform the "moral intimacies of care" that his job required. Analysis of the degree to which male nurses in wartime China performed the emotional labor described here awaits further research.

83. Chang Peng-yuan and Lo Jiu-rung, *Zhou Meiyu xiansheng fangwen jilu,* 58.

84. Yao Aihua, "Memoir of Yao Aihua," in Fang Jun, *Zuihou yi ci jijie* (The last concentration of troops) (Shenyang: Liaoning renmin chubanshe, 2012), 205.

85. Yang Shanyao, *Kangzhan shiqi de Zhongguo junyi* (China's military medicine during the War of Resistance) (Taipei: Academia Historica, 2015), 139–40, 152–53.

86. Ibid., 129, 157.

87. A 1933 survey in Dingxian calculated an infant mortality rate of 199 per 1,000. Cited in Merkel-Hess, "The Public Health of Village Private Life: Reform and Resistance in Early Twentieth Century Rural China," *Journal of Social History* 49, no. 4 (2016): 891.

88. While both of these stories appeared undated in the archives, they can be fairly accurately dated to the 1940s given the quality of the paper, the style of writing, the types of shorthand used (such as certain forms of simplified characters within traditional character writing that were common in the period), and the vocabulary the authors employed.

89. Merkel-Hess, *Rural Modern,* 35, 37, 100.

90. Ibid., 99, 101.

91. Zhou Liaoxun, *Gonggong weisheng* (Public health), n.d., 89-1-17, CMA, 1–3.

92. On earlier, Daoist meanings of *weisheng,* see Ruth Rogaski, *Hygienic Modernity: Meanings of Health and Disease in Treaty-Port China* (Berkeley: University of California Press, 2004), 22–47.

93. Zhou Liaoxun, *Gonggong weisheng,* 9–10.

94. Ibid., 15–18.

95. Xun Liu, *Daoist Modern: Innovation, Lay Practice, and the Community of Inner Alchemy in Republican Shanghai* (Cambridge, MA: Harvard University Asia Center, 2009).

96. Zhou Liaoxun, *Gonggong weisheng,* 19–28. For analysis of the overuse of the figure of four hundred million as the national population throughout the first half of the twentieth century, and the implications thereof, see Tong Lam, *A Passion for Facts: Social Surveys and the Construction of the Chinese Nation-State, 1900–1949* (Berkeley: University of California Press, 2011), 32–41.

97. Watt, *Saving Lives in Wartime China*, 23–24. For a specific example of outlawing cut melons and cold drinks to prevent cholera, see CBPH 1939 Summertime Cholera Prevention Plan, 1939, CMA, 162-1-20, 45–46.

98. Gu Qizhong, *Kepa de huoluan*, n.d., 89-1-17, CMA, 49b–50a.

99. Ibid., 51a.

100. Marta Hanson, *Speaking of Epidemics in Chinese Medicine: Disease and the Geographical Imagination in Late Imperial China* (New York: Routledge, 2011), 136, 141–43.

101. Gu, *Kepa de huoluan*, 51a.

102. Ibid., 51b–60b.

103. Zhou Hui'an, "Humanity's Silent Killer," n.d., 89-1-17, CMA.

104. Chen, *Medicine in Rural China*, 2.

105. Daniel Immerwahr, *Thinking Small: The United States and the Lure of Community Development* (Cambridge, MA: Harvard University Press, 2015). "The transnational practice of development as it emerged in the 1950s responded to the threat posed by popular mobilization in the global South." Tania Murray Li, *The Will to Improve: Governmentality, Development, and the Practice of Politics* (Durham, NC: Duke University Press, 2007), 8.

106. Merkel-Hess, "Public Health of Village Private Life," 895.

107. See, e.g., *Dagongbao*, nos. 12670, 12675, and 12727 (December 19, 1938; January 13, 1939; and February 2, 1939). On medical kits for soldiers, see Chou Chun-yen, "Funü yu kangzhan,"170.

108. Lee, *Revolution of the Heart*, 7, 8.

109. Ibid., 256.

110. Merkel-Hess, *Rural Modern*, 33.

111. One of the systems operated in "Free China" under the control of Chiang Kai-shek, the second in central China under the control of Wang Jingwei, and the third in Beijing under the control of the collaborationist government of Wang Kemin in Beijing. Parks M. Coble, *China's War Reporters: The Legacy of Resistance against Japan* (Cambridge, MA: Harvard University Press, 2015), 91.

112. Chou Chun-yen, "Funü yu kangzhan," 163.

113. *Xin shenghuo yundong cujin zonghui: Shangbing zhi you she zongshe qi nianlai gongzuo jianbao* (New Life Promotion Committee: Friends to Wounded Soldiers Society work report for the past seven years), January 1947, GMD Party Archives, 483/39.1,2,3, pp. 12, 20.

114. Qing, "Weilao fushang zhuangshi" (Comforting wounded heroes), *Funü shenghuo* (Women's lives) 8, no. 5 (December 1939): 14.

115. Ibid., 15.

116. Haili Kong, "Disease and Humanity: Ba Jin and His *Ward Four: A Novel of Wartime China,*" *Frontiers of Literary Studies in China* 6, no. 2 (2012): 201–2. Ba Jin stayed in Ward Three, a third-class ward, of the Central Hospital of Guiyang in May and June of 1944 (ibid., 203).

117. Ba Jin, *Ward Four*, 153, 89. In the preface Ba denotes the main character as "Lu XX" or "Mr. Lu," though in later revisions he gains a full name, Lu Huamin. Kong, "Disease and Humanity," 202.

118. Kong, "Disease and Humanity," 204.

119. Ibid. Ba Jin's direct quotes are from a 1961 article he wrote on the novel.

120. Ba Jin, *Ward Four*, 178.

121. Cited in Kong, "Disease and Humanity," 203.

122. Ibid.

123. Ba Jin, *Ward Four,* 215.

124. Ibid., 149.

125. Ibid., 159.

126. Ibid., 210–11.

127. Ibid., 22.

128. Ibid., 23.

129. Ka-Ming Wu, "Elegant and Militarized: Ceremonial Volunteers and the Making of New Woman Citizens in China," *Journal of Asian Studies* 77, no. 1 (February 2018): 205–23.

130. On Woman as figure of tradition in occupied Manchuria, see Prasenjit Duara, *Sovereignty and Authenticity: Manchukuo and the East Asian Modern* (Lanham, MD: Rowman and Littlefield, 2003), 131–69.

3. HEALING TO KILL THE TRUE INTERNAL ENEMY

Yao Aihua, "Memoir of Yao Aihua," in Fang Jun, *The Last Concentration of Troops (Zuihou yi ci jijie)* (Liaoning: Shenyang: Liaoning renmin chubanshe, 2012), 205.

1. Reflecting the fact that it began as a regional war, the Japanese originally called the "China Incident" (*Shina Jiken*) the "North China Incident" but changed the name after the Battle of Shanghai, one of the largest campaigns in the war. S. C. M. Paine, *The Wars for Asia: 1911–1949* (New York: Cambridge University Press, 2012), 7–8, 132.

2. Chou Chun-yen, "Funü yu kangzhan shiqi de zhandi jiuhu" / "Women and battlefield first aid during the Second Sino-Japanese War," *Jindai Zhongguo funüshi yanjiu / Research on Women in Modern Chinese History* 24 (December 2014): 208.

3. Ibid., 163–64.

4. Achille Mbembe, "Necropolitics," trans. Libby Meintjes, *Public Culture* 15, no. 1 (2003): 11–40.

5. John R. Watt, *Saving Lives in Wartime China: How Medical Reformers Built Modern Healthcare Systems amid War and Epidemics, 1928–1945* (Leiden: E. J. Brill, 2014), 4–5, 94, 98, 134–35, 223.

6. John R. Watt, *A Friend in Deed: ABMAC and the Republic of China, 1937–1987* (New York: American Bureau for Medical Advancement in China, 1992), 3.

7. Sean Hsiang-lin Lei, *Neither Donkey nor Horse: Medicine in the Struggle over China's Modernity* (Chicago: University of Chicago Press, 2014), 237–47.

8. On the AMA, see Yang Shanyao, *Kangzhan shiqi de Zhongguo junyi* (The Chinese military doctor in War of Resistance) (Taipei: Academia Historica, 2015). The personal relationship between Dr. Lim and Lu Zhide, a former student of his and head of the AMA, supported smooth coordination between the two systems.

9. J. Heng Liu, "Our Responsibilities in Public Health," *Chinese Medical Journal* 51, no. 6 (June 1937): 1039. This article was a transcript of the speech that Dr. Liu had delivered on April 2 of the same year to the Public Health section of the China Medical Association conference held in Shanghai.

10. Theodore H. White and Annalee Jacoby, *Thunder Out of China* (New York: Da Capo Press, 1946), 129.

11. Martha C. Nussbaum, *Political Emotions: Why Love Matters for Justice* (Cambridge, MA: Belknap Press of Harvard University Press, 2013), 206.

12. Alfred Kohlberg, "The Medical Relief Corps of the Chinese Red Cross," November 22, 1943, ABMAC, RBML, box 22.

13. Watt, *Saving Lives in Wartime China*, 132 graph 4.1

14. National Red Cross Society of China, Emergency Medical Service Training School Personnel Trained (From May 1938 to March 1941), ABMAC archives, RBML, box 23; Chang Peng-yuan, interviewer, and Lo Jiu-jung, recorder, *Zhou Meiyu xiansheng fangwen jilu* (The reminiscences of Professor Chow Mei-yu), Oral History Series no. 47 (Taipei: Academia Sinica Institute of Modern History, 1993), 54.

15. Watt, *Saving Lives in Wartime China*, 148, 280–81.

16. ABMAC, "Army Medical Service," in "A Survey of China's Medical and Health Problems and the Progress Made by the Chinese Government in Providing for the Health of the Nation," November 1943, CMB, RAC, box 9, folder 62, 1; Marshall C. Balfour Officer's Diary, October 3, 1943, record group 12.1, RFA, RAC, 50; Watt, *Saving Lives in Wartime China;* 160–67. Watt's book contains a much more detailed analysis of these events.

17. Yao Aihua, "Memoir of Yao Aihua," 209–10, 212.

18. Chang Peng-yuan and Lo Jiu-jung Lo, *Zhou Meiyu xiansheng fangwen jilu,* 43, 45; Watt, *Saving Lives in Wartime China,* 127.

19. Hsiung Ping-chen, interviewer, and Cheng Li-jung, recorder, *Yang Wenda xiansheng fangwen jilu (Reminiscences of Dr. Yang Wen-ta)* (Oral History Series no. 26) (Taipei: Academia Sinica Institute of Modern History, 1991), 31–32, 34. Yang's monthly salary was 62 yuan. On one prominent group of volunteer physicians from India, see Khwaja Ahmad Abbas, *And One Did Not Come Back! The Story of the Congress Medical Mission to China* (Bombay: Sound Magazine, 1944).

20. Chang Peng-yuan and Lo Jiu-jung Lo, *Zhou Meiyu xiansheng fangwen jilu,* 63–64.

21. Ibid., 65. The New Fourth Army Incident was a battle between Nationalist and Communist forces, with no agreement about which side was responsible for starting it.

22. Nussbaum, *Political Emotions,* 2. I insert "Communist" and "Nationalist" in place of "antiliberal" and "liberal" here only to make the larger point, *not* to argue that these terms in any way encapsulated a chief difference between the two parties, which were both at turns antiliberal and liberal in their own ways.

23. Quoted in Odd Arne Westad, *Decisive Encounters: The Chinese Civil War, 1946–1950* (Stanford, CA: Stanford University Press, 2003), 62.

24. Nussbaum, *Political Emotions,* 207.

25. Eugenia Lean, *Public Passions: The Trial of Shi Jianqiao and the Rise of Popular Sympathy in Republican China* (Berkeley: University of California Press, 2007), 211.

26. On Nationalist party operatives' constant surveillance, arrest, torture, and execution of Communists and suspected Communists, see Frederic Wakeman Jr., *Spymaster: Dai Li and the Chinese Secret Service* (Berkeley: University of California Press, 2003).

27. Quoted in Yang Shanyao, *Kangzhan shiqi de Zhongguo junyi,* 130.

28. Ibid. Chiang urged his military medicine officials to train such individuals so as to improve the NRA. It should be noted that Yang Shanyao takes a different approach in analyzing the conflict that led to Lim's loss of his two posts. He cites other features thereof, including most notably the tensions between the German-Japanese medical training of Army

Medical Administration (AMA) officers, and the Anglo-American training of Lim's people in the MRC and EMSTS. This tension grew into outright conflict when Dr. Liu Ruiheng, an ally of Lim's, as head of the Army Medical College from April 1935 to June 1937, changed its language of instruction from German to English by administrative fiat. Yang also notes the clash between general cultures: the AMA contained people of military background and perspective, while the MRC and EMSTS contained people from the public health and state medicine sectors (ibid., 100–103, 109, 113). John Watt also notes a further feature of this conflict: the intense jealousy of leaders of civilian health organizations over the amount of overseas donations that Lim's organizations received. (For more on this, see chap. 4.) This was the case for both Minister of Health P. Z. King (Jin Baoshan) and Sze Szeming (Shi Siming), general secretary of the Chinese Medical Association. See Marshall C. Balfour Officer's Diary, September 8, 1943, record group 12.1, RF, RAC, 40; and Edwin C. Lobenstine, interview with Szeming Sze, September 13, 1944, folder 1109, box 152, CMB, RAC, 2. It remains to be seen whether Nationalist Party rightists encouraged King and Sze to launch their smear campaigns.

29. Wang Jingwei is the most famous example. Unable to stomach his party's continuous killing of fellow Chinese, he eventually decided that an alliance with the Japanese would bring him closest to his goal of bringing swift peace to his homeland—an act for which he has been vilified ever since. See Rana Mitter, *Forgotten Ally: China's World War II, 1937–1945* (Boston: Houghton Mifflin, 2013), 197–210.

30. Yang Shanyao, *Kangzhan shiqi de Zhongguo junyi*, 155. This page contains a table from the Acadamia Historica archives of Taipei with statistics from the Ministry of War. These statistics, though likely incomplete, are reliable.

31. Ibid., 162; Lloyd E. Eastman, "Nationalist China during the Sino-Japanese War 1937–1945," in *The Cambridge History of China*, vol. 13, *Republican China 1912–1949, Part 2*, ed. John K. Fairbank and Albert Feuerwerker (Cambridge: Cambridge University Press, 1986), 573, 575.

32. ABMAC, "Army Medical Service," 2–3.

33. American Bureau for Medical Advancement in China, *Medicine on a Mission: A History of the American Bureau for Medical Aid to China, Inc., 1937–1954* (New York: ABMAC, 1954), sec. 2, p. 17.

34. Watt, *Saving Lives in Wartime China*, 4; Mitter, *Forgotten Ally*, 5.

35. Superintendent Yang Wenda, who saw thousands of hospitalized soldiers around the country, recalled in his oral history interviews that "more people died of illness than of battle wounds during the war." Hsiung Ping-chen and Cheng Li-jung, *Yang Wenda xiansheng fangwen jilu*, 36.

36. Andrew F. Trofa, Hannah Ueno-Olsen, Ruiko Oiwa, and Masanosuke Yoshikawa, "Dr. Kiyoshi Shiga: Discoverer of the Dysentery Bacillus," *Clinical Infectious Diseases* 29, no. 5 (November 1999): 1303–6.

37. The Chinese term for bacillary dysentery—*chili*, or "red diarrhea"—is a descriptive term for the blood present in the stool of dysentery sufferers. The Japanese use the same characters for their word, *sekiri*, and the term may be a return-graphic loan word.

38. Joshua H. Howard, *Workers at War: Labor in China's Arsenals, 1937–1953* (Stanford, CA: Stanford University Press, 2004), 131–32.

39. Nick Ragsdale, "Dysentery," in *Encyclopedia of Pestilence, Pandemics, and Plagues*, vol. 1, *A–M*, ed. Joseph P. Byrne (Westport, CT: Greenwood Press, 2008), 174–76.

40. Hsiung Ping-chen and Cheng Li-jung, *Yang Wenda xiansheng fangwen jilu*, 36.

41. White and Jacoby, *Thunder Out of China*, 138.

42. National Health Administration Medical and Epidemic Prevention Teams, eds. *Huoluan* (Cholera) (Chongqing: National Health Administration, 1940), 8–9.

43. Chang Peng-yuan and Lo Jiu-jung Lo, *Zhou Meiyu xiansheng fangwen jilu*, 50.

44. Hsiung Ping-chen and Cheng Li-jung, *Yang Wenda xiansheng fangwen jilu*, 36.

45. Watt, *Saving Lives in Wartime China*, 133–45, 175, 219, 242.

46. Ibid., 135, 210; National Health Administration, "The Initial Year of the National Institute of Health (April 1–December 31, 1941), Chungking, ABMAC box 21, Columbia University RBML, 9.

47. Robert L. Atenstaedt, *The Medical Response to the Trench Diseases in World War One* (Newcastle upon Tyne: Cambridge Scholars Publishing, 2011).

48. Zhao Chuan, *Taiwan laobing koushu lishi* (Oral histories of Taiwanese soldiers) (Guilin: Guangxi Normal University Press, 2013), 65.

49. Watt, *Saving Lives in Wartime China*, 133–34, 177. The NHA focused on controlling contamination from soldiers to civilians. See P. Z. King, "On the Experience of Establishing Delousing and Scabies Treatment Stations, September 23, 1943, in People's Political Council 3rd Meeting 2nd Session," in *Weishengshu da fuxun wen'an* (National Health Administration consultative response cases) (Chongqing: Datong Publishing House, 1943).

50. Chang Peng-yuan and Lo Jiu-jung Lo, *Zhou Meiyu xiansheng fangwen jilu*, 46, 49.

51. Diana Lary, *The Chinese People at War: Human Suffering and Social Transformation, 1937–1945* (New York: Cambridge University Press, 2010), 20, 32–33.

52. Part of the concern for soldiers' health was in fact concern for civilians; serving as mobile vectors, soldiers frequently brought disease into residential communities as they passed through or requested lodging or meals. See Ka-che Yip, "Disease and the Fighting Men: Nationalist Anti-Epidemic Efforts in Wartime China, 1937-1945," in *China and the Anti-Japanese War, 1937-1945: Politics, Cutlure, and Society,* ed. David P. Barrett and Larry N. Shyu (New York: Peter Lang, 2001), 171–72.

53. G. C. Marshall, *War Department Technical Bulletin: Scrub Typhus Fever (Tsutsugamushi Disease)* (Washington, DC: United States War Department, 1944), 1, folder 165, box 18, ser. 601, record group 1.1, Rockefeller Foundation Archives, RAC.

54. Dr. H. W. Tseng, "A Hospital Doctor Speaks," in *Looking After China's Civilians,* United China Relief Series, no. 6 (Chungking: China Publishing Company, 1941), 14.

55. Howard, "Workers at War," 244.

56. Isabel Brown Crook and Christina Kelley Gilmartin with Yu Xiji, *Prosperity's Predicament: Identity, Reform, and Resistance in Rural Wartime China,* comp. and ed. Gail Hershatter and Emily Honig (Lanham, MD: Rowman and Littlefield, 2013), 225–49.

57. Peng Chengfu, *Chongqing renmin dui Kangzhan de gongxian* (Chongqing people's contributions to the War of Resistance against Japan) (Chongqing: Chongqing Publishing House, 1995), 1–17; Wan Fang, Wan Fang, *Chuanhun: Sichuan Kangzhan dang'an shiliao xuanbian* (The soul of Sichuan: An edited collection of historical materials on the War of Resistance from the Sichuan Archives) (Chengdu: Sichuan Provincial Archives, 2005), 2–3; Yang Yulin. "Bingli yu liangshi: Sichuan sheng disan xingzheng duchaqu renmin dui Kangzhan zhong de zhuyao gongxian" (Military power and grain: Principal War of Resistance contributions from the people of Sichuan Province's Number Three

Administrative Superintendency), in *Sichuan Kangzhan dang'an yanjiu* (Research on the War of Resistance in Sichuan Archives), ed. Li Shigen (Chengdu: Southwest Jiaotong University Publishing House, 2005), 119, 121. Sichuan men had already been under the physical strain of war for years. Until at least 1935, during their territorial battles Sichuan warlords regularly sent press gangs into the countryside to recruit porters and fighters by force. See Margaret Timberlake Simkin Oral History, Claremont Graduate School Oral History Project, January 27, 1970, and December 10, 1971, Yale Day Divinity Library, record group 8, box 227, folder 6, 55; and Robert A. Kapp, *Szechwan and the Chinese Republic: Provincial Militarism and Central Power, 1911-1938* (New Haven, CT: Yale University Press, 1973), 10–11.

58. Miriam Gross, *Farewell to the God of Plague: Chairman Mao's Campaign to De-worm China* (Berkeley: University of California Press, 2016).

59. "Memorandum to American Red Cross and to American Bureau for Medical Aid to China," June 10, 1941, box 21, folder NHA 1940–1941, ABMAC.

60. ABMAC, "Army Medical Service," 2–3.

61. Lloyd Eastman, *Seeds of Destruction: Nationalist China in War and Revolution, 1937–1949* (Stanford, CA: Stanford University Press, 1984), 152–57; Charles F. Romanus and Riley Sunderland, *The China-Burma-India Theater: Time Runs Out in CBI*, United China Relief Series, no. 6 (Washington, DC: Chief Office of the Military History Department of the Army, 1959), 242, 371; Watt, *Saving Lives in Wartime China*, 131–32; White and Jacoby, *Thunder Out of China*, 136–48.

62. Hsiung Ping-chen and Cheng Li-jung, *Yang Wenda xiansheng fangwen jilu*, 33.

63. Lary, *Chinese People at War*, 160–61.

64. Zhao Chuan, *Taiwan laobing koushu lishi*, 64.

65. Eastman, *Seeds of Destruction*, 130; Mitter, *Forgotten Ally*, 379; Luo Zhuanxu, ed., *Chongqing kangzhan dashiji* (Grand record of Chongqing's War of Resistance) (Chongqing: Chongqing Publishing House, 1995), 3; Paine, *Wars for Asia*, 128–29.

66. Most Soviet aid, which included nearly one thousand planes and two thousand pilots, went to the NRA rather than the Communists. Eastman, "Nationalist China," 576. Communist guerrilla soldiers in North China captured some of this advanced weaponry from the IJA, chiefly machine guns and trench mortars. See Abbas, *And One Did Not Come Back!*, 109.

67. Mitter, *Forgotten Ally*, 106–07; Paine, *Wars for Asia*, 133, 202. Quite fortunately for China, the Allies had launched a massive bombing campaign against Japan, so in late 1944 the IJA called the entire campaign to a halt in order to prioritize defending the home islands. Paine, *Wars for Asia*, 203.

68. Parks M. Coble, *China's War Reporters: The Legacy of Resistance against Japan* (Cambridge, MA: Harvard University Press, 2015), 31–54; Mitter, *Forgotten Ally*, 160–64; Paine, *Wars for Asia*, 129.

69. Bob Tadashi Wakabayashi, "The Messiness of Historical Reality," in *The Nanking Atrocity, 1937–1938: Complicating the Picture*, ed. Bob Tadashi Wakabayashi (New York: Berghahn Books, 2007), 3.

70. The fire destroyed thirteen hospitals and a large portion of the city's grain reserves. Lary, *Chinese People at War*, 62–64.

71. Ibid., 60–61.

72. Micah S. Muscolino, *The Ecology of War in China: Henan Province, the Yellow River, and Beyond, 1938–1950* (New York: Cambridge University Press, 2015).

73. Mitter, *Forgotten Ally*, 106–07; Paine, *Wars for Asia*, 133.

74. Yao Aihua, "Memoir of Yao Aihua," 209.

75. Zhao Chuan, *Taiwan laobing koushu lishi*, 65.

76. White and Jacoby, *Thunder Out of China*, 133–34, 140. Although there are many problems with this journalistic book, which frequently employs false data to underscore its politically motivated argument, I employ it here since scholarship corroborates White and Jacoby on this point.

77. Watt, *Saving Lives in Wartime China*, 181–83, 189, 191, 193–94, 197.

78. Eastman, *Seeds of Destruction*, 151–52; Landdeck, "Under the Gun: Nationalist Military Service and Society in Wartime Sichuan, 1938–1945" (PhD diss., University of California, Berkeley, 2011). This event was reported in the evening edition of *Dagongbao* (French name *L'Impartiale*) (*Dagongwanbao*) on July 10, 1945.

79. Mitter, *Forgotten Ally*, 258–59.

80. Ibid., 332; Watt, *Saving Lives in Wartime China*, 170.

81. Zhao Chuan, *Taiwan laobing koushu lishi*, 65–66. Although lucky enough to escape the fate of a wild ghost (one unsettled in the afterlife because the body never received a proper burial), Pan never returned to his Sichuan home; the army flew him to Jiangsu, where he met up with an uncle in Nanjing and got a job in a munitions factory. When that factory moved to Taiwan in 1949, Pan moved with it and eventually married a Taiwanese woman.

82. Yao Aihua, "Memoir of Yao Aihua," 207.

83. Many theorists in anthropology, sociology, philosophy, and psychoanalysis write of this, but one foundational text is Emile Durkheim, *The Elementary Forms of the Religious Life*, trans. Joseph Ward Swain (London: Allen and Unwin, 1915). Durkheim argues that all societies, regardless of the complexity of their social organization, work to perpetuate, produce, and reproduce the social unit, to which death constitutes a threat. Hence, he posited that every human society possesses a means of repairing the damage that death does to the social through mortuary ritual.

84. Evelyn S. Rawski, "A Historian's Approach to Chinese Death Ritual," in *Death Ritual in Late Imperial and Modern China*, ed. James L. Watson and Evelyn S. Rawski (Berkeley: University of California Press, 1988), 27.

85. Stuart E. Thompson, "Death, Food, and Fertility," in *Death Ritual in Late Imperial and Modern China*, ed. James L. Watson and Evelyn S. Rawski (Berkeley: University of California Press, 1988), 84–85. See also the essays throughout this volume for details of proper funerary ritual, which of course varies across space and time in China, even if the ultimate aim of appeasing the dead to ensure their smooth transition into the afterlife and repairing the social community of the living remains constant.

86. Susan Naquin, "Funerals in North China: Uniformity and Variation," in *Death Ritual in Late Imperial and Modern China*, ed. James L. Watson and Evelyn S. Rawski (Berkeley: University of California Press, 1988), 47. Janet Theiss has written about how women in late imperial China who were raped committed suicide with agency, so as to simultaneously clear their family name from the shame and employ their power as vengeful ghosts to haunt and trouble their perpetrators. Janet Theiss, *Disgraceful Matters: The Politics of Chastity in Eighteenth-Century China* (Berkeley: University of California Press, 2004).

87. Myron L. Cohen, "Souls and Salvation in Popular Religion: Conflicting Themes in Chinese Popular Religion," in *Death Ritual in Late Imperial and Modern China,* ed. James L. Watson and Evelyn S. Rawski (Berkeley: University of California Press, 1988), 191. Cohen writes in reference to the late nineteenth through the early twentieth centuries. The belief that a person needed a complete body for safe transition to the afterlife made cremation immensely unpopular for all but staunch Buddhists throughout most of Chinese history and across the country. See Martin K. Whyte, "Death in the People's Republic of China," in *Death Ritual in Late Imperial and Modern China,* ed. James L. Watson and Evelyn S. Rawski (Berkeley: University of California Press, 1988), 292, esp. n. 8.

88. Cited in Lary, *Chinese People at War,* 143. See also ibid., 115–16, 180.

89. Rebecca Nedostup, "Burying, Repatriating, and Leaving the Dead in Wartime and Postwar China and Taiwan, 1937–1955," *Journal of Chinese History* 1 (2017): 137. The quote is from one such woman, Chu T'ien-hsin.

90. Frederic Wakeman Jr., "Mao's Remains," in *Death Ritual in Late Imperial and Modern China,* ed. James L. Watson and Evelyn S. Rawski (Berkeley: University of California Press, 1988), 260.

91. Yang Shanyao, *Kangzhan shiqi de Kangzhan junyi,* 175–84.

92. Watt, *Saving Lives in Wartime China,* 122–23, 126–29; Yang Shanyao, *Kangzhan shiqi de Kangzhan junyi,* 58. These two books provide much more detailed information on all military medical systems than the present work does. Watt focuses on Dr. Lim's organizations as well as the medical organizations in and around Yan'an, while Yang focuses on the AMA and its Army Medical College.

93. Chou Chun-yen, "Funü yu kangzhan," 150; Eastman, "Nationalist China," 574.

94. Yang Shanyao, *Kangzhan shiqi de Zhongguo junyi,* 128, 137.

95. Xie Bingying, *A Woman Soldier's Own Story,* trans. Lily Chia Brissman and Barry Brissman (New York: Berkeley Books, 2001), 273.

96. Laurie S. Stoff, "The Sounds, Odors, and Textures of Russian Wartime Nursing," in *Russian History through the Senses: From 1700 to the Present,* ed. Matthew P. Romaniello and Tricia Starks (London: Bloomsbury, 2016), 117.

97. This theory has come under much criticism, but it has also fueled hundreds of publications in psychology, principally by Paul Ekman. Foundational works are Paul Ekman and Wallace V. Friesen, "Constants across Cultures in the Face and Emotion," *Journal of Personality and Emotional Psychology* 17, no. 2 (1971): 124–29; and Paul Ekman, Wallace V. Friesen, and Phoebe Ellsworth, *Emotion in the Human Face: Guidelines for Research and an Integration of Findings* (New York: Pergamon Press, 1972).

98. Chou Chun-yen, "Funü yu kangzhan," 158–64.

99. The famous scholar and political thinker Liang Qichao most famously made such a case in his essay "Lun nüxue" (On women's education), *Shiwubao,* no. 23, April 1897.

100. Chou Chun-yen, "Funü yu kangzhan," 166. The students from Taiyuan went to Jehol to treat soldiers wounded in the North China Plain war that preceded the War of Resistance.

101. Dewen Zhang, "The Making of National Women: Gender, Nationalism and Social Mobilization in China's Anti-Japanese War of Resistance, 1937–1945" (PhD diss., Stony Brook University, 2013); Xie Bingying, *Woman Soldier's Own Story.*

102. Yao Aihua, "Memoir of Yao Aihua," 205, 207.

103. Xia Gaotian, "Problems with Wounded Soldiers and Refugees," essay no. 1 (n.p., Independent Publisher, November 1938), 615/460, GPA.

104. Yang Shanyao, *Kangzhan shiqi de Zhongguo junyi*, 141.

105. Cited in ibid., 138. Three hundred *li* is roughly equivalent to ninety-three miles.

106. Yao Aihua, "Memoir of Yao Aihua," 205. While under normal conditions tetanus is a noncommunicable disease, its causative agent, the bacterium *Clostridium tetani*, can move from one open wound to another when human bodies are in great physical proximity to one another, as wounded soldiers often were in makeshift hospitals.

107. Ibid., 205, 207.

108. *The Chinese Red Cross* (Nanjing: Executive Yuan News Bureau, 1947), 5, GPA 000/143.19; Watt, *Saving Lives in Wartime China*, 122–23.

109. "National Red Cross Society of China, Medical Relief Commission, Third Report, August-December 1938," ABMAC box 23, National Red Cross Society of China, Reports, RBML.

110. Lyle Stephenson Powell, *A Surgeon in Wartime China* (Lawrence: University of Kansas Press, 1946), 204–5.

111. Ji Hong, "Problems with Wounded Soldiers and Refugees," essay no. 2 (n.p.: Independent Publisher, November 1938), 615/460, GPA.

112. Benedict Anderson, *Imagined Communities: Reflections on the Origin and Spread of Nationalism*, 2nd ed. (London: Verso Press, 1991), 144.

113. Naoki Sakai, *Translation and Subjectivity: On Japan and Cultural Nationalism* (Minneapolis: University of Minnesota Press, 1997), 181.

114. Du Si, recorder, "Nü hushi de hua (Zuotan hui)" (Words from female nurses [Discussion forum]), *Funü shenghuo* (Women's lives) 8, no. 3 (November 1939): 13.

115. Crook and Gilmartin, *Prosperity's Predicament*, 225.

116. Chang Peng-yuan and Lo Jiu-jung Lo, *Zhou Meiyu xiansheng fangwen jilu*, 58.

117. Elaine Scarry, "Injury and the Structure of War," *Representations*, no. 10 (Spring 1985): 5.

118. Ibid., 20.

119. For a poignant story of how Japanese soldiers were trained to become killers in "trial[s] of courage," see Haruko Taya Cook and Theodore F. Cook, *Japan at War: An Oral History* (New York: W. W. Norton and Company, 1992): 41–43.

120. Du Si, "Nü hushi de hua." Emphasis added.

121. Yao Aihua, "Memoir of Yao Aihua," 205.

122. Xie Bingying, *Woman Soldier's Own Story*, 273. Xie originally published this work in two volumes, in 1936 and 1946, but they did not necessarily circulate widely until republished in Chengdu in 1985 and Beijing in 1994. Coble, *China's War Reporters*, 186–87. Fang Jun interviewed Yao Aihua in 2010, so Yao may well have renarrated her own past through the words of Xie Bingying.

123. Tani E. Barlow, *The Question of Women in Chinese Feminism* (Durham, NC: Duke University Press, 2004), 96–114, esp. 100 and 131.

124. Scarry, "Structure of War," 1. Nurses were far from alone in this work. In her article, Scarry analyzes many other means of obfuscating this violence.

125. Du Si, "Nü hushi de hua."

126. Ibid., 14.

127. Yao Aihua, "Memoir of Yao Aihua," 205.

128. Xie Bingying, *Woman Soldier's Own Story,* 270.

129. Ibid.

130. Only recently have mainland Chinese begun to acknowledge the fact that the Nationalist Party bore the greatest weight of the War of Resistance. Mitter, *Forgotten Ally,* 371–74.

131. Barbara H. Rosenwein, "Worrying about Emotions in History," *American Historical Review* 107, no. 3 (June 2002): 821–45, esp. 844–45; Barbara H. Rosenwein, *Emotional Communities in the Early Middle Ages* (Ithaca, NY: Cornell University Press, 2006); and Barbara H. Rosenwein, *Generations of Feeling: A History of Emotions, 600–1700* (Cambridge: Cambridge University Press, 2016). Rosenwein is a historian of medieval Europe, but her concept and method are more broadly applicable. On their applicability, see Rob Boddice, *The History of Emotions* (Manchester, UK: Manchester University Press, 2018), 77–83; Jan Plamper, *The History of Emotions: An Introduction* (Oxford: Oxford University Press, 2012), 67–71, esp. 69; and Barbara H. Rosenwein and Riccardo Cristiani, *What Is the History of Emotions?* (Cambridge: Polity, 2018), 39–45.

132. The concept of "nested wars" comes from Paine, *Wars for Asia,* 4–5.

133. Chang Peng-yuan and Lo Jiu-jung Lo, *Zhou Meiyu xiansheng fangwen jilu,* 27; Chou Chun-yen, "Funü yu kangzhan," 208–9.

4. AUTHORITY IN THE HALLS OF SCIENCE: WOMEN OF THE WARDS

Du Si, recorder, "Nü hushi de hua (Zuotan hui)" (Words from Female Nurses [Discussion forum]), *Funü shenghuo (Women's lives)* 8, no. 3 (November 1939): 13. Emphasis added.

1. Bridie Andrews, *The Making of Modern Chinese Medicine* (Vancouver: University of British Columbia Press, 2014), 118.

2. As noted in chap. 2, Xie Bingying asserted that nine out of ten women joined her Women's Auxiliary Corps to escape arranged marriages, which Xie herself had done. See Xie Bingying, A Woman Soldier's Own Story, trans. Lily Chia Brissman and Barry Brissman (New York: Berkeley Books, 2001), 52.

3. Andrews, *Modern Chinese Medicine,* 11.

4. Gyan Prakash advocates the use of "translation" rather than "adaptation" because it adequately "recognize[s] the renegotiation of knowledge and power forced upon Western science because its hegemony could not be established through imposition." Gyan Prakash, *Another Reason: Science and the Imagination of Modern India* (Princeton, NJ: Princeton University Press, 1999), 83.

5. Shing-ting Ling, "The Female Hand: The Making of Western Medicine for Women in China, 1880s–1920s" (PhD diss., Columbia University, 2015), 154–55. See also ibid., 26, 75–121, 147.

6. Women's access to scientific authority was challenged in other societies as well. See, e.g., Jenna Tonn, "Extralaboratory Life: Gender Politics and Experimental Biology at Radcliffe College, 1894–1910," *Gender & History* 29, no. 2 (August 2017): 329–58.

7. Arlie Russell Hochschild, *The Managed Heart: Commercialization of Human Feeling* (Berkeley: University of California Press, 2003), 7. Emphasis in the original. See also Michael Hardt and Antonio Negri, *Multitude: War and Democracy in the Age of Empire* (New York: Penguin Press, 2004), 111.

8. Eugenia Lean, *Public Passions: The Trial of Shi Jianqiao and the Rise of Popular Sympathy in Republican China* (Berkeley: University of California Press, 2007), 88–93.

9. Xie Bingying, *Woman Soldier's Own Story*, 276.

10. Antonia Finnane, *Changing Clothes in China: Fashion, History, Nation* (New York: Columbia University Press, 2008), 160.

11. Chang Peng-yuan, interviewer, and Lo Jiu-rung, recorder, *Zhou Meiyu xiansheng fangwen jilu* (The reminiscences of Professor Chow Mei-yu), Oral History Series no. 47 (Taipei: Academia Sinica Institute of Modern History, 1993), 103–04.

12. Yao Aihua, "Memoir of Yao Aihua," in Fang Jun, *Zuihou yi ci jijie* (The last concentration of troops) (Liaoning: Shenyang: Liaoning renmin chubanshe, 2012), 208, 211–12.

13. Margaret Humphreys, *Marrow of Tragedy: The Health Crisis of the American Civil War* (Baltimore: Johns Hopkins University Press, 2013), 50–51.

14. Barbara H. Rosenwein, *Emotional Communities in the Early Middle Ages* (Ithaca, NY: Cornell University Press, 2006), 2.

15. There are interesting parallels with Soviet women who fought in and commanded military divisions during World War II. Having psychological, emotional, and discursive access to the "new liberated Soviet womanhood," women in the Soviet Red Army "did not represent themselves as *women* enacting *male* roles," but as "women 'realizing their hidden female talents'" and living "a legitimate type of womanhood." Anna Krylova, *Soviet Women in Combat: A History of Violence on the Eastern Front* (Cambridge: Cambridge University Press, 2010), esp. 9–10, 12–14. The stories of the many women who fought with and cared for the communist guerrilla armies in North China would likely reflect the modes of self-identification most fitting for comparison with Soviet fighters. See Dewen Zhang, "The Making of National Women: Gender, Nationalism and Social Mobilization in China's Anti-Japanese War of Resistance, 1937–1945" (PhD diss., Stony Brook University, 2013).

16. Anna Krylova, "Gender Binary and the Limits of Poststructuralist Method," *Gender & History* 28, no. 2 (August 2016): 307–23, esp. 316.

17. Dorothy Ko, *Teachers of the Inner Chambers: Women and Culture in Seventeenth-Century China* (Stanford, CA: Stanford University Press, 1994), esp. 3–4.

18. Krylova, "Gender Binary," 318–20.

19. Dipesh Chakrabarty, *Provincializing Europe: Postcolonial Thought and Historical Difference* (Princeton, NJ: Princeton University Press, 2000).

20. This occurred in a variety of fields, including physical education, home economics, and medicine. See Zheng Wang, *Women in the Chinese Enlightenment: Oral and Textual Histories* (Berkeley: University of California Press, 1999); Helen M. Schneider, *Keeping the Nation's House: Domestic Management and the Making of Modern China* (Vancouver: University of British Columbia Press, 2011); and Connie A. Shemo, *The Chinese Medical Ministries of Kang Cheng and Shi Meiyu, 1872–1937: On a Cross-Cultural Frontier of Gender, Race, and Nation* (Bethlehem, MD: Lehigh University Press, 2011).

21. *Tienü* is frequently translated as "Iron Girls" (see, e.g., Zheng Wang, *Finding Women in the State: A Socialist Feminist Revolution in the People's Republic of China, 1949–1964* [Berkeley: University of California Press, 2016], 221–41), but *nü* clearly means "woman" or "women" and not "girl."

22. On medical uniforms and sartorial signaling of authority in women's medicine, see Ling, "Female Hand," 154.

23. This helps to explain why historians of medicine in China have largely neglected women's history. The overrepresentation of men in positions of prominence held even as many of those men learned from their mothers and grandmothers. See, e.g., Volker Scheid, *Currents of Tradition in Chinese Medicine, 1626–2006* (Seattle: Eastland Press, 2007), 369. The life story of the only documented literate female doctor in late imperial China, Tan Yunxian, also affirms that women in medical lineages played a key role in transmitting knowledge of healing. (Tan inherited her grandmother's medical library and learned much about the healing arts from her female elder.) See Tan Yunxian, *Miscellaneous Records of a Female Doctor,* trans. Lorraine Wilcox with Yue Lu (Portland, OR: Chinese Medicine Database, 2015).

24. John R. Watt, *Saving Lives in Wartime China: How Medical Reformers Built Modern Healthcare Systems amid War and Epidemics, 1928–1945* (Leiden: E. J. Brill, 2014), 174, 185, 228, 234 graph 6.5.

25. Albert E. Cowdrey, *Fighting for Life: American Military Medicine in World War II* (New York: Free Press, 1994), 336.

26. Chang Peng-yuan and Lo Jiu-rung, *Zhou Meiyu xiansheng fangwen jilu,* 100.

27. Sean Hsiang-lin Lei, *Neither Donkey nor Horse: Medicine in the Struggle over China's Modernity* (Chicago: University of Chicago Press, 2014), 223–57.

28. In his 1940 report to the China Medical Board, Chen Zhiqian, in his capacity as director of the Sichuan Provincial Health Administration (SPHA), described financial duress as the greatest strain of the war. See C. C. Chen to M. C. Balfour, November 6, 1940, folder 161, box 18, series 601, record group 1.1, RF, RAC.

29. "A Summary of the Proceedings of a Conference on Medicine and Public Health in China, Held in New York City under the Auspices of United China Relief on April 11–12, 1942," ABMAC records, box 28, folder "United China Relief—Medical Conference April 1942," RBML, 11–12, 14.

30. Executive Yuan Media Bureau, *Zhongguo hongshizihui* (The Chinese Red Cross) (Nanjing, 1947), 10, SML.

31. Khwaja Ahmad Abbas, *And One Did Not Come Back! The Story of the Congress Medical Mission to China* (Bombay: Sound Magazine, 1944), 38, 44.

32. American Friends Service Committee, *Under the Red and Black Star,* American Friends Service Committee Miscellaneous Pamphlets, n.d., BUTSL, 5, 9–10; American Friends Service Committee Annual Report, 1942, BUTSL, 7–8; A. Tegla Davies, *Friends Ambulance Unit: The Story of the F.A.U. in the Second World War, 1939–1946* (London: George Allen and Unwin, 1947).

33. Abbas, *And One Did Not Come Back;* Chang Peng-yuan and Lo Jiu-rung, *Zhou Meiyu xiansheng fangwen jilu,* 56, 61–63, 101; Watt, *Saving Lives in Wartime China,* 254–70.

34. John R. Watt, *A Friend in Deed: ABMAC and the Republic of China, 1937–1987* (New York: ABMAC, 1992), 2–5; American Bureau for Medical Advancement in China, *Medicine on a Mission: A History of the American Bureau for Medical Aid to China, 1937–1954* (New York: ABMAC Headquarters, 1954), sec. 1, p. 15.

35. *United China Relief Five Year Report, 1941–1945,* 1946, BUTSL, n.p. The precise amount given to China was $36,277,940.82.

36. American Bureau for Medical Advancement in China, *Medicine on a Mission,* sec. 1, p. 21.

37. Ibid., sec. 1, p. 6; sec. 2, pp. 1, 4, 14, 18–19. After creating detailed plans for penicillin production in China, it was determined that it was much more cost-effective to produce it in the United States and ship it to China. A small penicillin plant opened in a temple compound in Beijing in January 1947, with a daily production output of one hundred vials. Ibid., sec. 3, p. 10.

38. Finnane, *Changing Clothes in China,* 205, 208–9.

39. Caption text attached to photograph. Emphasis added. ABMAC Archives, Columbia University Rare Book & Manuscript Library, box 85, folder "Surgical Relief Supplies."

40. Helen Kennedy Stevens and Ruth H. Block, "The American Bureau for Medical Aid to China: A Survey of China's Medical and Health Problems and the Progress Made by the Chinese Government in Providing for the Health of the Nation," November 1943, folder 62, box 9, CMB, RAC, app.

41. Lei, *Neither Donkey Nor Horse,* 83. Lei points out that in the early twentieth century, Chinese educated in scientific medicine were much more strident critics of Chinese medicine than were foreigners. This was often the case in the war years as well.

42. American Bureau for Medical Advancement in China, *Medicine on a Mission,* sec. 2, p. 18.

43. Mary Brown Bullock, *The Oil Prince's Legacy: Rockefeller Philanthropy in China* (Stanford, CA: Stanford University Press, 2011), 19. The precise sum for medical projects in China was $32,810,322.33. "The Rockefeller Foundation Payments for Work in China, 1914–1951," p. 9, folder 133, box 13, ser. 601, record group 1, RF, RAC. Ten million dollars were given between 1939 and 1951; see Edwin C. Lobenstine to Szeming Sze, August 31, 1942, folder 1109, box 152, CMB, RAC.

44. Among these were Chen Zhiqian (C. C. Chen, PUMC class of 1929), head of the Mass Education Movement Department of Public Health (1931–37) and director of the Sichuan Provincial Health Administration (1938–45); Liu Ruiheng (J. Heng Liu, PUMC faculty in Surgery 1918–20; PUMC superintendent 1923–29), minister of health (1929–39) and surgeon general of the Chinese Army (1938–45); Lim Kho Seng (Robert Lim, director of the PUMC Department of Physiology, 1924–37), director of the Emergency Medical Service Training School and the Chinese Red Cross Medical Relief Corps (1938–42); Zhou Meiyu (PUMC School of Nursing class of 1930), chief of the Nursing Service of the Chinese Army Medical Corps; Yang Chongrui (Marion Yang, educated at various missionary schools, instructor at PUMC), head of the National Health Administration Division of Maternity and Child Health (1942–45); Nie Yuchan (Vera Nieh, PUMC School of Nursing class of 1926), assistant dean (1938–40) and dean (1940–46) of the PUMC School of Nursing; Zhu Zhanggeng (C. K. Chu, PUMC class of 1928), director of the Public Health Personnel Training Institute (PHPTI, 1939–41), vice-director (1941–42) and then director of the National Institute of Health (1942–43), and secretary of the Commission on Medical Education; Yang Wenda (PUMC class of 1937), superintendent of the Chinese Red Cross Medical Relief Corps headquarters hospital in Guiyang during the War of Resistance, and head of the Army Medical Administration during the Civil War; and Li Ting'an (Lei Ting On, PUMC Class of 1926, PUMC faculty in Public Health 1926–31), Shanghai commissioner of health (1934–37), NHA special commissioner for epidemic prevention in South China (1937–39), NHA chief of the Epidemic Prevention Corps (1939), director of the National Central University Medical College Department of Public Health (1939–41 and 1942–43),

director of the National Institute of Health (1941–42), and professor of public health at West China Union University (1944–46).

45. Hsiung Ping-chen, interviewer, and Cheng Li-jung, recorder, *Yang Wenda xiansheng fangwen jilu* (Reminiscences of Dr. Yang Wen-ta), Oral History Series no. 26 (Taipei: Academia Sinica Institute of Modern History, 1991), 17.

46. Bullock, *Oil Prince's Legacy,* 3.

47. Marcos Cueto, ed., *Missionaries of Science: The Rockefeller Foundation and Latin America* (Bloomington, IN: Indiana University Press, 1994). On JDR Sr.'s transformation from philanthropy focused on Baptist missionaries to philanthropy centered on scientific medicine, see Bullock, *Oil Prince's Legacy,* 13–14.

48. John Farley, *To Cast Out Disease: A History of the International Health Division of the Rockefeller Foundation, 1913–1951* (Oxford: Oxford University Press, 2003).

49. C. C. Chen, *Medicine in Rural China: A Personal Account* (Berkeley: University of California Press, 1989), 57; Lei, *Neither Donkey nor Horse,* 228–29; C. C. Chen, "A Statement of the Szechuan Provincial Health Administration," December 1, 1939, p. 1, folder 161, box 18, ser, 601, record group 1.1, RF, RAC. Although Chen Zhiqian assumed different posts after the war's end, the SPHA continued operation through 1948.

50. Ka-che Yip, *Health and National Reconstruction in Nationalist China: The Development of Modern Health Services, 1928–1937* (Ann Arbor, MI: University of Michigan Press, 1995).

51. Hsiung Ping-chen and Cheng Li-jung, *Yang Wenda xiansheng fangwen jilu,* 19; Chen, *Medicine in Rural China,* 33.

52. Li T'ing-an files, box 1760, folder 1, PUMC Archives, Peking Union Medical College, Beijing. Thanks to Liping Bu for pointing this out.

53. Chang Peng-yuan and Lo Jiu-rung, *Zhou Meiyu xiansheng fangwen jilu,* 9; Hsiung Ping-chen and Cheng Li-jung, *Yang Wenda xiansheng fangwen jilu,* 21.

54. Kate Merkel-Hess, *The Rural Modern: Reconstructing the Self and State in Republican China* (Chicago: University of Chicago Press, 2016), 150. Another group of Chinese medical elites, more prevalent in the Army Medical Administration, had been educated in German and Japanese schools that followed a different educational model. See Yang Shanyao, *Kangzhan shiqi de Zhongguo junyi* (China's military medicine during the War of Resistance) (Taipei: Academia Historica, 2015), 100–3, 109, 113.

55. Chang Peng-yuan and Lo Jiu-rung, *Zhou Meiyu xiansheng fangwen jilu,* 99.

56. Kathryn Montgomery, "Redescribing Biomedicine: Toward the Integration of East Asian Medicine into Contemporary Healthcare," in *Integrating East Asian Medicine into Contemporary Healthcare,* ed. Volker Scheid and Hugh MacPherson (Edinburgh: Churchill Livingstone, 2012), 229.

57. Bullock, *Oil Prince's Legacy,* 14.

58. The EMSTS had originally accepted high school graduates, for whom they provided three months of training before deploying them to the MRC or a hospital run by the NHA. Yang Shanyao, *Kangzhan shiqi de Zhongguo junyi* (China's military medicine during the War of Resistance) (Taipei: Academia Historica, 2015), 59.

59. Yao Aihua "Memoir of Yao Aihua," 212.

60. Ibid.

61. David Luesink, "Anatomy and the Reconfiguration of Life and Death in Republican China," *Journal of Asian Studies* 76, no. 4 (November 2017): 1010.

62. "Nursing Program: Nurses' Association of China, Chungking," in P. Z. King to Dr. George W. Bachman, September 15, 1942, ABMAC records, RBML, box 23, folder "Nurses Association of China," p. 3.

63. Ibid.

64. Ibid.

65. Ling, "Female Hand," cited text in unpaginated abstract. Ling grounds her study in the Hackett Medical Complex in Guangzhou, but her argument is more broadly applicable.

66. "Science Teaching Is Helping to Develop China's Leaders," n.d, UCC.

67. Watt, *Friend in Deed,* 3.

68. "Report of School of Nursing PUMC for the period of December 8, 1941, to June 30, 1944," folder 708, box 99, CMB, RAC, 13; Vera Nieh, "A Brief Account of the PUMC School of Nursing During and After World War II: A Message to its Alumnae," folder 711, box 99, CMB, RAC, 22.

69. Margaret Humphreys, "Women, War and Medicine," in *Marrow of Tragedy: The Health Crisis of the American Civil War* (Baltimore: Johns Hopkins University Press, 2013), 48–75. Although many blacks, both free and enslaved, performed much of the nursing labor for the Confederate Army during the American Civil War and continued to support their communities with hospital healthcare through the post-Reconstruction period, they had no opportunity for equity until the establishment of the Women's Auxiliary Army Corps in 1942. See Sarah Ann Johnson, "Healing in Silence: Black Nurses in Charleston, South Carolina, 1896–1948" (PhD diss., Medical University of South Carolina, 2008), esp. 113; and Barbara Lee Maling, "Black Southern Nursing Care Providers in Virginia during the American Civil War, 1861–1865" (PhD diss., University of Virginia, 2009). On Japanese nurses, see Aya Takahashi, *The Development of the Japanese Nursing Profession: Adopting and Adapting Western Influences* (New York: Routledge, 2004).

70. Du Si, "Nü hushi de hua," 13.

71. "Nursing Program: Nurses' Association of China, Chungking," in P. Z. King to Dr. George W. Bachman, September 15, 1942, ABMAC records, RBML, box 23, folder "Nurses Association of China," p. 1.

72. Irene Harris, 1943 Work Report from Chongqing, 1943, 1983.047C, 9–230, UCC.

73. C. M. Hoffman, "Canadian Medical Work in Chungking," *West China Missionary News* 39, no.10 (October 1937): 49.

74. Gladys Cunningham to Dr. Arnup, September 7, 1950, 1983.047C, 13–331, UCC.

75. *China Inland Mission Story for 1942-3 of the Hospital at Paoning, Szechwan, China* (Newington Green, London: China Inland Mission, 1942), 25, SOAS ASC, CIM box 19, file 418/16.

76. Alexander Stuart Allen, Report of Dr. A. Stewart Allen on the Investigation of Hospitals and Relief throughout China, 1946, 1983.047C, 11–274, UCC, 8.

77. Harris, 1943 Work Report from Chongqing.

78. I. C. Yuan to Alan Gregg, May 31, 1946, folder 708, box 99, CMB, RAC.

79. Yip, *Health and National Reconstruction,* 177.

80. *Dagongbao,* nos. 13709 (January 26, 1942). 13717 (February 3, 1942), and 13960 (October 4, 1942).

81. *Dagongbao,* no. 13797 (April 23, 1942).

82. Chang Peng-yuan and Lo Jiu-rung, *Zhou Meiyu xiansheng fangwen jilu,* 59. Zhou's monthly salary while stationed in Guiyang was 36.66 yuan.

83. Johnson, *Delivering Modernity*, 100–101.

84. Harris, 1943 Work Report from Chongqing; Allen, Report of Dr. A. Stewart Allen, 4.

85. "Zuijin yishi renyuan tongji" (The most recent statistics on medical personnel), *Xinan yixue zazhi* 4, no. 3 (March 15, 1944): n.p.

86. Chang Peng-yuan and Lo Jiu-rung, *Zhou Meiyu xiansheng fangwen jilu*, 27.

87. Chou Chun-yen, "Funü yu kangzhan shiqi de zhandi jiuhu" / "Women and battlefield first aid during the Second Sino-Japanese War," *Jindai Zhongguo funüshi yanjiu / Research on Women in Modern Chinese History* 24 (December 2014): 147.

88. Chang Peng-yuan and Lo Jiu-rung, *Zhou Meiyu xiansheng fangwen jilu*, 28.

89. Ibid., 27.

90. Chou Chun-yen, "Funü yu kangzhan," 208–9. Chou does note, however, that in the ensuing Civil War people with nursing training, regardless of their sex, were once again mobilized for military service.

91. Xie Bingying, *Woman Soldier's Own Story*, 273. Emphasis added.

92. Judith Butler, *Gender Trouble* (New York: Routledge, 1990).

93. Haiyan Lee, *Revolution of the Heart: A Genealogy of Love in China, 1900–1950* (Stanford, CA: Stanford University Press, 2007), 256–65; the citation is on p. 256.

94. Chang-tai Hung, *War and Popular Culture: Resistance in Modern China, 1937–1945* (Berkeley: University of California Press, 1994).

95. Hu Ying, *Burying Autumn: Poetry, Friendship, and Loss* (Cambridge, MA: Harvard University Asia Center, 2016).

96. Lean, *Public Passions*, 187–93, 210; the citation is on p. 192.

97. Xie Bingying, *Woman Soldier's Own Story*, 272.

98. Chou Chun-yen, "Funü yu kangzhan," 201.

99. Laurie S. Stoff, "The Sounds, Odors, and Textures of Russian Wartime Nursing," in *Russian History through the Senses: From 1700 to the Present*, ed. Matthew P. Romaniello and Tricia Starks (London: Bloomsbury, 2016), 122. On Japanese Red Cross nurses, see Takahashi, *Japanese Nursing Profession*, 82.

100. Yao Aihua, "Memoir of Yao Aihua," 205; Chang Peng-yuan and Lo Jiu-rung, *Zhou Meiyu xiansheng fangwen jilu*, 49.

101. "Fenfen qingying shadi" (One after another volunteering for military service to kill the enemy), *Funü shenghuo* (Women's lives) 9, no. 7 (August 1939): 8.

102. Nai Tian, "Beizhanchang shang de yihuo nübing" (A group of women soldiers on the northern battlefront), *Funü shenghuo* (Women's lives) 9, no. 7 (August 1939): 31–32.

103. David Strand, *An Unfinished Republic: Leading by Word and Deed in Modern China* (Berkeley: University of California Press, 2011), 127.

104. Nai, "Beizhanchang shang de yihuo nübing," 32.

105. Krylova, *Soviet Women in Combat*.

106. Still, it bears pointing out that the armed forces organized in the communist base at Yan'an more frequently accepted women into the military ranks, due to both the Communist Party's ideological commitment to women's liberation and the guerrilla army's desperate need for soldiers. See Pan Yihong, "Zhanzheng conglai buzhishi nanren de shiye: Jiedu Xinsijun nübing huiyilu" / "Never a Man's War: The Self-Reflections of the Women Soldiers of the New Fourth Army in the War of Resistance against Japan, 1937–1945," *Jindai Zhongguo funüshi yanjiu / Research on Women in Modern Chinese History* 24 (December 2014): 83–131.

107. Yao Aihua, "Memoir of Yao Aihua," 209.

108. Du Si, "Nü hushi de hua," 14. Emphasis added.

109. Chang Peng-yuan and Lo Jiu-rung, *Zhou Meiyu xiansheng fangwen jilu,* 49. Emphasis added.

110. On Hu Lanqi, the first woman to attain the rank of major general in the NRA, see Kristin Stapleton, "Hu Lanqi: Woman, Soldier, Heroine, and Survivor," in *The Human Tradition in Modern China,* ed. Kristin Stapleton and Kenneth J. Hammond (Lanham, MD: Rowman and Littlefield, 2008), 166.

111. Joan Judge, *The Precious Raft of History: The Past, the West, and the Woman Question in China* (Stanford, CA: Stanford University Press, 2008), 188.

112. Strand, *Unfinished Republic,* 111.

113. Hu Ying, *Burying Autumn,* 290–91, 330; Yao Aihua, "Memoir of Yao Aihua," 206.

114. Wang, *Women in the Chinese Enlightenment,* 22. Wang is referring to the women of the May Fourth generation who joined the CCP, a party that "demanded total submission of the individual." I relate this to the situation of women working as nurses in the NRA during the War of Resistance due to the similarities in their positionalities.

115. Joan Scott, "The Evidence of Experience," *Critical Inquiry* 17 (Summer 1991): 792–93. Thanks to James Nealy for calling this argument to my attention.

116. Watt, *Saving Lives,* 172. On the blood bank and African-Americans, see Wayne Soon, "Blood, Soymilk, and Vitality: The Wartime Origins of Blood Banking in China, 1943–1945," *Bulletin of the History of Medicine* 90, no. 3 (2016), 430–32.

117. Soon, "Blood, Soymilk, and Vitality," 436–39.

118. Quoted in ibid., 439.

119. Watt, *Saving Lives,* 173.

120. Helena Wong, "Report from the Donor's Clinic (September 1944), November 14, 1944, correspondence, ABMAC. Cited in Soon, "Blood, Soymilk, and Vitality," 439.

121. John Z. Bowers, *Western Medicine in a Chinese Palace: Peking Union Medical College, 1917–1951* (Philadelphia: Josiah Macy Jr. Foundation, 1972), 209; "Faculty and Teaching Staff of PUMC Nursing School in University Hospital, Chengtu," folder 1038, box 143, CMB, RAC, 1.

122. Houghton to Lobenstine, December 9, 1938, folder 707, box 99, CMB, RAC.

123. CEF to Dr. Wong Wen-hao, September 13, 1943, folder 1039, box 144, CMB, RAC; CEF cable to ECL, received September 20, 1943, folder 1039, box 144, CMB, RAC; "Report of School of Nursing"; Dewen Zhang, "Rockefeller Foundation and China's Wartime Nursing, 1937–1945," *Rockefeller Archive Center Research Reports Online,* 2009, http://www.rockarch. org/publications/resrep/zhang.pdf.

124. Ruth Ingram, "Report on Visit to the PUMC School of Nursing in the West China Union University Hospital, Chengtu," October 18–November 2, 1945, folder 1041, box 143, CMB, RAC, 2–3.

125. CEF to Vera Nieh and CEF to Y. T. Tsur, February 24, 1944, folder 1039, box 144, CMB, RAC. Tsur was a graduate of Yale University (class of 1909), had served as president of Hsiangya Medical College (Yale-in-China), and during the war built in Guizhou Province a successful boys' school and a large cultural compound comprising a library, a scientific training center for high school teachers, an exhibition hall for displaying native products, and an art museum. See Lyle Stephenson Powell, *A Surgeon in Wartime China* (Lawrence: University of Kansas Press, 1946), 127–29.

126. Vera Nieh cable to ECL, February 25, 1944, folder 1039, box 144, CMB, RAC.

127. Dr. Li Ting'an to Dr. Y. T. Tsur, confidential letter, March 3, 1944, folder 1040, box 143, CMB, RAC.

128. CEF letter no. 50, March 9, 1944, folder 1040, box 143, CMB, RAC; Dr. Li Ting-an to Mr. Earle Ballou, CMB, RAC; confidential letter, March 11, 1944, folder 1040, box 143, CMB, RAC.

129. CEF to Dr. Tsur, February 24, 1944, folder 1039, box 144, CMB, RAC.

130. Stephen Chang to ECL, March 18, 1944, 6, folder 1040, box 143, CMB, RAC.

131. CEF to Dr. Tsur, February 24, 1944, folder 1039, box 144, CMB, RAC.

132. Dr. Li Ting'an to Dr. Y. T. Tsur, confidential letter, March 3, 1944, folder 1040, box 143, CMB, RAC. After receiving academic awards and becoming a favored student of Dr. John B. Grant, director of the PUMC Department of Public Health, in 1944, Dr. Li assumed two posts at West China Union University—professor of public health, and superintendent of the University Hospital—in order to be of assistance to the PUMC School of Nursing faculty.

133. Faculty, PUMC School of Nursing to Dr. Y. T. Tsur, Chairman of PUMC Board of Trustees, March 20, 1944, folder 1040, box 143, CMB, RAC.

134. Dr. Y. T. Tsur to ECL, March 27, 1944, folder 1040, box 143, CMB, RAC.

135. Mei Yu Chou, A. C. Hsu, Chi Chen, Mary Sia, Katherine Yu, Lily Tseng, and Margaret Wang Sung to Y. T. Tsur, May 3, 1944, folder 1040, box 143, CMB, RAC.

136. *China Handbook, 1937–1943: A Comprehensive Survey of Major Developments in China in Six Years of War* (Chungking: Chinese Ministry of Information, July 1943), 667.

137. Sichuan Provincial Health Administration, *Health Statistics for all of Sichuan Province,* 1945, SPA, 113-1-118, 11.

138. In the fall of 1943, Claude Forkner also got into a deep conflict with Drs. I. C. Yuan, James Shen, and Y. L. Mei. See CEF to Lobenstine and Pearce, October 4, 1943, folder 221, box 32, CMB, RAC; CEF to CMB, October 18, 1943, folder 156, box 22, CMB, RAC; and CEF to CMB, November 12, 1943, folder 221, box 32, CMB, RAC. No sooner had he cleared up this dispute than another emerged with Dr. Chow Shou-kuai. See CEF to CMB, December 6, 1943, folder 221, box 32, CMB, RAC. The chief archivist for China materials at the Rockefeller Archive Center, Tom Rosenbaum, told me that Forkner repeatedly made social mistakes during his China Medical Board tenure (personal communication, December 2009). Dr. John Watt told me of Forkner's condescending attitude toward women in a personal communication, October 28, 2009.

139. Nieh to J. Heng Liu, cable received February 9, 1944, folder 1040, box 143, CMB, RAC; Nieh to ECL, cable received February 25, 1944, folder 1040, box 143, CMB, RAC. For the assessment that these two cables constituted an attack, see ECL to Wong Wen-hao, March 21, 1944, folder 1040, box 143, CMB, RAC.

140. See CEF to Dr. Tsur, February 24, 1944, folder 1039, box 144, CMB, RAC; and CEF cable to CMB, March 3, 1944, folder 1040, box 143, CMB, RAC.

141. Andrew Scull, *Hysteria: The Biography* (Oxford: Oxford University Press, 2009); Elaine Showalter, ed., *Daughters of Decadence: Women Writers of the Fin-de-Siècle* (New Brunswick, NJ: Rutgers University Press, 1993), ix–x.

142. Li Ting-an to CEF, April 20, 1944, folder 1040, box 143, CMB, RAC. In late March 1944, three well-known Chinese men—J. Heng Liu, Alfred Sze, and Hu Shih—decided to

send a personal message to Dean Nieh after attending a meeting of the PUMC Board of Trustees. See ECL to Wong Wen-hao, March 21, 1944, folder 1040, box 143, CMB, RAC. Soon thereafter, Li Ting-an wrote, "Since Miss Nieh is now quite silent, there has not arisen much difficulty for the past two weeks." See Li Ting-an to CEF, March 31, 1944, folder 1040, box 143, CMB, RAC. By April 20, Dean Nieh had left Chengdu for Chongqing and Guiyang, where she inspected other health administration facilities and got a rest from her duties. See Li Ting-an to Y. T. Tsur, April 20, 1944; and Li Ting-an to CEF, April 20, 1944; both folder 1040, box 143, CMB, RAC.

143. Li Ting-an to CEF, May 11, 1944, folder 1040, box 143, CMB, RAC; Li Ting-an to CEF, March 31, 1944, folder 1040, box 143, CMB, RAC; CEF to Dr. Wilford of United Hospital, October 17, 1943, folder 1038, box 143, CMB, RAC.

144. "Report of School of Nursing."

145. Ruth Ingram, daughter of medical missionary James H. Ingram of the American Board of Congregational Missions, was born in China and spoke fluent Mandarin Chinese. She served as dean of the PUMC School of Nursing until Gertrude Hodgman succeeded her in 1930. See Bowers, *Western Medicine*, 206–7.

146. Ingram, "Report on Visit," 1.

147. Students and faculty of the PUMC School of Nursing finally departed Chengdu for their return trip to Beijing on April 24, 1946. See Bowers, *Western Medicine*, 213.

148. Ingram, "Report on Visit," 1.

149. Ibid., 1, 3.

150. Ibid., 3–4.

151. Ibid., 3.

152. *Alumnae News*, no. 9, Alumnae Association of School of Nursing, PUMC, Peiping, October 1948, folder 711, box 99, CMB, RAC, 2; Vera Y. C. Nieh files, box 2437, folder 3, files 182, 204, and 214, PUMC.

153. I. C. Yuan to Alan Gregg, May 31, 1946, folder 708, box 99, CMB, RAC.

154. Bowers, *Western Medicine*, 214.

155. If Mao Zedong's personal physician Li Zhisui is to be believed, another possible explanation could be Mao's own admiration for scientific medicine. Li Zhisui, *The Private Life of Chairman Mao*, trans. Tai Hung-chao (New York: Random House, 1994).

156. Mary Augusta Brazelton, "Vaccinating the Nation: Public Health and Mass Immunization in Modern China, 1900–1960" (PhD diss., Yale University, 2015); Watt, *Saving Lives*, 221–22, 238.

157. Watt, *Saving Lives*, 248–49.

158. Sze-ming Sze, *The Origins of the World Health Organization: A Personal Memoir, 1945–1948* (Boca Raton, FL: L.I.S.Z. Publications, 1982).

159. Other leaders in wartime nursing had also moved to Taiwan (including Hsu Ai-Chu, who continued to serve as director of nursing at the NIH after its move to Taipei), so the Republic of China became a key center of nursing training within the Western Pacific Region (WPRO) of the World Health Organization. For example, in November 1952 nurses from Australia, Malaya, the Philippines, Japan, and Taiwan meeting in New Zealand convened the first WPRO nursing conference in Taipei. "Nursing Education Seminar Sponsored by World Health Organization Western Pacific Region, Taipei, Taiwan, November 1952," in *Seminars/Conferences Reports, WHO Regional Offices for the Western Pacific, 1952–1957*, WHO Library, Geneva.

160. In October 1969 the CMB funded the construction of a public health demonstration center in Seoul and sponsored a Korean faculty member's study trip to Taipei. M. Iliyas, M.D., Public Health Administrator, "Second Quarterly Field Report, Korea 0041 Training of Health and Medical Workers," 1 July 1969; "First Quarterly Field Report, Korea 0041 Training of Health and Medical Workers," 30 March 1969; both in KOR-HMD-001 1968–1970 HMD 1 Education & Training of Health Personnel (ROK/72/P02) A PRO.308, WHO, Geneva.

161. Rosalind Wang, "Nursing in China," *American Journal of Chinese Medicine* 2, no. 1 (1974): 45–47. For a detailed analysis of how the split into two Chinas affected the development of nursing, see Sonya Grypma and Cheng Zhen, "The Development of Modern Nursing in China," in *Medical Transitions in Twentieth-Century China*, ed. Bridie Andrews and Mary Brown Bullock (Bloomington: Indiana University Press, 2014), 308–16.

162. Registration of Nurses Associations in Various Cities and Provinces, SHA, October 1946–October 1948, 11.2.4321.

163. Zhang, "China's Wartime Nursing," 5.

164. Wang Xiuying, "Wu yi'er hushi jie ganyan" (Testimonials for Nurses' Day on May 12), *Chinese Nurses* 1, no. 2 (1947). Quoted in "Nursing Specialist Wang Xiuying," in Zhongguo xiandai yixue zhuanlue (Medical biographies of modern China) (Beijing: Kexue jishu wenxian chubanshe, 1984), 321.

165. Yao Aihua, "Memoir of Yao Aihua," 203–4, 213–14.

166. Patricia D'Antonio, Julie A. Fairman, and Jean C. Whelan, Introduction to *Routledge Handbook on the Global History of Nursing* (New York: Routledge, 2013), 6.

167. This was certainly the case for women in the American Civil War. See Jeanie Attie, "Warwork and the Crisis of Domesticity in the North," in *Divided Houses: Gender and the Civil War*, ed. Catherine Clinton and Nina Silber (Oxford: Oxford University Press, 1992), 247–49.

168. Rana Mitter, "Classifying Citizens in Nationalist China during World War II, 1937–1941," in "China in World War II, 1937–1945: Experience, Memory, and Legacy," special issue, *Modern Asian Studies* 45, no. 2 (2011): 273.

169. Christina Kelley Gilmartin, *Engendering the Chinese Revolution: Radical Women, Communist Politics, and Mass Movements in the 1920s* (Berkeley: University of California Press, 1995); Wang, *Women in the Chinese Enlightenment*, 22.

5. MOTHERS FOR THE NATION

CBPH Work Report, 1944, CMA, Chongqing, 66-1-2, 14.

1. John R. Watt, *Saving Lives in Wartime China: How Medical Reformers Built Modern Healthcare Systems amid War and Epidemics, 1928–1945* (Leiden: E. J. Brill, 2014), 68–69.

2. Isabel Brown Crook and Christina Kelley Gilmartin with Yu Xiji, *Prosperity's Predicament: Identity, Reform, and Resistance in Rural Wartime China*, comp. and ed. Gail Hershatter and Emily Honig (Lanham, MD: Rowman and Littlefield, 2013), 188.

3. In Nanjing, e.g., state-registered midwives attended 237 births in 1931–32, and 2,565 in 1934–35. State-registered midwives and nurses delivered 43 percent of the births at the Beijing First Health Station in the same time period. Nanjing's maternal mortality rate of 15.2 was on the high end of Yang Chongrui's estimate, but its infantile mortality rate of 168.4

per 1,000 was far below her national calculation of 200 to 250. See Watt, *Saving Lives in Wartime China*, 67.

4. Executive Committee and the Committee on Science and Publication of the Ninth Congress of the Far Eastern Association of Tropical Medicine, *A Glimpse of China* (Shanghai: Mercury Press, 1934), 75.

5. The repercussions of this social change are poorly documented and understudied.

6. During the Song dynasty (960–1279), elite male physicians developed gynecology (*fuke*) as a medical specialty grounded in the theory of women's bodies as ruled by blood and inherently weak, and in this way they claimed professional authority over the parturient female body. Although male gynecologists in the Ming (1368–1644) and Qing (1644–1911) dynasties challenged their predecessors' claim of female weakness, they continued the professionalization of this field of medicine. See Charlotte Furth, *A Flourishing Yin: Gender in China's Medical History* (Berkeley: University of California Press, 1999); and Yi-li Wu, *Reproducing Women: Medicine, Metaphor and Childbirth in Late Imperial China* (Berkeley: University of California Press, 2010).

7. Tani E. Barlow, *The Question of Women in Chinese Feminism* (Durham, NC: Duke University Press, 2004), 59.

8. Yun-Chen Chiang, "Womanhood, Motherhood and Biology: The Early Phases of *The Ladies' Journal*, 1915–25," *Gender and History* 18, no. 3 (November 2006): 519–45.

9. Joan Judge, "Citizens or Mothers of Citizens?: Gender and the Meaning of Modern Chinese Citizenship," in *Citizenship in Modern China*, ed. Elizabeth Perry and Merle Goldman (Cambridge, MA: Harvard University Asia Center, 2002): 23–43; Joan Judge, *The Precious Raft of History: The Past, the West, and the Woman Question in China* (Stanford, CA: Stanford University Press, 2008), 107–38; Helen M. Schneider, *Keeping the Nation's House: Domestic Management and the Making of Modern China* (Vancouver: University of British Columbia Press, 2011), esp. 23.

10. Scholars have noted that even women who hold to otherwise radical politics often readily embrace political representation through their role as mothers and wives. On revolutionary France, see Lynn Hunt, *The Family Romance of the French Revolution* (Berkeley: University of California Press, 1992), 123. On Meiji Japan, see Sharon H. Nolte and Sally Ann Hastings, "The Meiji State's Policy toward Women, 1890–1910," in *Recreating Japanese Women, 1600–1945*, ed. Gail Lee Bernstein (Berkeley: University of California Press, 1991), 169–70. On wartime Germany, see Claudia Koonz, *Mothers in the Fatherland: Women, the Family and Nazi Politics* (New York: St. Martin's Press, 1987). See also Judge, *Precious Raft of History*, 116.

11. Dr. F. C. Yen (Yan Fuqing), "The Importance of Woman and Child Welfare Work," *People's Tribune*, November 1938, ABMAC box 21, folder NHA 1940–1941, RBML, 2. Dr. Yan wrote, "Ever since the outbreak of hostilities, Chinese newspapers have carried frequent reports of the enemy abducting thousands of Chinese boys in the occupied area."

12. M. Colette Plum, "Unlikely Heirs: War Orphans during the Second Sino-Japanese War, 1937–1945" (PhD diss., Stanford University, 2006).

13. Kazuko Ono, *Chinese Women in a Century of Revolution, 1850–1950*, ed. Joshua A. Fogel. (Stanford, CA: Stanford University Press, 1989), 27.

14. M. Colette Plum, "Lost Childhoods in a New China: Child-Citizen-Workers at War, 1937–1945," *European Journal of East Asian Studies* 11, no. 2 (December 2012): 237–58.

15. Chart of Women's Organizations in Chongqing, May–July 1941, CMA, 51-2-564, 1–13.

16. Tang Guozhen, "Zhongguo funü weilao ziwei kangzhan jiangshi zonghui Zhanshi ertong baoyu hui gongzuo baogao" (National Association of Chinese Women for the Cheering and Comforting of the Officers and Soldiers of the War of Self-Defense and Resistance against Japan Wartime Association for Child Welfare work report), in *Funü tanhua hui gongzuo baogao* (Women's Conversational Committee work reports), ed. Women's Conversational Committee (n.p., 1938), 23. Although Tang does not specify, she was likely referring solely to male orphans since the language at the time assumed a male standard for all nouns, and only females needed qualifiers.

17. Plum, "Lost Childhoods," 238, 242–43.

18. Plum, "Unlikely Heirs," 103, 227–28, 241.

19. Chang Peng-yuan, interviewer, and Lo Jiu-jung, recorder, *Zhou Meiyu xiansheng fangwen jilu* (The reminiscences of Professor Chow Mei-yu), Oral History Series no. 47 (Taipei: Academia Sinica Institute of Modern History, 1993), 57–58.

20. Qing, "*Weilao fushang zhuangshi*" (Comforting wounded heroes), *Funü shenghuo* (Women's lives) 8, no. 5 (December 1939): 15.

21. Danke Li, *Echoes of Chongqing: Women in Wartime China* (Urbana and Chicago: University of Illinois Press, 2010), 102–6.

22. Ibid., 121–23.

23. Hui Nian, "Chongqing funü dui junshu de yijian" (Chongqing women's opinions on military families), *Funü shenghuo* (Women's lives) 8, no. 3 (Nov 1939): 7.

24. Parks M. Coble, *China's War Reporters: The Legacy of Resistance against Japan* (Cambridge, MA: Harvard University Press, 2015), 91.

25. Li, *Echoes of Chongqing*, 63.

26. For stories of two men kidnapped by Japanese troops, see R. Keith Schoppa, *In a Sea of Bitterness: Refugees during the Sino-Japanese War* (Cambridge, MA: Harvard University Press, 2011), 111–36.

27. Diana Lary, *The Chinese People at War: Human Suffering and Social Transformation, 1937–1945* (New York: Cambridge University Press, 2010), 118.

28. Lloyd E. Eastman, *Seeds of Destruction: Nationalist China in War and Revolution, 1937–1945* (Stanford, CA: Stanford University Press, 1984), 56, 64–65; Schoppa, *Sea of Bitterness*, 52.

29. Crook and Gilmartin, *Prosperity's Predicament*, 67, 77–78, 86.

30. Schneider, *Keeping the Nation's House*, 18.

31. Hui Nian, "Chongqing funü dui junshu de yijian," 7–8.

32. Crook and Gilmartin., *Prosperity's Predicament*, 87–88.

33. Li, *Echoes of Chongqing*, 61–64.

34. Announcement placed in the *Dagongbao*, no. 13514, July 15, 1941.

35. Li, *Echoes of Chongqing*, 86–87. Stories like Li Shuhua's corroborate Gail Hershatter's discovery that many rural women in the collective era—another period in Chinese history when women's domestic and reproductive labors were unrewarded—experienced extreme exhaustion during their reproductive years, and therefore supported the One Child Policy in the 1970s. Gail Hershatter, *The Gender of Memory: Rural Women and China's Collective Past* (Berkeley: University of California Press, 2011), 182–209.

36. Yao Aihua, "Memoir of Yao Aihua," in Fang Jun, *Zuihou yi ci jijie* (The last concentration of troops) (Shenyang: Liaoning renmin chubanshe, 2012), 212.

37. Cai Chusheng and Zheng Junli, *Yijiang chunshui xiang dongliu* (*The Spring River Flows East*) (Shanghai: Lianhua Film Company, 1947).

38. Tina Phillips Johnson, *Childbirth in Republican China: Delivering Modernity* (Lanham, MD: Lexington Books, 2011), xvii–xviii, xxv–xxvi.

39. For a fascinating story of how villagers in Yunnan resisted biomedical treatment in favor of traditional religious practices during a 1942 cholera epidemic, see Francis L. K. Hsu, *Religion, Science and Human Crises: A Study of China in Transition and Its Implications for the West* (London: Routledge and Kegan Paul, 1952).

40. Johnson, *Childbirth in Republican China*, 83.

41. Ibid., 81, 88; Marion Yang files, boxes 76 and 77, CMB, RAC.

42. Nina Rattner Gelbert, *The King's Midwife: A History and Mystery of Madame Du Coudray* (Berkeley: University of California Press, 1998).

43. American Bureau for Medical Advancement in China, *Medicine on a Mission: A History of the American Bureau for Medical Aid to China, 1937–1954* (New York: ABMAC Headquarters, 1954), sec. 2, p. 8.

44. Tina Phillips Johnson, "Yang Chongrui and the First National Midwifery School: Childbirth Reform in Early Twentieth-Century China," *Asian Medicine* 4, no. 2 (2008): 288.

45. Yang Chongrui, Midwifery Bag "A" Type for Maternity Assistants—Old type Midwiver [*sic*] or short course trained, n.d., CMB I, RAC, box 77, folder 539; Johnson, *Childbirth in Republican China*, 56–57.

46. Johnson, *Childbirth in Republican China*, xvii.

47. National Institute of Health (Geleshan, Chongqing), Public Health Calendar, 1943, National Library of Medicine.

48. Yao Aihua, "Memoir of Yao Aihua," 210.

49. Hsiao Li Lindsay, *Bold Plum: With the Guerrillas in China's War against Japan* (Morrisville, NC: Lulu Press, 2007), 152–65.

50. CBPH Work Report, January–June 1940, CMA, 66-1-3, 171; CBPH Work Report, 1940, CMA, 66-1-3, "Table of Private and Public Hospitals in Chongqing Proper and in the Suburbs," August 1940, CMA, 66-1-3, 198; CBPH Work Report, September 1940–February 1941, CMA, 66-1-3, 198.

51. "Report of Szechuan Provincial Health Administration For the Year of 1941," folder 2719, box 218, series 3, record group 5.3, IHBA, 8.

52. CBPH Work Report, September 1940–February 1941, CMA, 66-1-3, 200.

53. CBPH Work Report, January–June 1940, CMA, 66-1-3, 172; CPBH Work Report, September 1940–February 1941, CMA, 66-1-3, 199.

54. CBPH Work Report, 1938, CMA, 66-1-2, 189.

55. CPBH Work Report, September 1940–February 1941, CMA, 66-1-3, 214. In 1940, the clinics and mobile medic teams combined provided 15,275 smallpox inoculations and 19,149 preventive vaccinations. See CBPH Work Report, September 1940–February 1941, CMA, 66-1-3, 200.

56. CBPH Work Report, January–June 1940, CMA, 66-1-3, 185.

57. CBPH Work Report, September 1940–February 1941, CMA, 66-1-3, 217.

58. CBPH Work Report, May 15–21, 1944, CMA, 0066-1-2, 66, 78; CBPH, Survey of Public and Private Health Organizations in Chongqing, 1944, CMA, 66-1-9(1), 1–4.

59. CBPH Work Report, 1943, CMA, 66-1-2, 206–7. The bureau had originally budgeted 505,640 yuan for the hospital's equipment and construction, but spent only 266,860, and began the 1944 fiscal year with 238,600 yuan left over in this line of the budget.

60. CBPH Work Report, October 1946, AH, 90–183, 1b.

61. Watt, *Saving Lives in Wartime China*, 227.

62. Johnson, "Yang Chongrui," 286.

63. Watt, *Saving Lives in Wartime China*, 283–88.

64. China Women's Welfare Society, *Sinian lai zhi peidu funü fuli she* (The past four years in the Women's Welfare Society of the Wartime Capital) (Nanjing: China Women's Welfare Society, 1946), 2–3. The group had wanted to raise 900,000 yuan: 560,000 yuan for construction, and an additional 340,000 yuan for monthly operational costs.

65. Johnson, "Yang Chongrui," 293.

66. Du Si, recorder, "Nü hushi de hua (Zuotan hui)" (Words from female nurses [Discussion forum]), *Funü shenghuo* (Women's lives) 8, no. 3 (November 1939): 14.

67. Ibid.

68. Bishan's 1945 budget was over one million yuan, and the county reported a total of seventy-two medical personnel, whereas Chengdu had twenty-three. See 1945 Complete Statistical Health Report Compiled by the Sichuan Provincial Health Administration, 1945, SPA, 113-1-118, 4, 7–10, 15–21, 105–8; "Report on Health Improvements in This Province," 1940, SPA, 113–116, 10; "Resume of Activities in January to August, 1940," folder 161, box 18, ser. 601, record group 1.1, RF, RAC, 2; Crook and Gilmartin, *Prosperity's Predicament*, 188–89.

69. Kate Merkel-Hess challenges this narrative in her recent book, *The Rural Modern: Reconstructing the Self and State in Republican China* (Chicago: University of Chicago Press, 2016).

70. Bishan CHC Work Report, July 1944, SPA, 113-1-694; Watt, *Saving Lives in Wartime China*, 228.

71. Bishan County Health Center Report on Personnel Training, February 1942, SPA, 96–100.

72. Michael Hardt and Antonio Negri, *Multitude: War and Democracy in the Age of Empire* (New York: Penguin Press, 2004), 108.

73. Bishan CHC Work Report, January–June 1940, SPA, 113-1-129, 84–85.

74. Ibid., n.p. Women constituted 61 percent of outpatients during the reporting period—an astonishingly high number given that in other counties and cities men regularly outnumbered women as recipients of hospital care.

75. 1945 Complete Statistical Health Report Compiled by the Sichuan Provincial Health Administration, 1945, SPA, 113-1-118, 98–99.

76. Ibid., 90–92.

77. Bishan CHC Work Reports, March and April 1943, SPA, 113-1-926, 16, 22. The scabies treatment station at the Bishan bus terminal cost the CHC a total of 1,039 yuan, a cost offset only slightly by 60 yuan in donations.

78. Watt, *Saving Lives in Wartime China*, 95n69. A school health survey conducted in Chongqing in March 1945 found that nearly 65 percent of schoolchildren suffered from

trachoma—the highest incidence of any one disease among over five thousand children surveyed. Zhou Yong, ed., *Chongqing tongshi* (A comprehensive history of Chongqing), vol. 3 (Chongqing: Chongqing Press, 2002), 1145. A 1940 survey of schoolchildren in Xinglong found that 60 percent suffered from eye troubles, mostly trachoma. Crook and Gilmartin, *Prosperity's Predicament*, 200, 204n30; Ka-che Yip, *Health and National Reconstruction in Nationalist China: The Development of Modern Health Services, 1928–1937* (Ann Arbor, MI: University of Michigan Press, 1995), 81.

79. Johnson, *Childbirth in Republican China*, 85; Watt, *Saving Lives in Wartime China*, 228.

80. Bishan CHC Work Report, March 1943, SPA, 113-1-926, 20.

81. Fang Xiaoping, *Barefoot Doctors and Western Medicine in China* (Rochester, NY: University of Rochester Press, 2012).

82. Crook and Gilmartin, *Prosperity's Predicament*, 173–74, 268.

83. Ibid., 199–200.

84. Ibid., 201–2.

85. CBPH Work Report, 1940, 197.

86. CBPH Work Report, 1944, CMA, 66-1-2, 34, 48. These statistics were reported only from July through December 1944, and the number of male and female residents at the hospital is a combination of those reported separately for July through September (266 men and 108 women) and for October through December (168 men and 36 women).

87. Chongqing Municipal Hospital, Patient Statistics and Work Report, January 1944–June 1945, CMA, 165-2-5. There are, in fact, two exceptions to this statement: statistics for May and June 1945. This is solely because the hospital's Obstetrics and Gynecology Department opened on May 1, and hundreds of women came to the hospital for its services (318 women in May; 708 in June). By taking these numbers out of the aggregate, I calculated the *non*-OB-GYN numbers for all eighteen months, rather than allowing the last two months to skew the remaining sixteen months' statistics.

88. Ibid.

89. CBPH Work Report, January–June 1940, CMA, 66-1-3, 172; CBPH Work Report, July–September 1944, CMA, 66-1-2, 21; CBPH Work Report, October–December 1944, CMA, 66-1-2, 58; CBPH Work Report, October 1946, AH, 90-183, 14b, 15a.

90. Johnson, *Childbirth in Republican China*, 20–22, 24. Helen Schneider also notes a trend of bourgeois women distinguishing themselves from either lower- or very upper-class women through their consumption habits. Schneider, *Keeping the Nation's House*, 14.

91. Helen M. Schneider, "Mobilising Women: The Women's Advisory Council, Resistance and Reconstruction during China's War with Japan," *European Journal of East Asian Studies* 11, no. 2 (December 2012): 213–36.

92. Lo Jiu-jung, Yu Chien-ming, and Chiu Hei-yuan, eds., *Fenghuo suiyue xia de Zhongguo funü fangwen jilu* (Twentieth-century wartime experiences of Chinese women: An oral history) (Taipei: Academia Sinica Institute of Modern History, 2004), 5–21. Unfortunately, Zhang does not mention the name of this establishment, which could have been one of the eight clinics operated by the CBPH or a private clinic.

93. *Dagongbao*, nos. 13685 (January 3, 1942), 13687 (January 5, 1942), 13754 (March 12, 1942), and 14079 (January 31, 1943).

94. *Dagongbao,* nos. 12658B (December 12, 1938), 12693 (January 6, 1939), 12725 (February 7, 1939), 13687 (January 5, 1942), 13721 (February 7, 1942), 13755 (March 13, 1942), and 13796 (April 23, 1942).

95. *Dagongbao,* nos. 12688 (January 1, 1939) and 13717 (February 3, 1942).

96. *Dagongbao,* nos. 14076 (January 28, 1943) and 14078 (January 30, 1943).

97. *Dagongbao,* no. 14197 (June 1, 1943).

98. *Dagongbao,* no. 13831 (May 28, 1942).

99. Crook and Gilmartin, *Prosperity's Predicament,* 203.

100. American Bureau for Medical Advancement in China, *Medicine on a Mission,* sec. 2, pp. 8–9.

101. On transformations in Ayurvedic practice due to doctors' vernacularization of specific technologies, see Projit Bihari Mukharji, *Doctoring Traditions: Ayurveda, Small Technologies, and Braided Sciences* (Chicago: University of Chicago Press, 2016).

102. Marshall C. Balfour Officer's Diary, May 29, 1939, RF Archives, RG 12.1, RAC, 30; letter from C. H. Huang, January 20, 1943, NHA files, folder 682, box 95, CMB, RAC; Mary Brown Bullock, *An American Transplant: The Rockefeller Foundation and Peking Union Medical College* (Berkeley: University of California Press, 1980), 194.

103. *Funü Xinyun* (Women's New Life Movement), an organ of the WAC, was published monthly in Chongqing from late 1938 through July 1948.

104. American Bureau for Medical Advancement in China, *Medicine on a Mission,* sec. 2, p. 8.

105. Yang Chongrui, *Zhufu xuzhi: Jiating weisheng ji jiazheng gaiyao* (What a housewife must know: An outline of family hygiene and home economics) (Nanjing: NHA, 1940 [1934]), 1–2, 17.

106. Ibid., 23.

107. Ibid., 18.

108. Ibid., 23, 26. Presumably, Yang used "venereal disease" (*hualiubing*) here to reference HSV-1, the herpes simplex virus known as orolabial herpes and manifesting on the facial lips. The linguistic slip probably originated from the fact that HSV-1 belongs to the same viral family, *Herpesviridae,* as HSV-2, the source of most genital herpes.

109. Schneider, *Keeping the Nation's House,* 9.

110. Song Meiling, *Madame Chiang Kai-shek on the New Life Movement* (Shanghai: China Weekly Review Press, 1937), 69.

111. Yang Chongrui and Wang Shijin, *Fuying weisheng xue* (The study of maternal and children's health) (Chongqing: National Institute of Health, 1944), 153.

112. Ibid., 1. On the translation of *minzu,* a Sino-Japanese-European loanword (Liu, *Translingual Practice: Literature, National Culture, and Translated Modernity: China, 1900–1937* [Stanford, CA: Stanford University Press, 1995], 292), as "nation-race," see Andrew D. Morris, *Marrow of the Nation: A History of Sport and Physical Culture in Republican China* (Berkeley: University of California Press, 2004), 102.

113. Margaret Jolly, "Introduction: Colonial and Postcolonial Plots in the History of Maternities and Modernities," in *Maternities and Modernities: Colonial and Postcolonial Experiences in Asia and the Pacific,* ed. Margaret Jolly and Kalpana Ram (Cambridge: Cambridge University Press, 1998), 2.

114. Crook and Gilmartin, *Prosperity's Predicament,* 173–74, 268.

115. Yang Chongrui and Wang Shijin, *Fuying weisheng xue*, 1.

116. On the introduction of a new understanding, developed in the early twentieth century, of birth as a medical event and the birthing woman as patient, see Johnson, *Childbirth in Republican China*, xv–xvi; and Brigitte Jordan, *A Crosscultural Investigation of Childbirth in Yucatan, Holland, Sweden, and the United States* (Prospect Heights, IL: Waveland Press, 1993), 45.

117. Yang Chongrui and Wang Shijin, *Fuying weisheng xue*, 2–3.

118. Furth, *Flourishing Yin;* Wu, *Reproducing Women.*

119. Yang Chongrui, *Zhufu xuzhi*, 27.

120. Wu, *Reproducing Women.*

121. Tong Lam, *A Passion for Facts: Social Surveys and the Construction of the Chinese Nation-State, 1900–1949* (Berkeley: University of California Press, 2011).

122. Yang Chongrui and Wang Shijin, *Fuying weisheng xue*, 3, 20.

123. For a discussion of the "Europe *manqué*" dynamic in scholarship, see Kenneth Pomeranz, *The Great Divergence: China, Europe, and the Making of the Modern World Economy* (Princeton, NJ: Princeton University Press, 2001), 207.

124. Yang Chongrui and Wang Shijin, *Fuying weisheng xue*, 4–6.

125. Rebecca Nedostup, *Superstitious Regimes: Religion and the Politics of Chinese Modernity* (Cambridge, MA: Harvard University Asia Center, 2009), 114–15.

126. Juliette Yuehtsen Chung, *Struggle for National Survival: Chinese Eugenics in a Transnational Context, 1896–1945* (New York: Routledge, 2002); Johnson, *Childbirth in Republican China*, 36, 38–42.

127. Sean Hsiang-lin Lei, *Neither Donkey nor Horse: Medicine in the Struggle over China's Modernity* Chicago: (University of Chicago Press, 2014), 223–57.

128. Yang Chongrui and Wang Shijin, *Fuying weisheng xue*, 5.

129. A similar phenomenon occurred in nineteenth-century Boston and changed the orientation of certain women's groups. Sarah Deutsch, "Learning to Talk More Like a Man: Boston Women's Class-Bridging Organizations, 1870–1940," *American Historical Review* 97, no. 2 (April 1992): 379–404.

130. Schneider, *Keeping the Nation's House*, 5.

131. Stephen Shapin, *A Social History of Truth: Civility and Science in Seventeenth-Century England* (Chicago: University of Chicago Press, 1994). See also Shing-ting Ling, "The Female Hand: The Making of Western Medicine for Women in China, 1880s–1920s" (PhD diss., Columbia University, 2015), esp. 26.

132. Fang Xiaoping, *Barefoot Doctors.*

133. C. C. Chen in collaboration with Frederica M. Bunge, *Medicine in Rural China: A Personal Account* (Berkeley: University of California Press, 1989), 94.

134. Ibid., 90–91. Although Chen's memoir was published in 1989, many of the quotes in the passage on MCH work were taken directly from a report he wrote in October 1936, suggesting more strongly that he (and possibly other health workers) held these attitudes at the time. See Kate Merkel-Hess, "The Public Health of Village Private Life: Reform and Resistance in Early Twentieth Century Rural China," *Journal of Social History* 49.4 (2016): 891, 902n79.

135. Merkel-Hess, "Public Heath of Village Private Life," 892.

136. Ibid., 896.

137. Irene Ssu-chin Liu Hou, ed., *Liu Ruiheng boshi yu Zhongguo yiyao ji weisheng shiye* (Dr. J. Heng Liu and medical and health development in China) (Taipei: Taiwan Commercial Press, 1989), 296.

138. ECL interview with Szeming Sze, September 13, 1944, folder 1109, box 152, CMB, RAC, 2.

139. Szeming Sze, *The Origins of the World Health Organization: A Personal Memoir, 1945–1948* (Boca Raton, FL: L.I.S.Z. Publications, 1982).

140. Johnson, *Childbirth in Republican China*, 180n41.

CONCLUSION

Yu Yun, trans., "Zuo 'hushi' shi zhanshi funü baoxiao guojia zui gaogui de shiye" (Being a "nurse" is wartime women's most noble profession to repay the country), *Funü gongming* (Women's echo) 13, no. 6 December 1944): 56.

1. Though it would be impossible to cite all scholarship on female nurses during wartime, prominent examples include Kara Dixon Vuic, "Wartime Nursing and Power," in *Routledge Handbook on the Global History of Nursing,* ed. Patricia D'Antonio, Julie A. Fairman, and Jean C. Whelan (New York: Routledge, 2013), 22–34; Margaret Humphreys, *Marrow of Tragedy: The Health Crisis of the American Civil War* (Baltimore: Johns Hopkins University Press, 2013); and Aya Takahashi, *The Development of the Japanese Nursing Profession: Adopting and Adapting Western Influences* (New York: Routledge, 2004). On the role of female nurses in national crisis, see Nancy K. Bristow, *American Pandemic: The Lost Worlds of the 1918 Influenza Pandemic* (Oxford: Oxford University Press, 2012).

2. The need for constant emotional work to create the political community—suppression of base emotions such as greed, shame, and disgust, coupled with cultivation of compassion and sympathy for others—is one of the central points in Martha C. Nussbaum's *Political Emotions: Why Love Matters for Justice* (Cambridge, MA: Belknap Press of Harvard University Press, 2013).

3. See, e.g., Timothy Brook, *Collaboration: Japanese Agents and Local Elites in Wartime China* (Cambridge, MA: Harvard University Press, 2007); Christian Henriot and Yeh Wen-hsin, eds., *In the Shadow of the Rising Sun: Shanghai under Japanese Occupation* (Cambridge: Cambridge University Press, 2004); and Lee McIsaac, "The Limits of Chinese Nationalism: Workers in Wartime Chongqing, 1937–1945" (PhD diss., Yale University, 1994).

4. Rana Mitter, *Forgotten Ally: China's World War II, 1937–1945* (Boston: Houghton Mifflin Harcourt, 2013), 378. See also Rana Mitter, "Classifying Citizens in Nationalist China during World War II, 1937–1941," in "China in World War II, 1937–1945: Experience, Memory, and Legacy," special issue, Modern Asian Studies 45, no. 2 (2011): 243–75.

5. Dai Yingcong, *The Sichuan Frontier and Tibet: Imperial Strategy in the Early Qing* (Seattle: University of Washington Press, 2009).

6. Robert A. Kapp, *Szechwan and the Chinese Republic: Provincial Militarism and Central Power, 1911–1938* (New Haven, CT: Yale University Press, 1973), 7, 15. Pinyin Romanization added.

7. Missionaries who came into Sichuan from other parts of China were shocked by the prevalent number of corpses visible in the streets, noting that this was the sordid outcome

of nearly twenty years of constant warfare. See, e.g., Esther Tappert Mortenson, Letter home from Chongqing, October 26, 1937, Esther Tappert Mortenson Papers, record group 21, box 4, folder 57, DDDL.

8. Luo Zhuanxu, ed., *Chongqing Kangzhan dashiji* (Grand record of Chongqing's War of Resistance) (Chongqing: Chongqing Publishing House, 1995), 16. After Liu's death at the Wanguo Hospital in Wuhan, his body was carried to Chongqing, where he was posthumously named Supreme Commander of the Nationalist Army and given a state burial. Since Liu enjoyed much more local power in Sichuan than did Chiang Kai-shek, his widow and close associates suspected malfeasance in his death, but no proof has yet surfaced. On the latter point see Kapp, *Szechwan and the Chinese Republic*, 139.

9. Di Wang notes that the Paoge rose to local dominance in Sichuan as an anti-Manchu, Han-nativist group in the early Qing dynasty, and that it played a key role in the 1911 Revolution, which toppled this dynasty. Di Wang, *Violence and Order on the Chengdu Plain: The Story of a Secret Brotherhood in Rural China, 1939–1949* (Stanford, CA: Stanford University Press, 2018), 40–41, 49.

10. G. William Skinner, *Rural China on the Eve of Revolution: Sichuan Fieldnotes, 1949–1950*, ed. Stevan Harrell and William Lavely (Seattle: University of Washington Press, 2017), 237.

11. Troops of the former strolled into a silent provincial capital on December 25–26, 1949, while the PLA troops enjoyed the fanfare of an organized parade and hastily pasted banners in Gaodianzi, but "the crowd seemed to be apathetic." Township leaders in Gaodianzi did feed PLA soldiers, less out of any concern for the men than to keep them from stealing from the villagers as the NRA soldiers were doing. Ibid., 147–49, 153, 156.

12. Kapp, *Szechwan and the Chinese Republic*, 140–41.

13. While stationed in rural Sichuan for fieldwork in late 1949, William Skinner met a soldier from Guangdong who had learned to speak the language of Hunan and Hubei as well as traveled all over the country while in the army. Skinner, *Rural China*, 157.

14. Ruth Rogaski, *Hygienic Modernity: Meanings of Health and Disease in Treaty-Port China* (Berkeley: University of California Press, 2004), 225–53, esp. 250. On "always already," see Paul Ricoeur, *Time and Narrative*, vol. 1, trans. Kathleen McLaughlin and David Pellauer (Chicago: University of Chicago Press, 1984), 57.

15. Key works include Christina Kelley Gilmartin, *Engendering the Chinese Revolution: Radical Women, Communist Politics, and Mass Movements in the 1920s* (Berkeley: University of California Press, 1995); Gail Hershatter, *The Gender of Memory: Rural Women and China's Collective Past* (Berkeley: University of California Press, 2011) (on rural women's lives under collectivization and the denial of the economic and political value of women's domestic labors of textile production and childrearing); Dorothy Ko, *Teachers of the Inner Chambers: Women and Culture in Seventeenth-Century China* (Stanford, CA: Stanford University Press, 1994), esp. 1–5; and Zheng Wang, *Finding Women in the State: A Socialist Feminist Revolution in the People's Republic of China, 1949–1964* (Berkeley: University of California Press, 2016).

16. Here I follow the lead of Elizabeth J. Remick, "Introduction to the *JAS* at AAS Roundtable on 'Sexuality and the State in Asia,'" *Journal of Asian Studies* 71, no. 4 (November 2012): 919–27, esp. 921.

17. All of these items come directly from a 1953 report in the Shanghai Municipal Archive, cited in full in Zheng Wang, "Gender and Maoist Urban Reorganization," in *Gender in Motion: Divisions of Labor and Cultural Change in Late Imperial and Modern China*, ed. Bryna Goodman and Wendy Larson (Lanham, MD: Rowman and Littlefield, 2005), 195–96.

18. Wang, "Gender and Maoist Urban Reorganization," 195.

19. Zhao Ma, *Runaway Wives, Urban Crimes, and Survival Tactics in Wartime Beijing, 1937–1949* (Cambridge, MA: Harvard University Asia Center, 2015), 329.

20. Ibid., 317, 331.

21. Ibid., 329–30. Ma cites the particular story of one woman here but indicates that she is an exemplar of a broader trend.

22. Wang, "Gender and Maoist Urban Reorganization," 195.

23. Ibid., 190, 191, 201.

24. Ma, *Runaway Wives*, 329; Wang, "Gender and Maoist Urban Reorganization," 204.

25. Wang, "Gender and Maoist Urban Reorganization," 200, 204. For analysis of the convergence of "two potentially separate emotional communities," see Barbara H. Rosenwein, "Worrying about Emotions in History," *American Historical Review* 107, no. 3 (June 2002): 843–45; the citation is on p. 844.

26. Zhao Ma, *Runaway Wives*, 331.

27. See Wang, "Gender and Maoist Urban Reorganization," 200–203, for the story of the working-class woman Zhang Xiulian, who narrated her work as a resident representative as a story of personal liberation.

28. Zhao Ma, *Runaway Wives*, 330.

29. Kate Merkel-Hess, "The Public Health of Village Private Life: Reform and Resistance in Early Twentieth Century Rural China," *Journal of Social History* 49, no. 4 (2016): 896.

30. Isabel Brown Crook and Christina Kelley Gilmartin with Yu Xiji, *Prosperity's Predicament: Identity, Reform, and Resistance in Rural Wartime China*, comp. and ed. Gail Hershatter and Emily Honig (Lanham, MD: Rowman and Littlefield, 2013), 268.

31. Merkel-Hess, "Public Health of Village Private Life," 897.

32. In many ways women's experiences during the War of Resistance echoed those of women who operated as nurses and soldiers in the 1911 Revolution and the Northern Expedition (1926–1928). See Gilmartin, *Engendering the Chinese Revolution*.

33. Emily Honig and Gail Hershatter, *Personal Voices: Chinese Women in the 1980s* (Stanford, CA: Stanford University Press, 1988), 25. Cited in Wang, *Finding Women in the State*, 230.

34. Wang, *Finding Women in the State*, 232–33.

35. Ibid., 230, 236.

36. Barbara Mittler, *A Continuous Revolution: Making Sense of Cultural Revolution Culture* (Cambridge, MA: Harvard University Asia Center, 2012), 7.

37. The working-class aesthetic that valorizes female strength should not be conflated with the *jianmei* (robust beauty) aesthetic of the 1930s, which celebrated the healthy female body partly as a counterpoint to "Sick Woman" discourse, but also as tied to the ideal of the "revolutionary" body of the Communist woman that circulated at the same time. See An-

tonia Finnane, *Changing Clothes in China: Fashion, History, Nation* (New York: Columbia University Press, 2008), 169–70; and Yunxiang Gao, "Nationalist and Feminist Discourses on *Jianmei* (Robust Beauty) during China's 'National Crisis' in the 1930s," *Gender and History* 18, no. 3 (November 2006): 546–73.

38. Barbara H. Rosenwein, "Worrying about Emotions," 843–45.

39. Yao Aihua, "Memoir of Yao Aihua," in Fang Jun, *Zuihou yi ci jijie* (The last concentration of troops) (Liaoning: Shenyang: Liaoning renmin chubanshe, 2012), 204.

GLOSSARY OF PERSONAL NAMES AND TERMS

Personal Names

Ba Jin	巴金
Bai Qiu'en (Norman Bethune)	白求恩
Bao Huaguo	包華國
Cai Chusheng	蔡楚生
Chang Gexin	暢革新
Chen Hui	陳惠
Chen Yuanchao	陳遠超
Chen Zhiqian (C.C. Chen)	陳志潛
Cheng Zerun	程澤潤
Deng Xihou	登錫侯
Deng Yingchao	鄧穎超
Ding Ling	丁玲
Fang Yuyong (Bang Wooyong)	方禹鏞
Feng Yuxiang	馮玉祥
Gu Qizhong	顧綺仲
Guo Zhaoxi	郭櫂西
He Xiangning	何香凝
Hu Lanqi	胡蘭畦
Hu Shi	胡適
Hua Tuo	華陀

Huan Shi'an	宦世安
Huang Ruozhen (Helena Wong)	黃若珍
Jiang Lan	江蘭
Jiao Yitang	焦易堂
Jin Baoshan (P. Z. King)	金寶善
Kang Cheng (Ida Kahn)	康成
Kang'er	抗兒
Kang Youwei	康有為
Ke Dihua (Dwarkanath Shantaram Kotnis)	柯棣華
Kitasato Shibasaburo	北里柴三郎
Kong Xiangxi (H. H. Kung)	孔祥熙
Lao She	老舍
Liang Guifang	梁閨放
Liang Qichao	梁啟超
Liang Shiqiu	梁實秋
Liang Zheng	梁拯
Liang Zhenglun (Alexander Stuart Allen)	梁正倫
Liao Junming	寥君明
Li Dianju	李殿舉
Li Dequan	李德荃
Li Jixing	李繼興
Li Hua	李華
Li Shifang	李世芳
Li Shiwei	李士偉
Li Ting'an (Lei Ting On)	李廷安
Li Zongren	李宗仁
Lin Kesheng (Lim Kho Seng; Robert "Bobby" K. S. Lim)	林可勝
Lin Wenqing (Lim Boon Keng)	林文慶
Lin Yutang	林語堂
Liu Qiying	劉崎應
Liu Ruiheng (J. Heng Liu)	劉瑞恆
Liu Xiang	劉湘
Liu Yongmao	劉永楙
Lu Jin	陸晉
Lu Zhide (Dick Loo; C. T. Loo)	盧致德
Lu Zuofu	盧作孚

Ma Haide (Shafick George Hatem)	馬海德
Ma Jiaji	馬家驥
Mei Yilin (sobriquet Yinqing)	梅貽琳（字吟青）
Mei Yiqi	梅貽琦
Nagayo Sensai	長與專齊
Nie Yuchan (Vera Y. C. Nieh)	聶毓禪
Pan Yintang	潘銀堂
Qiu Jin	秋瑾
Shi Liang	史良
Shi Meiyu (Mary Stone)	石美玉
Shi Siming (Sze Szeming)	施思明
Shiga Kiyoshi	志賀潔
Shimoda Utako	下田歌子
Song Ailing	宋藹齡
Song Jiashu (Charlie Soong)	宋嘉樹
Song Meiling (Jiang furen)	宋美齡 (蔣夫人)
Song Qingling	宋慶齡
Sufen	素芬
Tang Guozhen	唐國楨
Tang Shaoqian	唐紹潛
Tao Xingzhi	陶行知
Wang Jingwei	汪精衛
Wang Lanfang	王蘭芳
Wang Liujie	汪六皆
Wang Shijin	王詩錦
Wang Shixiong	王士雄
Wang Xiuying	王琇瑛
Wang Zuxiang	王祖祥
Wu Huaibai	吳懷白
Wu Liande (Wu Lien-teh)	伍連德
Wu Zheying	伍哲英
Xie Bingying	謝冰瑩
Xie Yunhua (Mary Sia Yun-Hua)	謝蘊華
Xiong Liaosheng	熊寥笙
Xue Yue	薛岳
Yan Fuqing (F. C. Yen)	顏福慶

Yan Yangchu (James "Jimmy" Y.C. Yen)	晏陽初
Yang Chongrui (Marion Yang)	楊崇瑞
Yang Sen	楊森
Yang Tingmei	楊廷美
Yang Xuegao	楊學高
Yao Aihua	姚愛華
Yu Wei	郁維
Zhang Lianghui	張良惠
Zhang Rongzhen	張蓉楨
Zhang Yaoxian	張耀先
Zhang Zhongliang	張忠良
Zhang Zonglin	張宗麟
Zhao Fengqiao	趙峰樵
Zheng Hongfu	鄭洪福
Zheng Junli	鄭君里
Zheng Tuixian	鄭推先
Zhou Liaoxun	周瞭熏
Zhou Meiyu	周美玉
Zhou Muying	周穆英
Zhou Shanpei	周善培
Zhou Yichun (Y.T. Tsur)	周貽春
Zhu Baotian	朱寶鈿
Zhu Xiuzhen	朱秀珍
Zhu Zhanggeng (C.K. Chu)	朱章庚

Terms

aiguo	愛國
baidai bing	白帶病
Baigu ta	白骨塔
baihua	白話
bairihou	百日喉
baojia	保甲
baojian yuan	保健院
Beibei (Beipei)	北碚
bei bu zisheng	悲不自勝
Beijing xiehe yixueyuan	北京協和醫學院

bieluosha	瘰螺痧
bingren	病人
Bishan xian	璧山縣
bu zun weisheng guiding	不尊衛生規定
Chanfuke Yiyuan	產婦科醫院
changjue	猖獗
Changning zhen	長凝鎮
chiku	吃苦
chiku nailao fucong zhihui	吃苦耐勞服從指揮
chili	赤痢
Chongqing funü fuli she	重慶婦女福利社
Chongqing kuanren yiyuan	重慶寬仁醫院
Chongqing renji yiyuan	重慶仁濟醫院
Chongqing shimin yiyuan	重慶市民醫院
Chongqingshi funü hui	重慶市婦女會
Chongqingshi fanghu tuan	重慶市防護團
Chongqingshi fangkongdong guanlichu	重慶市防空洞管理處
Chongqingshi fangkong silingbu	重慶市防空司令部
Chongqingshi jiuhu dui	重慶市救護隊
Chongqingshi linshi canyihui	重慶市臨時參議會
Chongqingshi qudi laji qingjie guize	重慶市取締垃圾清潔規則
Chongqingshi weishengju	重慶市衛生局
Chongqingshi xialing weisheng yundong cujin weiyuanhui	重慶市夏令衛生運動促進委員會
Chongqingshi xin shenghuo yundong cujinhui	重慶市新生活運動促進會
chouqi hengbi	臭氣衡鼻
chouyaoshui	臭藥水
chuanran bing	傳染病
chuqing	除清
cixiang de yisheng	慈祥的醫生
Dagongbao	大公報
daode/de	道德／德
diaojiaolou	吊腳樓
diaojiaosha	吊腳痧

Dingxian	定縣
Disi bingshi	第四病室
Dongya bingfu/fu	東亞病夫 / 婦
ernü yingxiong	兒女英雄
fa guonan cai	發國難財
fasha	發痧
fanghai weisheng an	妨害衛生案
fangshi xiang	訪視箱
fei jiehe	肺結核
Feiliaoye gonghui	肥料業工會
feiyan	肺炎
fucong jingshen	服從精神
fuke	婦科
funü neng ding banbiantian	婦女能頂半邊天
Funü Xinyun	婦女新運
Funü xin shenghuo yundong zhidao weiyuanhui	婦女新生活運動指導委員會
Funü zazhi	婦女雜誌
fuying baojiansuo	婦嬰保健所
Fuying weisheng gaiyao	婦嬰衛生概要
Fuying weisheng jiangzuo	婦嬰衛生講座
Fuying weisheng xue	婦嬰衛生學
gei xiyi jiule huilai	給西醫救了回來
Geleshan	歌樂山
Gong'anju	公安局
Gongce yunshu guanlichu	公廁運輸管理處
gongde	公德
gonggong weisheng	公共衛生
gongwu gongyi gongde weisheng	公物公益公德衛生
Gongwuju	工務局
Gongyi jiuhudui	公誼救護隊
gongyi zhidu	公醫制度
guasha	刮痧
guanggun	光棍
guanxin min mo	關心民瘼
Guofang yixueyuan	國防醫學院

Guofang zuigao weiyuanhui	國防最高委員會
guofu	國父
guojia	國家
guojia minzu guannian	國家民族觀念
guojing	國警
Guoli tongji daxue fushe gaoji hushi zhiye xuexiao	國立同濟大學附設高級護士職業學校
Guoli zhongyang gaoji hushi zhiye xuexiao	國立中央高級護士職業學校
Guoli zhongyang gaoji zhuchan zhiye xuexiao	國立中央高級助產職業學校
guomin	國民
Guomin canzhenghui	國民參政會
guomin zhi mu	國民之母
guoshu	國術
guoyi yundong	國醫運動
guxiang	故鄉
hao duizhang	好隊長
haonan bu dangbing	好男不當兵
Hechuan	合川
heirebing	黑熱病
Hei shizi	黑石子
hezuo yi jiushi jiuren	合作以救世救人
Hongwanzihui	紅卍字會
Hongyan	紅岩
hualiubing	花柳病
Huangdi neijing	黃帝內經
huanjing weisheng	環境衛生
huanwo heshan	還我河山
huchan	胡產
huliela	虎列拉
hushi	護士
huiqi	穢氣
huoluan	霍亂
Huoluan lun	霍亂論
jiapo renwang	家破人亡

jiaqiang minzu liliang	加強民族力量
Jiarong	嘉戎
jianju hanjian, suqing Gongdang	檢舉漢奸，肅清共黨
jianqiang wo houfang Kangzhan nengli	健強我後方抗戰能力
jian shu fu	撿鼠伕
jiaochangsha	攪「絞」腸痧
Jiaoyubu yixue jiaoyu weiyuanhui	教育部醫學教育委員會
Jiepou shiti guize	解剖屍體規則
jieshengpo	接生婆
jihe yanshuo	集合言說
jiji shusan	積極疏散
jinguo famei	巾幗髮眉
jinguo yingxiong	巾幗英雄
jinyinhua	金銀花
jinzhong baoguo	盡忠報國
jiuguo de shenglijun	救國的生力軍
Junyishu	軍醫署
juweihui	居委會
kanhu	看護
Kangzhan daodi	抗戰到底
KangRi zhanzheng	抗日戰爭
Kangzhan peng	抗戰棚
Kepa de huoluan	可怕的霍亂
kexuehua	科學化
kouji jing	口籍警
Kuanren gaoji hushi zhiye xuexiao	寬仁高級護士職業學校
Kuanren nan yiyuan	寬仁男醫院
Kuanren nü yiyuan	寬仁女醫院
lengku wuqing	冷酷無情
Leshan	樂山
liyi zhiyuan	禮儀志願
liuli shisuo	流離失所
louxiang ji qiongku juhu zhi exi wuran chu	陋巷及窮苦居戶之惡習污染處
Lugouqiao shibian	蘆溝橋事變
Lun nüxue	論女學

luohou	落後
mingyi	名醫
minsheng	民生
minzu	民族
mofan gongce	模範公廁
Nan'an	南岸
nangeng nüzhi	男耕女織
Nanmin zhoukan	難民週刊
panmin ruguo	叛民辱國
Paoge	袍哥
paolu chouwei chuanbo bingzheng	拋露臭味傳播病症
pengmin	棚民
Pingmin jiaoyu cujin hui	平民教育促進會
Pingmin qianzi ke	平民千字課
poyou nanzi feng	頗有男子風
qianxin wanku	千辛萬苦
qiangpo zhushe	強迫注射
qiangzu jianguo	強族建國
Qilu (Cheeloo) Medical College	齊魯大學
qingdao fu	清道伕
qingjie fu	清潔伕
qingjie zongdui	清潔總隊
qipao	旗袍
Qudi tinggui zhanxing zhangcheng	取締停櫃暫行章程
rebing	熱病
rendan	仁丹
Renji gaoji hushi zhiye xuexiao	仁濟高級護士職業學校
Renji yiyuan	仁濟醫院
renyi daxiaobian	任意大小便
ren you di geng you fan chi	人有地耕有飯吃
rongyu junren	榮譽軍人
ruyi	儒醫
sanduo	三多
sharen ruma	殺人如麻
shaqiwan	痧氣丸
shazhao	紗罩

shangfeng	傷風
Shapingba-Ciqikou	沙坪壩—磁器口
shifanqu	示範區
shirong	市容
Shiwubao	時務報
shizong	失蹤
shuang	孀
shusan qu	疏散區
Sichuan sheng weishengchu	四川省衛生處
sixiang chunzheng	思想純正
Songpan	松潘
taidu wenrou	態度溫柔
taijiao	胎教
Taierzhuang	台兒莊
tiaofen renfu	挑糞人夫
tienü	鐵女
tiyu	體育
tongqing	同情
tuhao	土豪
wawa bing	娃娃兵
wei guojia shijie mouqiu fuli	為國家世界謀求福利
weihu shehui de zhixu	維護社會的秩序
wei Kangzhan jianguo zhi zuida sunshi	為抗戰建國之最大損失
wei renmin fuwu	為人民服務
weisheng (Jp. eisei)	衛生
Weisheng bu	衛生部
Weisheng fagui	衛生法規
Weishengshu	衛生署
wen, wenhua, wenming	文，文化，文明
wenbing	溫病
wudao kouwai	勿倒口外
Wufu Gong	五福宮
Wugong xian	武功縣
Wuhua	五花
wujia kegui	無家可歸
wushu	武術

xiajiangren	下江人
xianbing	憲兵
xiangcun jianshe	鄉村建設
xianqi liangmu (Jp. *ryosai kenbo*)	賢妻良母
xian weishengyuan	縣衛生院
xialing weisheng	夏令衛生
xiao'erke	小兒科
xiaozhang	校長
Xikang	西康
xin funü	新婦女
Xinhua ribao	新華日報
Xin shenghuo yundong	新生活運動
Xin shenghuo yundong cujinhui	新生活運動促進會
Xin shenghuo yundong cujin zonghui funü zhidao weiyuanhui	新生活運動促進總會婦女指導委員會
Xinglongxiang	興隆鄉
Xinzheng	新政
Xinan lianda	西南聯大
xinfa jiesheng	新法接生
xueliu chenghe	血流成河
yang	陽
Yibin	宜賓
yida dongya bingfu jincheng jian'er zhi mudi	以達東亞病夫儘成健兒之目的
Yijiang chunshui xiang dong liu	一江春水向東流
yilü shixing qiangpo zhushe	一律施行強迫注射
yin	陰
yixiao lieqiang	貽笑列強
you huitian zhili	有回天之力
you shang guoti	有傷國體
youshengxue	優生學
youtu youxie, mian xia bi jian, pi gan yan xian, shouzhi jiaozhi quan fa zhouwen	又吐又瀉，面狹鼻尖，皮乾眼陷，手指腳趾全發皺紋
Yuecuo yueyong	越挫越勇
zengqiang guojia jianshe, shuli jianquan jiazu	增強國家建設，樹立健全家族

zengqiang kangjian liliang	增強抗建力量
zengqiang zhanli	增強戰力
Zhanshi ertong baoyuhui	戰時兒童保育會
Zhanshi weisheng renyuan xunliansuo (EMSTS)	戰時衛生人員訓練所
Zhanshi yiliao yaopin jingli weiyuanhui	戰時醫療藥品經理委員會
Zhenji weiyuanhui	賑濟委員會
Zhongguo fuli hui	中國福利會
Zhongguo funü weilao ziwei Kangzhan jiangshi zonghui	中國婦女慰勞自衛抗戰將士總會
Zhongguo fuying weisheng guoqu yu xianzai	中國婦嬰衛生過去與現在
Zhongguo hongji yiyuan	中國宏濟醫院
Zhongguo hongshizihui jiuhu zongdui (CRC MRC)	中國紅十字會救護總隊
Zhongguo yixue lishihui (China Medical Board)	中國醫學理事會
Zhonghua hushi hui (NAC)	中華護士會
Zhongyang guoyiguan (CINM)	中央國醫館
Zhongyang shangbing guanlichu	中央傷兵管理處
Zhongyang weisheng shiyan yuan (NIH)	中央衛生實驗院
zhuchanshi	助產士
Zhufu xuzhi: Jiating weisheng ji jiazheng gaiyao	主婦須知：家庭衛生及家政概要
zhuyi qingjie	注意清潔
zuo yuezi	坐月子

BIBLIOGRAPHY

Abbreviations for Archives and Libraries

AH   Academia Historica Archives (*Guoshiguan*), Xindian, Taiwan
BUTSL   Burke Union Theological Seminary Library, Columbia University, New York City
CMA   Chongqing Municipal Archives, Chongqing
CMB   China Medical Board, Incorporated, Archives, Rockefeller Archive Center, Tarrytown, New York
DDDL   Dale Day Divinity Library, Yale University, New Haven, Connecticut
GPA   Guomindang Party Archives, Taipei, Taiwan
IHBA   International Health Board Archives, Rockefeller Archive Center, Tarrytown, New York
LOC   United States Library of Congress, Washington, DC
NLM   National Library of Medicine, Bethesda, Maryland
NML   Nanjing Municipal Library, Nanjing, Jiangsu
NYAM   New York Academy of Medicine, New York
RAC   Rockefeller Archive Center, Tarrytown, New York
PUMC   Peking Union Medical College Archives, Beijing
RBML   Rare Book and Manuscript Library, Columbia University, New York City
RFA   Rockefeller Foundation Archives, Rockefeller Archive Center, Tarrytown, New York
SML   Shanghai Municipal Library, Shanghai
SHA   Second Historical Archives of China, Nanjing
SOAS ASC   School of Oriental and African Studies Archives and Special Collections, London
SPA   Sichuan Provincial Archives, Chengdu, Sichuan
UCC   United Church of Canada Archives, Toronto, Ontario
WHO   World Health Organization Archives, Geneva, Switzerland

Abbreviations for organizations
ABMAC   American Bureau for Medical Aid to China
CBPH   Chongqing Bureau of Public Health
CIM   China Inland Mission
NHA   National Health Administration
RF   Rockefeller Foundation

Primary Sources
Abbas, Khwaja Ahmad. *And One Did Not Come Back! The Story of the Congress Medical Mission to China.* Bombay: Sound Magazine, 1944.
Alumnae News no. 9. Alumnae Association of School of Nursing, PUMC, Peiping, October 1948, folder 711, box 99, CMB, RAC.
American Bureau for Medical Advancement in China. *Medicine on a Mission: A History of the American Bureau for Medical Aid to China, 1937–1954.* New York: ABMAC Headquarters, 1954.
Ba Jin. *Ward Four: A Novel of Wartime China,* 2nd ed. Translated by Haili Kong and Howard Goldblatt. San Francisco: China Books, 2012. Originally published as *Disi bingshi* (Shanghai: Liangyou Publishing House, 1946).
Balfour, Marshall C. MCB Officer's Diaries. May 1939, 1943, 1944, 1945. Record group 12.1, RFA, RAC.
Bensheng tuijin weisheng baogao (Report on health improvements in this province). 1940. SPA, 113–16.Bishan County Health Center Report on Personnel Training. February 1942. SPA, 96–100.
Bishan County Health Center Work Reports. SPA, 113–1 series.
Cai Chusheng and Zheng Junli. *Yijiang chunshui xiang dongliu (The Spring River Flows East).* Shanghai: Lianhua Film Company, 1947.
CBPH Work Report, October 1946. 90–183, AH.
CBPH Work Reports, 1938–1945. 66–1 series, CMA.
Chongqingshi feiliaoye yunshu gonghui zhi Sichuan shengzhengfu zhuxi zhi qingyuanshu (Petition from the Chongqing Municipal Night Soil Porters' Professional Labor Union to the Sichuan Provincial Governor). March 1940. SPA, 59–60.
Chongqingshi ge funü tuanti yilanbiao (Chart of Women's Organizations in Chongqing). May–July 1941. CMA, 51-2-564.
Chongqingshi gong sili weisheng jiguan diaocha biao (CBPH Survey of Public and Private Health Organizations in Chongqing). 1944. CMA, 66-1-9(1).
Chongqingshi jiaowai gongsili yiyuan zhensuo yilanbiao (Chart of Public and Private Hospitals in Chongqing Suburbs). August 1940. CMA, 66-1-3, 182–83.
Chongqingshi weishenju 1939 nian xiaji fangzhi huoluan shishi banfa (CBPH 1939 Summertime Cholera Prevention Plan). 1939. CMA, 162-1-20, 45–46; also SPA, 113-1-639.
Chongqingshi yisheng yaojisheng zhuchanshi yilanbiao (Survey of physicians, pharmacists, and midwives in Chongqing City), February 1939. SPA, 113-1-637.
Chang Peng-yuan, interviewer, and Lo Jiu-jung, recorder. *Zhou Meiyu xiansheng fangwen jilu* (The reminiscences of Professor Chow Mei-yu). Oral History Series no. 47. Taipei: Academia Sinica Institute of Modern History, 1993.
Chen, C.C., in collaboration with Frederica M. Bunge. *Medicine in Rural China: A Personal Account.* Berkeley: University of California Press, 1989.

——. Periodic reports from the Sichuan Provincial Health Administration. 1939–1945. Folders 2718–21, box 218, series 3, record group 5, IHBA; folder 2680, box 142, RAC.

——. Letter to M. C. Balfour. November 6, 1940. Folder 161, box 18, series 601, record group 1.1, RFA, RAC.

Chen Lifu. *Suidao zhixi an shen weiyuan baogao fabiao* (Tunnel Asphyxiation Case Investigative Committee report). 1941. AH.

China Handbook, 1937–1943: A Comprehensive Survey of Major Developments in China in Six Years of War. Chungking: Chinese Ministry of Information, July 1943.

China Information Committee. *China after Four Years of War.* Chongqing: China Publishing Company, 1941.

China Women's Welfare Society. *Sinian lai zhi peidu funü fuli she* (The past four years in the Women's Welfare Society of the Wartime Capital). Nanjing: China Women's Welfare Society, 1946.

Chinese Medical Journal. 1937–1945. NYAM and BUTSL.

Chongqing Bureau of Police records on crimes against hygiene. 1942–1947. 61–15 series, CMA.

Chongqing Municipal Government. *Chongqingshi tongji tiyao* (A summary of Chongqing statistics). Chongqing: Chongqing Municipal Government, 1942.

Chongqing Municipal Hospital Patient Statistics and Work Report, January 1944–June 1945. CMA, 165-2-5.

Chongqing Women's Federation, *Chongqingshi funü hui liangnianlai zhi gongzuo baogao* (Chongqing Women's Federation work report for the past two years). Chongqing: Chongqing Women's Federation, 1942.

Chou Mei Yu, A. C. Hsu, Chi Chen, Mary Sia, Katherine Yu, Lily Tseng, and Margaret Wang Sung to Y. T. Tsur, May 3, 1944. folder 1040, box 143, CMB, RAC.

Cleanliness Regulations Outlawing Trash in Chongqing (*Chongqingshi qudi laji qingjie guize*). August 1939. CMA, 61–15-5091.

Dagongbao (*L'Impartiale*). Newspaper issues. Harvard-Yenching Library.

Davies, A. Tegla. *The Friends' Ambulance Unit: The Story of the F.A.U. in the Second World War, 1939–1946.* London: George Allen and Unwin, 1947.

Ding Rongcan. "Peidu fangkong shilüe" (A brief history of air raid defense in the wartime capital). August 8, 1985. AH.

Du Si, recorder. "Nü hushi de hua (Zuotan hui)" (Words from female nurses [Discussion forum]). *Funü Shenghuo* (Women's lives) 8, no. 3 (November 1939): 13–15.

Eskelund, Karl. *My Chinese Wife.* London: George G. Harrap, 1946.

Executive Committee and the Committee on Science and Publication of the Ninth Congress of the Far Eastern Association of Tropical Medicine. *A Glimpse of China.* Shanghai: Mercury Press, 1934.

Executive Yuan Media Bureau. *Zhongguo hongshizihui* (The Chinese Red Cross). Nanjing, August 1947. SML.

Faculty, PUMC School of Nursing to Dr. Y. T. Tsur, Chairman of PUMC Board of Trustees, March 20, 1944. Folder 1040, box 143, CMB, RAC.

Faculty and Teaching Staff of PUMC Nursing School in University Hospital, Chengtu, folder 1038, box 143, CMB, RAC.

Fairbank, John K., and T. L. Yuan. Confidential memo to China Medical Board, Inc., March 3, 1943. Folder 158, box 23, CMB, RAC.

Fangkongdong gongchengchu qing quid shimin renyi yingdao laji yu ge dasuidao zhi qidong-zhong yi an (Air Raid Shelter Engineering Office requests the prohibition of residents from discarding trash in the air passageways of underground shelters). February 9 1942. CMA, 61-15-1148.

Forkner, Claude E. Cable to CMB, March 3, 1944. Folder 1040, box 143, CMB, RAC.

———. Letter to Chen Lifu, July 12, 1943. Folder 156, box 22, CMB, RAC.

———. Letter to Dr. Tsur, February 24, 1944. Folder 1039, box 144, CMB, RAC.

———. Letter to Dr. Wong Wen-hao, September 13, 1943. Folder 1039, box 144, CMB, RAC.

———. Letter to Edwin C. Lobenstine & Miss Pearce, May 23, 1943. Folder 1038, box 144, CMB, RAC.

———. Letter to Mr. Chang Wen-po, San Mi Chu Yi Ching Nien Tuan, July 28, 1943. Folder 156, box 22, CMB, RAC.

Gonggong laji xiang tuxiang ji zhengchi qingjie huiyi jilu gei Chongqingshi Jingchaju dishi fenju de jinji mingling (Urgent Order to No. 10 Chongqing Police District Regarding Public Trash-Can Designs). June 4, 1946. CMA, 61-15-1409.

Guanyu diaocha Yang Guosheng qingdao fenbian yu jingli qingxing de qiancheng (Reports on investigating the situation of Yang Guosheng dumping excrement into the drinking well). June 25, 1948. CMA, 61-15-4994.

Guest, Freddie. *Escape from the Bloodied Sun.* London: Jarrolds, 1956.

Han Suyin. *Destination Chungking: An Autobiography.* Boston: Little, Brown, and Company, 1942.

Hsiung Ping-chen, interviewer, and Cheng Li-jung, recorder. *Yang Wenda xiansheng fangwen jilu* (*Reminiscences of Dr. Yang Wen-ta*). Oral History Series no. 26. Taipei: Academia Sinica Institute of Modern History, 1991.

Huang Yanfu and Wang Xiaoning, eds. *Mei Yiqi riji: 1941–1946* (Mei Yiqi's Diary: 1941–1946). Beijing: Qinghua University Press, 2001.

Hui Nian, "Chongqing funü dui junshu de yijian" (Chongqing women's opinions on military families). *Funü shenghuo* (Women's lives) 8, no. 3 (Nov 1939): 7–8.

Ingram, Ruth. "Report on Visit to the PUMC School of Nursing in the West China Union University Hospital, Chengtu." October 18–November 2, 1945. Folder 1041, box 143, CMB, RAC.

Ji Hong. "Problems with Wounded Soldiers and Refugees." Essay no. 2. N.p.: Independent Publisher, November 1938. 615/460, GPA.

Kilborn, Omar L. *Our West China Mission: Being a Somewhat Extensive Summary by the Missionaries on the Field of Work during the First Twenty-Five Years of the Canadian Methodist Mission in the Province of Szechwan, Western China.* Toronto: Missionary Society of the Methodist Church, 1920.

King, P.Z. "*Guanyu shezhi jiansao zhijie zhan zhi jingguo*" (On the experience of establishing delousing and scabies treatment stations), September 23, 1943. In "People's Political Council 3rd Meeting 2nd Session." In *Weishengshu da fuxun wen'an* (National Health Administration consultative response cases). Chongqing: Datong Publishing House, 1943.

———. "China's Civilian Health." In *Looking after China's Civilians,* United China Relief Series, no. 6. Chungking: China Publishing Company, 1941.

———. "Public Health During 1940–42," ABMAC archives, box 21, NHA, P.Z. King, 1942–43, RBML; and "Report of Anti-Epidemic Activities, NHA, January 1, 1942–June 30, 1943," ABMAC archives, box 20, NHA General, RBML.

Kohlberg, Alfred. "The Medical Relief Corps of the Chinese Red Cross." November 22, 1943. ABMAC archives, RBML, box 22.

Li T'ing-an [Lei Ting On] files. PUMC, Beijing, box 1760, folder 1.

——. Letters to CEF, March–May 1944. Folder 1040, box 143, CMB, RAC.

——. Letter to Y. T. Tsur, April 20, 1944. Folder 1040, box 143, CMB, RAC.

Liang Qichao. "Lun nüxue" (On women's education). *Shiwubao* (1897).

Lin, Adet, Anor Lin, and Meimei Lin. *Dawn over Chungking.* New York: John Day, 1941.

Lindsay, Hsiao Li. *Bold Plum: With the Guerrillas in China's War against Japan.* Morrisville, NC: Lulu Press, 2007.

Liu, J. Heng. "Our Responsibilities in Public Health." *Chinese Medical Journal* 51, no. 6 (June 1937): 1039–42.

Liu Hou, Irene Ssu-chin, ed. *Liu Ruiheng boshi yu Zhongguo yiyao ji weisheng shiye* (Dr. J. Heng Liu and medical and health development in China). Taipei: Taiwan Commercial Press, 1989.

Lo Jiu-jung, Yu Chien-ming, and Chiu Hei-yuan, eds. *Fenghuo suiyue xia de Zhongguo funü fangwen jilu* (Twentieth-century wartime experiences of Chinese women: An oral history). Taipei: Academia Sinica Institute of Modern History, 2004.

Lobenstine, Edwin C. Interview with Wilbur A. Sawyer, Dr. Szeming Sze, and Dr. L. E. Powers, January 20, 1945. Folder 1109, box 152, CMB, RAC.

——. Interview with Szeming Sze, September 13, 1944. Folder 1109, box 152, CMB, RAC, 2.

——. Letter to Szeming Sze, August 31, 1942, folder 1109, box 152, CMB, RAC.

Marshall, G. C. *War Department Technical Bulletin: Scrub Typhus Fever (Tsutsugamushi Disease).* Washington, DC: United States War Department, 1944. Folder 165, box 18, ser. 601, record group 1.1, RFA, RAC.

Mei Yilin to [Mayor] Bao Huaguo, August 29, 1940. CMA, 60–1-682.

Muerville, R. de. *La Chine du Yang-tse.* Paris: Payot, 1946.

Mortenson, Esther Tappert. Letter from Chongqing, October 26, 1937. Box 4, folder 57, record group 21, YDDL.

Nai Tian. "Beizhanchang shang de yihuo nübing" (A group of women soldiers on the northern warfront). *Funü shenghuo* (Women's lives) 9, no. 7 (August 1939): 31–32.

National Health Administration. *Jiuzhong fading chuanranbing qianshuo* (A brief introduction to the nine notifiable contagious diseases). Nanjing: National Health Administration, 1937.

National Health Administration Medical and Epidemic Prevention Teams, eds. *Huoluan* (Cholera). Chongqing: National Health Administration, 1940.

National Institute of Health. Public Health Calendar, 1943, NLM.

National Red Cross Society of China. "Emergency Medical Service Training School Personnel Trained (From May 1938 to March 1941)." ABMAC archives, RBML, box 23.

Nieh Yu-chan. "A Brief Account of the PUMC School of Nursing During and After World War II: A Message to its Alumnae." Folder 711, box 99, CMB.

——. Cable to ECL [Edwin C. Lobenstine], February 25, 1944. Folder 1039, box 144, CMB, RAC.

——. "*Wei Xie qian xiaozhang Yunhua dingqi juxing zhuidiaohui qishi*" (Letter to plan a memorial service in honor of Past Principal Sia Yun-hua), March 9, 1947. PUMC, folder 1195.

"Nursing Education Seminar Sponsored by World Health Organization Western Pacific Region, Taipei, Taiwan, November 1952." In *Seminars/Conferences Reports, WHO Regional Offices for the Western Pacific, 1952–1957.* WHO Library.

Pao San-shi. "ABMAC Report on EMSTS of Ministry of War." January 1942. ABMAC archives, EMSTS file, Columbia RBML, box 2.

Payne, Robert. *Chinese Diaries 1941–1946.* 2nd ed. New York: Weybright and Talley, 1970 [1945].

Peck, Graham. *Through China's Wall.* Boston: Houghton Mifflin Company, 1940.

People's Political Council 3rd Meeting 2nd Session. *Weishengshu da fuxun wen'an* (National Health Administration consultative responses). Chongqing: Datong Publishing House, 1943.

Powell, Lyle Stephenson. *A Surgeon in Wartime China.* Lawrence: University of Kansas Press, 1946.

Qing. "Weilao fushang zhuangshi" (Comforting wounded heroes). *Funü shenghuo* (Women's lives) 8, no. 5 (December 1939): 15–16.

Qingchu guomin zhengfu duimian renxingdao shang laji de mingling (Order to clean garbage off the sidewalk facing national government offices). May 1944. CMA, 61–15–5051, 395(2).

Report from Leslie G. Kilborn, December 26, 1937. Folder 193, box 21, series 601, RG 1.1, RFA, RAC.

Report of Committee on Health and Medical Care submitted to the Commission on Investigation and Planning of Relief and Rehabilitation of the Executive Yuan, July 1, 1944. Folder 156, box 22, CMB, RAC, 32.

Report of School of Nursing PUMC for the period of December 8, 1941 to June 30, 1944. Folder 708, box 99, CMB, RAC.

Shezhi Chongqginshi Jingchaju dishi fenju guannei laji xiang de cheng (Letter regarding trash can placement in the domain of the No. 10 Police District). May 1940. CMA, 61–15–5091.

Sichuan Provincial Health Administration County Health Center Reports, 1939–1945. 113–1 series, SPA.

Sichuan Provincial Health Administration Health Statistics for Sichuan Province, 1939–1945. 113–1 series, SPA.

Sichuan sheng shengshu ge jiguan gongwuyuan zhanshi yiyao shengyu sangzang buzhufei lingfa ji baoxiao banfa (Measures for reporting and dispersing medical, birth, and burial wartime assistance funds to civil employees in Sichuan provincial organizations). SPHA, 113–1–1076, 38, 105, 293.

Simpkin, Margaret Timberlake. Oral History. Claremont Graduate School Oral History Project. January 27, 1970 and December 10, 1971. Yale Day Divinity Library, Record Group 8, box 227, folder 6.

Sinton, J. R. Papers, Chungking Diary, December 8, 1941–April 19, 1946. SOAS ASC, CIM Personal Papers, box 2, folder CIM/PP 20 Sinton Papers.

Song Meiling. *Madame Chiang Kai-shek on the New Life Movement.* Shanghai: China Weekly Review Press, 1937.

Stampar, Andrija. "Report by Dr. A. Stampar on His Missions to China." *Quarterly Bulletin of the Health Organization* 5, no. 4 (December 1936): 1090–1126.

Stevens, Helen Kennedy, and Ruth H. Block. "The American Bureau for Medical Aid to China: A Survey of China's Medical and Health Problems and the Progress Made by the

Chinese Government in Providing for the Health of the Nation." November 1943. Folder 62, box 9, CMB, RAC.

Stilwell, Joseph Warren. *The Stilwell Papers*. Edited by Theodore H. White. New York: W. Sloane Associates, 1948.

Sze Sze-ming. *China's Health Problems*. Washington, DC: Chinese Medical Association, 1943. Copy at RAC.

Tang Guozhen. "Zhongguo funü weilao ziwei kangzhan jiangshi zonghui Zhanshi ertong baoyu hui gongzuo baogao" (National Association of Chinese Women for the Cheering and Comforting of the Officers and Soldiers of the War of Self-Defense and Resistance against Japan Wartime Association for Child Welfare work report). In *Funü tanhua hui gongzuo baogao* (Women's Conversational Committee work report). Edited by the Women's Conversational Committee. N.p., 1938.

Tseng, H. W. "A Hospital Doctor Speaks." In *Looking After China's Civilians*, United China Relief Series, no. 6 (Chungking: China Publishing Company, 1941), 12–15.

Wang, Rosalind. "Nursing in China." *American Journal of Chinese Medicine* 2, no. 1 (1974): 45–47.

Wang Xiuying. "Wu yi'er hushi jie ganyan" (Testimonials for Nurses' Day on May 12). *Chinese Nurses* 1, no. 2 (1947). Quoted in "Nursing Specialist Wang Xiuying." In *Zhongguo xiandai yixue zhuanlue* (Medical biographies of modern China), 321. Beijing: Kexue jishu wenxian chubanshe, 1984.

Weishengshu buzhu ge jiaohui yiyuan ji sili yiyuan zhiliao shangbing junmin feizhigei banfa (Regulations for reimbursement by the Military Medical Administration of mission and private hospitals for the medical treatment of wounded soldiers). N.d. CMA, 81–4-73.

Weishengshu gongying zhongyang ge jiguan yiliao yaopin banfa (Regulations for the NHA providing all central government organizations with medical treatment and medicines). October 26, 1944. AH, 01–939.

White, Theodore H., and Annalee Jacoby. *Thunder Out of China*. New York: Da Capo Press, 1946.

Xia Gaotian. "*Shangbing wenti yu nanmin wenti* (Problems with wounded soldiers and refugees). N.p.: Independent Publisher, November 1938. 615/460, GPA.

Xiao Li-ju, ed. *The Chiang Kai-shek Collections: The Chronological Events*. Vol. 43, *January–June 1940*. Taipei: Academia Sinica Institute of Modern History, 2010.

Yang Chongrui. *Fuying weisheng jiangzuo* (Lectures on Maternal and Child Fealth). N.p.: New Life Movement Women's Advisory Council Press, 1945.

———. Midwifery Bag "A" Type for Maternity Assistants—Old type Midwiver [*sic*] or short course trained. N.d. CMB, RAC, box 77, folder 539.

———. *Zhufu xuzhi: Jiating weisheng ji jiazheng gaiyao* (What a housewife must know: An outline of family hygiene and home economics). Nanjing: NHA, 1940 (1934).

Yang Chongrui and Wang Shijin. *Fuying weisheng xue* (The study of maternal and children's health). Chongqing: National Institute of Health, 1944.

Yao Aihua. "Memoir of Yao Aihua." In Fang Jun, *Zuihou yi ci jijie* (The last concentration of troops), 201–14. Shenyang: Liaoning renmin chubanshe, 2012.

Yen Fu-ching. Letters to Chongqing Municipal Government, June 30–July 16, 1938. CMA, 66-1-6, 32–44.

———. "The Importance of Woman and Child Welfare Work." *People's Tribune*, November 1938. ABMAC archives, box 21, folder "NHA 1940–1941," RBML.

Yen Fu-ching to Mayor Jiang, November 18, 1938. CMA, 53-1-386.

Yiyuan mingcheng yilanbiao (Hospital Name Chart). June 5, 1944. SPA, 113-1-1076.

Yu Yun, trans. "Zuo 'hushi' shi zhanshi funü baoxiao guojia zui gaogui de shiye" (Being a 'nurse' is wartime women's most noble profession to repay the country). *Funü gongming* (Women's echo) 13, no. 6 (December 1944): 56–57.

Yuan, I. C. Letter to Alan Gregg, May 31, 1946, folder 708, box 99, CMB, RAC.

Zhao Chuan. *Taiwan laobing koushu lishi* (Oral histories of Taiwanese soldiers). Guilin: Guangxi Normal University Press, 2013.

Zhou Huanqiang, ed. *Chongqing shizhi, disan juan* (Chongqing municipal gazetteer, volume three). Chongqing: Southwest Normal University Publishing House, 2004.

Secondary Sources

Abbas, Khwaja Ahmad. *And One Did Not Come Back! The Story of the Congress Medical Mission to China.* Bombay: Sound Magazine, 1944.

Anderson, Benedict. *Imagined Communities: Reflections on the Origin and Spread of Nationalism.* 2nd ed. London: Verso Press, 1991.

Andrews, Bridie. *The Making of Modern Chinese Medicine, 1850–1960.* Vancouver: University of British Columbia Press, 2014.

———. "Tuberculosis and the Assimilation of Germ Theory in China." *Journal of the History of Medicine and Allied Sciences* 52, no. 1 (1997): 114–57.

Andrews, Bridie, and Andrew Cunningham, eds. *Western Medicine as Contested Knowledge.* Manchester, UK, and New York: Manchester University Press, 1997.

Arnold, David. *Colonizing the Body: State Medicine and Epidemic Disease in Nineteenth-Century India.* Berkeley: University of California Press, 1993.

Atenstaedt, Robert L. *The Medical Response to the Trench Diseases in World War One.* Newcastle upon Tyne, UK: Cambridge Scholars Publishing, 2011.

Attie, Jeanie. "Warwork and the Crisis of Domesticity in the North." In *Divided Houses: Gender and the Civil War,* edited by Catherine Clinton and Nina Silber, 247–59. Oxford: Oxford University Press, 1992.

Barlow, Tani E. *The Question of Women in Chinese Feminism.* Durham, NC: Duke University Press, 2004.

Barnes, Nicole Elizabeth. "Disease in the Capital: Nationalist Health Services and the 'Sick (Wo)man of East Asia' in Wartime Chongqing." *European Journal of East Asian Studies* 11 (December 2012): 286–87.

———. "The Rockefeller Foundation's China Medical Board and Medical Philanthropy in Wartime China, 1938–1945." *Rockefeller Archive Center Research Reports Online,* 2009. www.rockarch.org/publications/resrep/barnes.php.

———. "Serving the People: Chen Zhiqian and the Sichuan Provincial Health Administration, 1939–1949." In *China and the Globalization of Biomedicine,* edited by David Luesink, William H. Schneider, and Zhang Daqing. Rochester, NY: University of Rochester Press, 2018.

Barnes, Nicole Elizabeth, and John R. Watt. "The Influence of War on China's Modern Health Systems." In *Medical Transitions in Twentieth-Century China,* edited by Bridie Andrews and Mary Brown Bullock, 227–42. Bloomington: Indiana University Press, 2014.

Barrett, David P., and Larry N. Shyu, eds. *China in the Anti-Japanese War, 1937–1945: Politics, Culture, Society.* New York: Peter Lang, 2000.

Bashford, Alison. *Imperial Hygiene: A Critical History of Colonialism, Nationalism, and Public Health.* New York: Palgrave Macmillan, 2004.

_____. "Medicine, Gender and Empire." In *Gender and Empire: The Oxford History of the British Empire,* edited by Philippa Levine, 113–33. Oxford: Oxford University Press, 2004.

Benedict, Carol. *Bubonic Plague in Nineteenth-Century China.* Stanford, CA: Stanford University Press, 1996.

Blécort, Willem de, and Cornelie Usborne, eds. *Cultural Approaches to the History of Medicine: Mediating Medicine in Early Modern and Modern Europe.* New York: Palgrave Macmillan, 2004.

Boddice, Rob. *The History of Emotions.* Manchester, UK: Manchester University Press, 2018.

Bolton, Sharon C. "Me, Morphine, and Humanity: Experiencing the Emotional Community in Ward 8." In *The Emotional organization: Passions and Power,* edited by Stephen Fineman, 15–25. Oxford: Blackwell, 2008.

Bowers, John Z. *Western Medicine in a Chinese Palace: Peking Union Medical College, 1917–1951.* Philadelphia: Josiah Macy, Jr. Foundation, 1972.

Bray, Francesca. *Technology and Gender: Fabrics of Power in Late Imperial China.* Berkeley: University of California Press, 1997.

Brazelton, Mary Augusta. "Vaccinating the Nation: Public Health and Mass Immunization in Modern China, 1900–1960." PhD diss., Yale University, 2015.

Bristow, Nancy K. *American Pandemic: The Lost Worlds of the 1918 Influenza Pandemic.* Oxford: Oxford University Press, 2012.

Brook, Timothy. *Collaboration: Japanese Agents and Local Elites in Wartime China.* Cambridge, MA: Harvard University Press, 2007.

Buhler-Wilkerson, Karen. *False Dawn: The Rise and Decline of Public Health Nursing, 1900–1930.* New York: Garland Publishing, 1989.

———. *No Place Like Home: A History of Nursing and Home Care in the United States.* Baltimore: Johns Hopkins University Press, 2001.

Bullock, Mary Brown. *An American Transplant: The Rockefeller Foundation and Peking Union Medical College.* Berkeley: University of California Press, 1980.

———. *The Oil Prince's Legacy: Rockefeller Philanthropy in China.* Stanford, CA: Stanford University Press, 2011.

Chakrabarty, Dipesh. "Postcoloniality and the Artifice of History: Who Speaks for 'Indian' Pasts?" In *A Subaltern Studies Reader, 1986–1995,* edited by Ranajit Guha, 263–93. Delhi: Oxford University Press, 1998.

———. *Provincializing Europe: Postcolonial Thought and Historical Difference.* Princeton, NJ: Princeton University Press, 2000.

Chang, Jui-te. "Chiang Kai-shek's Coordination by Personal Directives." In *China at War: Regions of China, 1937–1945,* edited by Stephen R. MacKinnon, Diana Lary, and Ezra F. Vogel, 65–87. Stanford, CA: Stanford University Press, 2007.

Chatterjee, Partha. *The Nation and Its Fragments: Colonial and Postcolonial Histories.* Princeton, NJ: Princeton University Press, 1993.

Chen, Janet Y. *Guilty of Indigence: The Urban Poor in China, 1900–1953.* Princeton, NJ: Princeton University Press, 2012.

Chen Kaiyi. "Missionaries and the Early Development of Nursing in China." *Nursing History Review* 4 (1996): 124–49.

Chen Lansun and Kong Xiangyun. *Xiajiangren de gushi* (Tales of downriver people). Hong Kong: Tianma Library Publishers, 2005.

Chen Ruoshui. "Guanyu Huaren shehui wenhua xiandaihua de jidian xingsi: Yi gongde wenti weizhu" (Some reflections on Chinese society, culture, and modernization: Focusing on the question of public virtue), 57–78. In *Gonggong yishi yu Zhongguo wenhua* (Public consciousness and Chinese culture). Taipei: Linjing chubanshe, 2005.

Chiang Yung-chen. "Womanhood, Motherhood and Biology: The Early Phases of *The Ladies' Journal*, 1915–25." In *Gender and History* 18, no. 3 (November 2006): 519–45.

Chongqing Municipal Bureau of Statistics, eds. *Chongqing tongji nianjian* (Chongqing statistical yearbook). Beijing: China Statistics Press, 2010.

Chou Chun-yen. "Funü yu kangzhan shiqi de zhandi jiuhu" / "Women and Battlefield First Aid during the Second Sino-Japanese War." *Jindai Zhongguo funüshi yanjiu / Research on Women in Modern Chinese History* 24 (December 2014): 133–220.

Chu, Samuel C. "The New Life Movement, 1934–1937." In *Researches in the Social Sciences on China,* edited by John E. Lane, 2–13. New York: Columbia University Press, 1957.

Chung, Juliette Yuehtsun. *Struggle for National Survival: Eugenics in Sino-Japanese Contexts, 1896–1945.* New York: Routledge, 2002.

Clegg, Arthur. *Aid China, 1937–1949: A Memoir of a Forgotten Campaign.* Beijing: New World Press, 1989.

Coble, Parks M. *China's War Reporters: The Legacy of Resistance against Japan.* Cambridge, MA: Harvard University Press, 2015.

Cochran, Sherman. *Chinese Medicine Men: Consumer Culture in China and Southeast Asia.* Cambridge, MA: Harvard University Press, 2006.

Cook, Haruoko Tfaya, and Theodore F. Cook. *Japan at War: An Oral History.* New York: W. W. Norton, 1992.

Crook, Isabel Brown, and Christina Kelley Gilmartin with Yu Xiji. *Prosperity's Predicament: Identity, Reform, and Resistance in Rural Wartime China.* Compiled and edited by Gail Hershatter and Emily Honig. Lanham, MD: Rowman and Littlefield, 2013.

Cueto, Marcos, ed. *Missionaries of Science: The Rockefeller Foundation and Latin America.* Bloomington: Indiana University Press, 1994.

Dai Yingcong. *The Sichuan Frontier and Tibet: Imperial Strategy in the Early Qing.* Seattle: University of Washington Press, 2009.

D'Antonio, Patricia, Julie A. Fairman, and Jean C. Whelan, eds. *Routledge Handbook on the Global History of Nursing.* New York: Routledge, 2013.

Davenport, Horace W. *Robert Kho Seng Lim, 1897–1969: A Biographical Memoir.* Washington, DC: National Academy of Sciences, 1980.

Deutsch, Sarah. "Learning to Talk More Like a Man: Boston Women's Class-Bridging Organizations, 1870–1940." *American Historical Review* 97, no. 2 (April 1992): 379–404.

Diamant, Neil J. *Revolutionizing the Family: Politics, Love, and Divorce in Urban and Rural China, 1949–1968.* Berkeley: University of California Press, 2000.

Dikötter, Frank. *The Discourse of Race in Modern China.* London: Hurst and Company, 1992.

Ding Yiyun. "Traditionalism and Wartime Education: The New Life Movement, 1934–1935." Paper presented at the annual meeting of the American Historical Association, January 2018.

Dirlik, Arif. *Anarchism in the Chinese Revolution*. Berkeley: University of California Press, 1991.

———. "The Ideological Foundations of the New Life Movement: A Study in Counterrevolution." *Journal of Asian Studies* 34, no. 4 (August 1975): 945–80.

Dower, John W. *Embracing Defeat: Japan in the Wake of World War II*. New York: W. W. Norton, 1999.

Duara, Prasenjit. *Culture, Power, and the State: Rural North China, 1900–1942*. Stanford, CA: Stanford University Press, 1988.

———. *Rescuing History from the Nation: Questioning Narratives of Modern China*. Chicago: Chicago University Press, 1995.

———. *Sovereignty and Authenticity: Manchukuo and the East Asian Modern*. Lanham, MD: Rowman and Littlefield, 2003.

Durkheim, Emile. *The Elementary Forms of the Religious Life*. Translated by Joseph Ward Swain. London: Allen and Unwin, 1915.

Eastman, Lloyd E. "Nationalist China during the Sino-Japanese War 1937–1945." In *The Cambridge History of China*, vol. 13, *Republican China 1912–1949, Part 2*, edited by John K. Fairbank and Albert Feuerwerker, 547–608. Cambridge: Cambridge University Press, 1986.

———. *Seeds of Destruction: Nationalist China in War and Revolution, 1937–1945*. Stanford, CA: Stanford University Press, 1984.

Edwards, Louise. "Policing the Modern Woman in Republican China." *Modern China* 26, no. 2 (2000): 115–47.

Eifring, Halvor, ed. *Minds and Mentalities in Traditional Chinese Literature*. Beijing: Culture and Art Publishing House, 1999.

Ekman, Paul, and Wallace V. Friesen. "Constants across Cultures in the Face and Emotion." *Journal of Personality and Emotional Psychology* 17, no. 2 (1971): 124–29.

Ekman, Paul, Wallace V. Friesen, and Phoebe Ellsworth. *Emotion in the Human Face: Guidelines for Research and an Integration of Findings*. NY: Pergamon Press, 1972.

Elman, Benjamin A. *On Their Own Terms: Science in China, 1550–1900*. Cambridge, MA: Harvard University Press, 2005.

Fang Jun. *Zuihou yi ci jijie* (The last concentration of troops). Shenyang: Liaoning renmin chubanshe, 2012.

Fang Xiaoping. *Barefoot Doctors and Western Medicine in China*. Rochester, NY: University of Rochester Press, 2012.

Farquhar, Judith, and Marta Hanson, eds. "Empires of Hygiene." Special issue, *Positions: East Asia Cultures Critique* 6, no. 3 (Winter 1998).

Feng Yurong, ed. *Guomin zhengfu Chongqing peidu shi* (History of the Nationalists in the wartime capital Chongqing). Chongqing: Southwest Normal University Press, 1993.

Ferlanti, Federica. "The New Life Movement at War: Wartime Mobilisation and State Control in Chongqing and Chengdu, 1938–1942." *European Journal of East Asian Studies* 11 (December 2012): 187–212.

Finnane, Antonia. *Changing Clothes in China: Fashion, History, Nation*. New York: Columbia University Press, 2008.

Foucault, Michel. *The Birth of the Clinic: An Archaeology of Medical Perception*. Translated by A. M. Sheridan Smith. 2nd ed. New York: Vintage Books, 1994.

———. *Discipline and Punish: The Birth of the Prison*. Translated by Alan Sheridan. 2nd ed. New York: Vintage Books, 1995.

Fu Jia-Chen. "Scientizing Relief: Nutritional Activism from Shanghai to the Southwest, 1937–1945." In *European Journal of East Asian Studies* 11, no. 2 (December 2012): 259–82.

Fukuda, Mahito H. "Public Health in Modern Japan: From Regimen to Hygiene." In *The History of Public Health and the Modern State*, edited by Dorothy Porter, 385–402. Amsterdam: Rodopi, 1994.

Furth, Charlotte. *A Flourishing Yin: Gender in China's Medical History, 960–1665*. Berkeley: University of California Press, 1999.

Gao Yunxiang. "Nationalist and Feminist Discourses on *Jianmei* (Robust Beauty) during China's 'National Crisis' in the 1930s." *Gender and History* 18, no. 3 (November 2006): 546–73.

Gelbert, Nina Rattner. *The King's Midwife: A History and Mystery of Madame du Coudray*. Berkeley: University of California Press, 1998.

Gillette, Maris. "Exploring Personal Meanings of State-Society Relations in China." *Urban Anthropology and Studies of Cultural Systems and World Economic Development* 33, nos. 2/3/4 (Summer, Fall, and Winter 2004): 283–320.

Gilmartin, Christina Kelley. *Engendering the Chinese Revolution: Radical Women, Communist Politics, and Mass Movements in the 1920s*. Berkeley: University of California Press, 1995.

Gluck, Carol. "The End of Elsewhere: Writing Modernity Now." *American Historical Review* 116, no. 3 (June 2011): 676–87.

Goodman, Jordan, Anthony McElligott, and Lara Marks, eds. *Useful Bodies: Humans in the Service of Medical Science in the Twentieth Century*. Baltimore: Johns Hopkins University Press, 2003.

Gross, Miriam. *Farewell to the God of Plague: Chairman Mao's Campaign to Deworm China*. Berkeley: University of California Press, 2016.

Grypma, Sonya. *Healing Henan: Canadian Nurses at the North China Mission, 1888–1947*. Vancouver: University of British Columbia Press, 2008.

———. "Neither Angels of Mercy nor Foreign Devils: Revisioning Canadian Missionary Nurses in China, 1935–1947." *Nursing History Review* 12 (2004): 97–119.

Grypma, Sonya, and Zhen Cheng. "The Development of Modern Nursing in China." In *Medical Transitions in Twentieth-Century China*, edited by Bridie Andrews and Mary Brown Bullock, 297–316. Bloomington: Indiana University Press, 2014.

Guha, Ranajit. *Elementary Aspects of Peasant Insurgency in Colonial India*. Delhi: Oxford University Press, 1983.

Hadley, M.B., L.S. Blum, S. Mujaddid, S. Parveen, S. Nuremowla, M.E. Haque, and M. Ullah. "Why Bangladeshi Nurses Avoid 'Nursing': Social and Structural Factors on Hospital Wards in Bangladesh." *Social Science and Medicine* 64, no. 6 (March 2007): 1166–77.

Hanson, Marta E. *Speaking of Epidemics in Chinese Medicine: Disease and the Geographic Imagination in Late imperial China*. New York: Routledge, 2011.

———. "Robust Northerners and Delicate Southerners: The Nineteenth-Century Invention of a Southern Medical Tradition." *positions: East Asia cultures critique* 6, no. 3 (1998): 515–50.

Hardt, Michael, and Antonio Negri. *Multitude: War and Democracy in the Age of Empire*. New York: Penguin Press, 2004.

Harrell, Paula. *Sowing the Seeds of Change: Chinese Students, Japanese Teachers, 1895–1905*. Stanford, CA: Stanford University Press, 1992.

Hayot, Eric. *The Elements of Academic Style: Writing for the Humanities*. New York: Columbia University Press, 2014.

Henriot, Christian, and Yeh Wen-hsin, eds. *In the Shadow of the Rising Sun: Shanghai under Japanese Occupation*. Cambridge: Cambridge University Press, 2004.

Henry, Todd A. *Assimilating Seoul: Japanese Rule and the Politics of Public Space in Colonial Korea, 1910–1945*. Berkeley: University of California Press, 2014.

Hershatter, Gail. *The Gender of Memory: Rural Women and China's Collective Past*. Berkeley: University of California Press, 2011.

———. "Making the Visible Invisible: The Fate of 'The Private' in Revolutionary China." In *Wusheng zhi sheng (I): Jindai Zhongguo de funü yu guojia (1600–1950)* (Voices amid silence: Women and the nation in modern China), ed. Fangshang Lu. Taipei: Academia Sinica Institute of Modern History, 2003.

Hippler, Thomas. *Governing from the Skies: A Global History of Aerial Bombing*. New York: Verso, 2017.

Hochschild, Arlie Russell. "Introduction: An Emotions Lens on the World." In *Theorizing Emotions: Sociological Exploration and Applications*, edited by Debra Hopkins, Jochen Kleres, Helena Flam, and Helmut Kizmics, 29–37. Frankfurt am Main: Campus, 2009.

———. *The Managed Heart: Commercialization of Human Feeling*. Berkeley: University of California Press, 2003.

Honig, Emily, and Gail Hershatter. *Personal Voices: Chinese Women in the 1980s*. Stanford, CA: Stanford University Press, 1988.

Howard, Joshua H. "Chongqing's Most Wanted: Worker Mobility and Resistance in China's Nationalist Arsenals, 1937–1945." *Modern Asian Studies* 37, no. 4 (2003): 955–97.

———. *Workers at War: Labor in China's Arsenals, 1937–1953*. Stanford, CA: Stanford University Press, 2004.

———. "Workers at War: Labor in the Nationalist Arsenals of Chongqing, 1937–1949." PhD diss., University of California at Berkeley, 1998.

Hsiung, James C., and Steven I. Levine, eds. *China's Bitter Victory: The War with Japan, 1937–1945*. Armonk, NY: M. E. Sharpe, 1992.

Hsu, Frances L. K. *Religion, Science and Human Crises: A Study of China in Transition and Its Implications for the West*. London: Routledge and Kegan Paul, 1952.

Hu Cheng. "The Modernization of Japanese and Chinese Medicine (1914–1931)." *Chinese Studies in History* 47, no. 4 (Summer 2014): 78–94.

Huang Jinlin. *Lishi, Shenti, Guojia: Jindai Zhongguo de shenti xingcheng, 1895–1937* (History, body, nation: The formation of the modern Chinese body). Beijing: New Star Press, 2006.

Humphreys, Margaret. *Marrow of Tragedy: The Health Crisis of the American Civil War*. Baltimore: Johns Hopkins University Press, 2013.

Hung Chang-tai. *War and Popular Culture: Resistance in Modern China, 1937–1945*. Berkeley: University of California Press, 1994.

Hunt, Lynn. *The Family Romance of the French Revolution*. Berkeley: University of California Press, 1992.

Iijima Wataru. "The Establishment of Japanese Colonial Medicine: Infectious and Parasitic Disease Studies in Taiwan, Manchuria, and Korea under Japanese Rule before WWII." *Aoyama rekishigaku* (Aoyama University historical studies), no. 28 (March 2010): 77–106.

Immerwahr, Daniel. *Thinking Small: The United States and the Lure of Community Development.* Cambridge, MA: Harvard University Press, 2015.

Janetta, Ann. *The Vaccinators: Smallpox, Medical Knowledge, and the "Opening" of Japan.* Stanford, CA: Stanford University Press, 2007.

Jewkes, Rachel, Naeemah Abrahams, and Zodumo Mvo. "Why Do Nurses Abuse Patients? Reflections from South African Obstetric Services." *Social Science and Medicine* 47, no. 11 (1998): 1781–95.

Johnson, Sarah Ann. "Healing in Silence: Black Nurses in Charleston, South Carolina, 1896–1948." PhD diss., Medical University of South Carolina, 2008.

Johnson, Tina Phillips. *Childbirth in Republican China: Delivering Modernity.* Lanham, MD: Lexington Books, 2011.

———. "Yang Chongrui and the First National Midwifery School: Childbirth Reform in Early Twentieth-Century China." *Asian Medicine* 4, no. 2 (2008): 280–302.

Jolly, Margaret. "Introduction: Colonial and Postcolonial Plots in the History of Maternities and Modernities." In *Maternities and Modernities: Colonial and Postcolonial Experiences in Asia and the Pacific,* edited by Margaret Jolly and Kalpana Ram, 1–24. Cambridge: Cambridge University Press, 1998.

Jones, Colin, and Roy Porter, eds. *Reassessing Foucault: Power, Medicine and the Body.* London and New York: Routledge, 1994.

Jordan, Brigitte. *A Crosscultural Investigation of Childbirth in Yucatan, Holland, Sweden, and the United States.* Prospect Heights, IL: Waveland Press, 1993.

Judge, Joan. "Citizens or Mothers of Citizens? Gender and the Meaning of Modern Chinese Citizenship." In *Citizenship in Modern China,* edited by Elizabeth Perry and Merle Goldman, 23–43. Cambridge, MA: Harvard University Asia Center, 2002.

———. *The Precious Raft of History: The Past, the West, and the Woman Question in China.* Stanford, CA: Stanford University Press, 2008.

Kapp, Robert A. "Chungking as a Center of Warlord Power, 1926–1937." In *The Chinese City between Two Worlds,* edited by Mark Elvin and G. William Skinner, 143–70. Stanford, CA: Stanford University Press, 1974.

———. *Szechwan and the Chinese Republic: Provincial Militarism and Central Power, 1911–1938.* New Haven, CT: Yale University Press, 1973.

Ko, Dorothy. *Teachers of the Inner Chambers: Women and Culture in Seventeenth-Century China.* Stanford, CA: Stanford University Press, 1995.

———. "Thinking about Copulating: An Early-Qing Confucian Thinker's Problem with Emotions and Words," in *Remapping China: Fissures in Historical Terrain,* edited by Gail Hershatter, Emily Honig, Jonathan N. Lipman, and Randall Stross, 59–75. Stanford, CA: Stanford University Press, 1996.

Kong Haili. "Disease and Humanity: Ba Jin and His *Ward Four: A Novel of Wartime China,*" *Frontiers of Literary Studies in China* 6, no. 2 (2012): 198–207.

Koonz, Claudia. *Mothers in the Fatherland: Women, the Family and Nazi Politics.* New York: St. Martin's Press, 1987.

Krylova, Anna. "Gender Binary and the Limits of Poststructuralist Method," *Gender & History* 28, no. 2 (August 2016): 307–23.

———. *Soviet Women in Combat: A History of Violence on the Eastern Front.* Cambridge: Cambridge University Press, 2010.

Kutcher, Norman. "The Skein of Chinese Emotions History." In *Doing Emotions History*, edited by Susan J. Matt and Peter N. Stearns, 57–73. Urbana and Chicago: University of Illinois Press, 2013.

Lam Tong. *A Passion for Facts: Social Surveys and the Construction of the Chinese Nation-State, 1900–1949*. Berkeley: University of California Press, 2011.

———. "Policing the Imperial Nation: Sovereignty, International Law, and the Civilizing Mission in Late Qing China," *Comparative Studies in Society and History* 52.4 (2015): 881–908.

Landdeck, Kevin P. "Chicken-Footed Gods or Village Protectors? Wartime Conscription and Community in Sichuan's Villages." Paper presented at the annual meeting of the Association for Asian Studies, Toronto, Ontario, March 15–18, 2012.

———. "Under the Gun: Nationalist Military Service and Society in Wartime Sichuan, 1938–1945." PhD diss., University of California at Berkeley, 2010.

Lang, Olga. *Chinese Family and Society*. New Haven, CT: Yale University Press, 1946.

Lary, Diana. *The Chinese People at War: Human Suffering and Social Transformation, 1937–1945*. New York: Cambridge University Press, 2010.

———. *Warlord Soldiers: Chinese Common Soldiers, 1911–1937*. Cambridge: Cambridge University Press, 1985.

———. "Writing and War: Silence, Disengagement, and Ambiguity." *Journal of Literature and Trauma Studies* 2, nos. 1–2 (Spring/Fall 2013): 45–62.

Lary, Diana, and Stephen R. MacKinnon, eds. *Scars of War: The Impact of Warfare on Modern China*. Vancouver: University of British Columbia Press, 2001.

Latour, Bruno. *The Pasteurization of France*. Cambridge, MA: Harvard University Press, 1988.

Lean, Eugenia. *Public Passions: The Trial of Shi Jianqiao and the Rise of Popular Sympathy in Republican China*. Berkeley: University of California Press, 2007.

Lee Haiyan. *Revolution of the Heart: A Genealogy of Love in China, 1900–1950*. Stanford, CA: Stanford University Press, 2007.

Lei, Sean Hsiang-lin. "Habituating Individuality: Framing Tuberculosis and Its Material Solutions in Republican China." *Bulletin for the History of Medicine* 84 (2010): 248–79.

———. *Neither Donkey nor Horse: Medicine in the Struggle over China's Modernity*. Chicago: University of Chicago Press, 2014.

———. "Sovereignty and the Microscope: Constituting Notifiable Infectious Diseases and Containing the Manchurian Plague (1910–11). In *Health and Hygiene in Chinese East Asia: Policies and Publics in the Long Twentieth Century*, edited by Angela Ki Che Leung and Charlotte Furth, 73–106. Durham, NC: Duke University Press, 2010.

Leung, Angela Ki Che. *Leprosy in China: A History*. New York: Columbia University Press, 2009.

Leung, Angela Ki Che, and Charlotte Furth, eds. *Health and Hygiene in Chinese East Asia: Policies and Publics in the Long Twentieth Century*. Durham, NC: Duke University Press, 2010.

Lewis, Milton J., and Kerrie L. MacPherson, eds. *Public Health in Asia and the Pacific: Historical and Comparative Perspectives*. New York: Routledge, 2008.

Li Danke. *Echoes of Chongqing: Women in Wartime China*. Urbana and Chicago: University of Illinois Press, 2010.

Li Zhisui, *The Private Life of Chairman Mao*. Translated by Tai Hung-chao. New York: Random House, 1994.

Ling Shing-ting. "The Female Hand: The Making of Western Medicine for Women in China, 1880s–1920s." PhD diss., Columbia University, 2015.

Lipkin, Zwia. *Useless to the State: "Social Problems" and Social Engineering in Nationalist Nanjing, 1927–1937.* Cambridge, MA: Harvard University Asia Center, 2006.

Liu, Lydia H. *Translingual Practice: Literature, National Culture, and Translated Modernity: China, 1900–1937.* Stanford, CA: Stanford University Press, 1995.

Liu, Michael Shiyung. *Prescribing Colonization: The Role of Medical Practices and Policies in Japan-Ruled Taiwan, 1895–1945.* Ann Arbor, MI: Association for Asian Studies, 2009.

Liu Xun. *Daoist Modern: Innovation, Lay Practice, and the Community of Inner Alchemy in Republican Shanghai.* Cambridge, MA: Harvard University Press, 2009.

Lo Jiu-jung, Yu Chien-ming, and Chiu Hei-yuan, eds., *Fenghuo suiyue xia de Zhongguo funü fangwen jilu* (Twentieth-century wartime experiences of Chinese women: An oral history). Taipei: Academia Sinica Institute of Modern History, 2004.

Lo Ming-cheng M. *Doctors within Borders: Profession, Ethnicity, and Modernity in Colonial Taiwan.* Berkeley: University of California Press, 2002.

Luesink, David. "Anatomy and the Reconfiguration of Life and Death in Republican China." *Journal of Asian Studies* 76, no. 4 (November 2017): 1009–34.

Lu Ping, "De Xiansheng he Sai Xiansheng zhiwai de guanhuai: Cong Mu Guniang de tichu kan Xinwenhua yundong shiqi daode geming de zouxiang" (Beyond Mr. Democracy and Mr. Science: The introduction of Miss Moral and the trend of moral revolution in the New Culture Movement). *Lishi yanjiu* (Historical research) 2006, no. 1: 79–95.

Luo Zhuanxu, ed. *Chongqing Kangzhan dashiji* (Grand record of Chongqing's War of Resistance). Chongqing: Chongqing Publishing House, 1995.

Ma Zhao. *Runaway Wives, Urban Crimes, and Survival Tactics in Wartime Beijing, 1937–1949.* Cambridge, MA: Harvard University Asia Center, 2015.

MacKinnon, Stephen R. "The Tragedy of Wuhan, 1938." *Modern Asian Studies* 30, no. 4 (1996): 931–43.

———. *Wuhan, 1938: War, Refugees, and the Making of Modern China.* Berkeley: University of California Press, 2008.

Stephen R. MacKinnon, Diana Lary, and Ezra F. Vogel, eds. *China at War: Regions of China, 1937–1945.* Stanford, CA: Stanford University Press, 2007.

MacPherson, Kerrie L. *A Wilderness of Marshes: The Origins of Public Health in Shanghai, 1843–1893.* Hong Kong: Oxford University Press, 1987.

Maling, Barbara Lee. "Black Southern Nursing Care Providers in Virginia during the American Civil War, 1861–1865." PhD diss., University of Virginia, 2009.

May-ling Soong Chiang. *War Messages and Other Selections by Madame Chiang Kai-shek.* Hankow [Hankou]: China Information Committee, 1938.

McIsaac, Mary Lee. "The City as Nation: Creating a Wartime Capital in Chongqing." In *Remaking the Chinese City: Modernity and National Identity, 1900–1950,* edited by Joseph W. Esherick, 174–91. Honolulu: University of Hawai'i Press, 1999.

———. "The Limits of Chinese Nationalism: Workers in Wartime Chongqing, 1937–1945." PhD diss., Yale University, 1994.

Merkel-Hess, Kate. "A New Woman and Her Warlord: Li Dequan, Feng Yuxiang, and the Politics of Intimacy in Twentieth-Century China." *Frontiers of History in China* 11, no. 3 (2016): 431–57.

———. "The Public Health of Village Private Life: Reform and Resistance in Early Twentieth Century Rural China." *Journal of Social History* 49, no. 4 (2016): 881–903.

———. *The Rural Modern: Reconstructing the Self and State in Republican China*. Chicago: University of Chicago Press, 2016.

Mitchell, Timothy. "Society, Economy, and the State Effect." In *State/Culture: State-Formation after the Cultural Turn*, edited by George Steinmetz, 76–97. Ithaca, NY: Cornell University Press, 1999.

Mitter, Rana. "Classifying Citizens in Nationalist China during World War II, 1937–1941." In "China in World War II, 1937–1945: Experience, Memory, and Legacy," special issue, *Modern Asian Studies* 45, no. 2 (March 2011): 243–75.

———. *Forgotten Ally: China's World War II, 1937–1945*. Boston: Houghton Mifflin Harcourt, 2013.

Mittler, Barbara. *A Continuous Revolution: Making Sense of Cultural Revolution Culture*. Cambridge, MA: Harvard University Asia Center, 2012.

Montgomery, Kathryn. "Redescribing Biomedicine: Toward the Integration of East Asian Medicine into Contemporary Healthcare." In *Integrating East Asian Medicine into Contemporary Healthcare*, edited by Volker Scheid and Hugh MacPherson, 229–34. Edinburgh: Churchill Livingstone, 2012.

Morris, Andrew D. *Marrow of the Nation: A History of Sport and Physical Culture in Republican China*. Berkeley: University of California Press, 2004.

Mukharji, Projit Bihari. *Doctoring Traditions: Ayurveda, Small Technologies, and Braided Sciences*. Chicago: University of Chicago Press, 2016.

Murray Li, Tania. *The Will to Improve: Governmentality, Development, and the Practice of Politics*. Durham, NC: Duke University Press, 2007.

Muscolino, Micah S. *The Ecology of War in China: Henan Province, the Yellow River, and Beyond, 1938–1950*. New York: Cambridge University Press, 2015.

Nedostup, Rebecca. "Burying, Repatriating, and Leaving the Dead in Wartime and Postwar China and Taiwan, 1937–1955." *Journal of Chinese History* 1 (2017): 111–39.

———. *Superstitious Regimes: Religion and the Politics of Chinese Modernity*. Cambridge, MA: Harvard University Asia Center, 2009.

Niewyk, Donald L. *The Columbia Guide to the Holocaust*. New York: Columbia University Press, 2000.

Nolte, Sharon H., and Sally Ann Hastings. "The Meiji State's Policy toward Women, 1890–1910." In *Recreating Japanese Women, 1600–1945*, edited by Gail Lee Bernstein, 151–74. Berkeley: University of California Press, 1991.

Nussbaum, Martha C. *Political Emotions: Why Love Matters for Justice*. Cambridge, MA: Belknap Press of Harvard University Press, 2013.

Ono, Kazuko. *Chinese Women in a Century of Revolution, 1850–1950*. Edited by Joshua A. Fogel. Stanford, CA: Stanford University Press, 1989.

Overy, Richard. *The Bombing War: Europe 1939–1945*. New York: Penguin Books, 2013.

———. *Russia's War: A History of the Soviet Effort, 1941–1945*. London: Allen Lane, 1998.

Paine, S. C. M. *The Wars for Asia, 1911–1949*. New York: Cambridge University Press, 2012.

Pan Yihong. "Zhanzheng conglai buzhishi nanren de shiye: Jiedu Xinsijun nübing huiyilu" / "Never a Man's War: The Self-Reflections of the Women Soldiers of the New Fourth Army in the War of Resistance against Japan, 1937–1945." In *Jindai Zhongguo funüshi yanjiu / Research on Women in Modern Chinese History* 24 (December 2014): 83–131.

Peng Chengfu. *Chongqing renmin dui kangzhan de gongxian* (Chongqing people's contributions to the War of Resistance). Chongqing: Chongqing Publishing House, 1995.

Plamper, Jan. *The History of Emotions: An Introduction.* Oxford: Oxford University Press, 2012.

Plum, M. Colette. "Lost Childhoods in a New China: Child-Citizen-Workers at War, 1937–1945." *European Journal of East Asian Studies* 11 (December 2012): 237–58.

———. "Unlikely Heirs: War Orphans during the Second Sino-Japanese War, 1937–1945." PhD diss., Stanford University, 2006.

Pomeranz, Kenneth. *The Great Divergence: China, Europe, and the Making of the Modern World Economy.* Princeton, NJ: Princeton University Press, 2000.

Porter, Dorothy, ed. *The History of Public Health and the Modern State.* Amsterdam and Atlanta: Editions Rodopi, 1994.

Prakash, Gyan. *Another Reason: Science and the Imagination of Modern India.* Princeton, NJ: Princeton University Press, 1999.

Ragsdale, Nick. "Dysentery." In *Encyclopedia of Pestilence, Pandemics, and Plagues,* vol. 1, A–M, edited by Joseph P. Byrne, 174–76. Westport, CT: Greenwood Press, 2008.

Ramsey, Matthew. "Public Health in France." In *The History of Public Health and the Modern State,* edited by Dorothy Porter, 45–117. Amsterdam: Rodopi, 1994.

Ran Minhui and Li Huiyu. *Minguo shiqi baojia zhidu yanjiu* (Research on the Baojia system in the Republican era). Chengdu: Sichuan University Press, 2005.

Reddy, William M. *The Navigation of Feeling: A Framework for the History of Emotions.* Cambridge: Cambridge University Press, 2001.

Reeves, Caroline Beth. "Grave Concerns: Bodies, Burial, and Identity in Republican China." In *Cities in Motion: Interior, Coast, and Diaspora in Transnational China,* edited by Sherman Cochran and David Strand, 27–52. Berkeley: University of California Press, 2007.

———. "The Power of Mercy: The Chinese Red Cross Society, 1900–1937." PhD diss., Harvard University, 1998.

Remick, Elizabeth J. "Introduction to the *JAS* at AAS Roundtable on 'Sexuality and the State in Asia.'" *Journal of Asian Studies* 71, no. 4 (November 2012): 919–27.

Renan, Ernest. "What Is a Nation?" Translated by Martin Thom. In *Nation and Narration,* edited by Homi K. Bhabha, 8–21. New York: Routledge, 1990 (1882).

Ricoeur, Paul. *Time and Narrative.* Vol. 1. Translated by Kathleen McLaughlin and David Pellauer. Chicago: University of Chicago Press, 1984.

Rogaski, Ruth. *Hygienic Modernity: Meanings of Health and Disease in Treaty-Port China.* Berkeley: University of California Press, 2004.

Romanus, Charles F., and Riley Sunderland. *The China-Burma-India Theater: Time Runs Out in CBI.* U.S. Army in World War II. Washington, DC: Chief Office of the Military History Department of the Army, 1959.

Rosen, George. "The Fate of the Concept of Medical Police, 1780–1890." *Centaurus* 5, no. 2 (June 1957): 97–113. Republished, 1980.

———. *A History of Public Health.* New York: MD Publications, 1958.

Rosenwein, Barbara H. *Emotional Communities in the Early Middle Ages*. Ithaca, NY: Cornell University Press, 2006.

―――. *Generations of Feeling: A History of Emotions, 600–1700*. Cambridge: Cambridge University Press, 2016.

―――. "Worrying about Emotions in History." *American Historical Review* 107, no. 3 (June 2002): 821–45.

Rosenwein, Barbara H., and Riccardo Cristiani. *What Is the History of Emotions?* Cambridge: Polity, 2018.

Rostker, Bernard D. *Providing for the Casualties of War: The American Experience through World War II*. Santa Monica, CA: RAND Corporation, 2013.

Rowe, William T. *Crimson Rain: Seven Centuries of Violence in a Chinese County*. Stanford, CA: Stanford University Press, 2007.

Sakai Naoki. *Translation and Subjectivity: On Japan and Cultural Nationalism*. Minneapolis: University of Minnesota Press, 1997.

Scarry, Elaine. "Injury and the Structure of War." *Representations* 10 (Spring 1985): 1–51.

Schneider, Helen M. *Keeping the Nation's House: Domestic Management and the Making of Modern China*. Vancouver: University of British Columbia Press, 2011.

―――. "Mobilising Women: The Women's Advisory Council, Resistance and Reconstruction during China's War with Japan." *European Journal of East Asian Studies* 11, no. 2 (December 2012): 213–36.

Schoppa, R. Keith. *In a Sea of Bitterness: Refugees during the Sino-Japanese War, 1937–1945*. Cambridge, MA: Harvard University Press, 2011.

Scull, Andrew. *Hysteria: The Biography*. Oxford: Oxford University Press, 2009.

Shapin, Steven. *A Social History of Truth: Civility and Science in Seventeenth-Century England*. Chicago: University of Chicago Press, 1994.

Shemo, Connie A. *The Chinese Medical Ministries of Kang Cheng and Shi Meiyu, 1872–1937: On a Cross-Cultural Frontier of Gender, Race, and Nation*. Bethlehem, MD: Lehigh University Press, 2011.

Shi Xia. *At Home in the World: Women and Charity in Late Qing and Early Republican China*. New York: Columbia University Press, 2018.

Showalter, Elaine, ed. *Daughters of Decadence: Women Writers of the Fin-de-Siècle*. New Brunswick, NJ: Rutgers University Press, 1993.

Sichuan Chongqing Cultural History Research Committee, eds. *Chongqing kangzhan jishi, 1937–1945* (A record of Chongqing events in the War of Resistance, 1937–1945). Chongqing: Chongqing Publishing House, 1985.

Sih, Paul K. T. *Nationalist China during the Sino-Japanese War*. New York: Exposition Press, 1977.

Skinner, G. William. *Marketing and Social Structure in Rural China*. Ann Arbor, MI: Association for Asian Studies, 1965.

―――. *Rural China on the Eve of Revolution: Sichuan Fieldnotes, 1949–1950*. Edited by Stevan Harrell and William Lavely. Seattle: University of Washington Press, 2017.

Smedley, Agnes. *China Fights Back: An American Woman with the Eighth Route Army*. London: Victor Gollancz, 1938.

Soon, Wayne. "Blood, Soymilk, and Vitality: The Wartime Origins of Blood Banking in China, 1943–1945." *Bulletin of the History of Medicine* 90. no. 3 (2016): 424–54.

Stapleton, Kristin. *Civilizing Chengdu: Chinese Urban Reform, 1895–1937.* Cambridge, MA: Harvard University Press, 2000.

———. "Hu Lanqi: Woman, Soldier, Heroine, and Survivor." In *The Human Tradition in Modern China,* edited by Kristin Stapleton and Kenneth J. Hammond, 157–76. Lanham, MD: Rowman and Littlefield, 2008.

———. "Warfare and Modern Urban Administration in Chinese Cities." In *Cities in Motion: Interior, Coast, and Diaspora in Transnational China,* edited by Sherman Cochran and David Strand, 53–77. Berkeley: University of California Press, 2007.

Stevens, Sarah Elizabeth. "Hygienic Bodies and Public Mothers: The Rhetoric of Reproduction, Fetal Education, and Childhood in Republican China." In *Mapping Meanings: The Field of New Learning in Late Qing China,* edited by Michael Lackner and Natascha Vittinghoff, 659–84. Leiden: E. J. Brill, 2004.

Stoff, Laurie S. "The Sounds, Odors, and Textures of Russian Wartime Nursing." In *Russian History through the Senses: From 1700 to the Present,* edited by Matthew P. Romaniello and Tricia Starks, 117–40. London: Bloomsbury, 2016.

Strand, David. *Rickshaw Beijing: City People and Politics in the 1920s.* Berkeley: University of California Press, 1989.

———. *An Unfinished Republic: Leading by Word and Deed in Modern China.* Berkeley: University of California Press, 2011.

Strobel, Margaret. *European Women and the Second British Empire.* Bloomington: Indiana University Press, 1991.

Sze, Szeming. *The Origins of the World Health Organization: A Personal Memoir, 1945–1948.* Boca Raton, FL: L.I.S.Z. Publications, 1982.

Takahashi, Aya. *The Development of the Japanese Nursing Profession: Adopting and Adapting Western Influences.* New York: Routledge, 2004.

Tan Yunxian. *Miscellaneous Records of a Female Doctor.* Translated by Lorraine Wilcox with Yue Lu. Portland, OR: Chinese Medicine Database, 2015.

Thaxton, Ralph A., Jr. *Catastrophe and Contention in Rural China: Mao's Great Leap Forward Famine and the Origins of Righteous Resistance in Da Fo Village.* Cambridge and New York: Cambridge University Press, 2008.

Theiss, Janet. *Disgraceful Matters: The Politics of Chastity in Eighteenth-Century China.* Berkeley: University of California Press, 2004.

Thompson, Malcolm. "Foucault, Fields of Governability, and the Population-Family-Economy Nexus in China." *History and Theory* 51, no. 1 (2012): 42–62.

Tonn, Jenna. "Extralaboratory Life: Gender Politics and Experimental Biology at Radcliffe College, 1894–1910." *Gender & History* 29, no. 2 (August 2017): 329–58.

Tow, Edna. "The Great Bombing of Chongqing and the Anti-Japanese War, 1937–1945." In *The Battle for China: Essays on the Military History of the Sino-Japanese War of 1937–1945,* edited by Mark Peattie, Edward Drea, and Hans van de Ven, 256–82. Stanford, CA: Stanford University Press, 2011.

Trofa, Andrew F., Hannah Ueno-Olsen, Ruiko Oiwa, and Masanosuke Yoshikawa. "Dr. Kiyoshi Shiga: Discoverer of the Dysentery Bacillus." *Clinical Infectious Diseases* 29, no. 5 (November 1999): 1303–6.

Tsin, Michael. "Imagining 'Society' in Early Twentieth-Century China." In *Imagining the People: Chinese Intellectuals and the Concept of Citizenship, 1890–1920,* edited by Joshua A. Fogel and Peter G. Zarrow, 212–31. Armonk, NY: M. E. Sharpe, 1997).

Vuic, Kara Dixon. "Wartime Nursing and Power." In *Routledge Handbook on the Global History of Nursing*, edited by Patricia D'Antonio, Julie A. Fairman, and Jean C. Whelan, 22–34. New York: Routledge, 2013.

Wakabayashi, Bob Tadashi, ed. *The Nanking Atrocity, 1937–1938: Complicating the Picture*. New York: Berghahn Books, 2007.

Wakeman, Frederic E., Jr. "Licensing Leisure: The Chinese Nationalists' Attempts to Regulate Shanghai, 1927–1949." In Frederic E. Wakeman Jr. *Telling Chinese History: A Selection of Essays*. Selected and edited by Lea H. Wakeman. Berkeley: University of California Press, 2009.

———. "Occupied Shanghai: The Struggle between Chinese and Western Medicine." In *China at War: Regions of China, 1937–1945*, edited by Stephen R. MacKinnon, Diana Lary, and Ezra F. Vogel, 265–87. Stanford, CA: Stanford University Press, 2007.

———. *Spymaster: Dai Li and the Chinese Secret Service*. Berkeley: University of California Press, 2003.

Wall, Rosemary, and Anne Marie Rafferty. "Nursing and the 'Hearts and Minds' Campaign (1948–1958): The Malayan Emergency." In *Routledge Handbook on the Global History of Nursing*, edited by Patricia D'Antonio, Julie A. Fairman, and Jean C. Whelan, 218–36. New York: Routledge, 2013.

Wan Fang, *Chuanhun: Sichuan Kangzhan dang'an shiliao xuanbian* (The soul of Sichuan: An edited collection of historical materials on the War of Resistance from the Sichuan Archives). Chengdu: Sichuan Provincial Archives, 2005.

Wang Di. *Street Culture in Chengdu: Public Space, Urban Commoners, and Local Politics in Chengdu, 1870–1930*. Stanford, CA: Stanford University Press, 2003.

———. *The Teahouse: Small Business, Everyday Culture, and Public Politics in Chengdu, 1900–1950*. Stanford, CA: Stanford University Press, 2008.

———. *Violence and Order on the Chengdu Plain: The Story of a Secret Brotherhood in Rural China, 1939-1949*. Stanford, CA: Stanford University Press, 2018.

Wang Zheng. *Finding Women in the State: A Socialist Feminist Revolution in the People's Republic of China, 1949–1964*. Berkeley: University of California Press, 2016.

———. "Gender and Maoist Urban Reorganization." In *Gender in Motion: Divisions of Labor and Cultural Change in Late Imperial and Modern China*, edited by Bryna Goodman and Wendy Larson, 189–209. Lanham, MD: Rowman and Littlefield, 2005.

———. *Women in the Chinese Enlightenment: Oral and Textual Histories*. Berkeley: University of California Press, 1999.

Wasserstrom, Jeffrey N. *Student Protests in Twentieth-Century China: The View from Shanghai*. Stanford, CA: Stanford University Press, 1991.

Watson, James L., and Evelyn S. Rawski, eds. *Death Ritual in Late Imperial and Modern China*. Berkeley: University of California Press, 1988.

Watt, John R. "Breaking into Public Service: The Development of Nursing in Modern China, 1870–1949." *Nursing History Review* 12 (2004): 67–96.

———. *A Friend in Deed: ABMAC and the Republic of China, 1937–1987*. New York: American Bureau for Medical Advancement in China, 1992.

———. *Saving Lives in Wartime China: How Medical Reformers Built Modern Healthcare Systems amid War and Epidemics, 1928–1945*. Leiden: E. J. Brill, 2014.

Weindling, Paul. "Public Health in Germany." In *The History of Public Health and the Modern State*, edited by Dorothy Porter, 119–30. Amsterdam: Rodopi, 1994.

Westad, Odd Arne. *Decisive Encounters: The Chinese Civil War, 1946–1950.* Stanford, CA: Stanford University Press, 2003.

———. *Restless Empire: China and the World since 1750.* New York: Basic Books, 2012.

Wilson, Ara. "Intimacy: A Useful Category of Transnational Analysis." In *The Global and The Intimate: Feminism in Our Time,* edited by Geraldine Pratt and Victoria Rosner, 31–56. New York: Columbia University Press, 2012.

Wood, Frances. *The Lure of China: Writers from Marco Polo to J. G. Ballard.* New Haven, CT: Yale University Press, 2009.

Wu, Ka-ming. "Elegant and Militarized: Ceremonial Volunteers and the Making of New Woman Citizens in China." *Journal of Asian Studies* 77, no. 1 (February 2018): 205–23.

Wu, Yi-Li. *Reproducing Women: Medicine, Metaphor, and Childbirth in Late Imperial China.* Berkeley: University of California Press, 2010.

Yang Shanyao. *Kangzhan shiqi de Zhongguo junyi* (China's military medicine during the War of Resistance). Taipei: Academia Historica, 2015.

Yang Yulin. "Bingli yu liangshi: Sichuan sheng disan xingzheng duchaqu renmin dui Kangzhan zhong de zhuyao gongxian" (Military power and grain: Principal War of Resistance contributions from the people of Sichuan Province's Number Three Administrative Superintendency). In *Sichuan Kangzhan dang'an yanjiu* (Research on the War of Resistance in Sichuan Archives), edited by Li Shigen, 16–29. Chengdu: Southwest Jiaotong University Publishing House, 2005.

Yip, Ka-che. "Disease and the Fighting Men: Nationalist Anti-Epidemic Efforts in Wartime China, 1937–1945." In *China in the Anti-Japanese War, 1937–1945: Politics, Culture, and Society,* edited by David P. Barrett and Larry N. Shyu, 171–88. New York: Peter Lang, 2001.

———. *Health and National Reconstruction in Nationalist China: The Development of Modern Health Services, 1928–1937.* Ann Arbor, MI: University of Michigan Press, 1995.

Zhang Dewen. "The Making of National Women: Gender, Nationalism and Social Mobilization in China's Anti-Japanese War of Resistance, 1937–1945." PhD diss., Stony Brook University, 2013.

Zhang Jin. *Quanli, chongtu, yu biange: 1926–1937 nian Chongqing chengshi xiandaihua yanjiu* (Power, conflict, and reform: The modernization of Chongqing, 1926–1937). Chongqing: Chongqing Publishing House, 2003.

Zhou Meiyu. *Zhongguo junhu jiaoyu fazhan shi* (History of the development of military nursing education). Taipei: Jianhe yinshua chang, 1985.

Zhou Yong, ed. *Chongqing tongshi* (A comprehensive history of Chongqing), vol. 3. Chongqing: Chongqing Publishing House, 2002.

INDEX